SOCIAL WORK IN HEALTH EMERGENCIES

This is the first comprehensive book that provides accessible, international knowledge for practitioners, students and academics about social work in health emergencies and spans fields of practice across world regions with particular reference to the COVID-19 pandemic.

Divided into three sections:

- *Regional, Historical and Social Work Perspectives* takes a journey through world regions during the first six months of the pandemic as it unfolded, explores the lessons found in the history of pandemics and situates public health social work practice in the values of the profession. Situating the diversity of challenges and opportunities in context, in turn, influences current and future social work practice.
- *Social Work Practice, Issues and Responses* explores social work practice innovations and responses across eleven key practice fields. International authors feature social work responses during the COVID-19 health emergency from different regions of the world.
- *Preparing for the Future* analyses broader concepts, innovations and the implications for future practices as social work enters a new era of service delivery. The 20 chapters explore the convergence of pandemic, politics and planet which is critiqued within a framework of the profession's ethics and values of human dignity, human rights and social justice. Social work's place in public health is firmly situated and built on the premise that the value social work brings to the table deserves recognition and should be documented to inform the development of the profession and future practice and how social work must carry lessons forward to prepare for the next pandemic.

The book is relevant to a wide range of audiences, including practitioners, educators and students in social work, human services, international development and public health, as well as policy makers and researchers.

Patricia Fronek is an Associate Professor in social work, academic and researcher in the School of Health Sciences and Social Work, Griffith University, Australia. Currently, she is the Director of the Bachelor of Social Work Program, a member of Griffith University's Law Futures Research Centre, and is Special Advisor to Child Identity Protection (CHIP). Social justice, human rights, ethics and professional practice are core to her practice and research over the last forty years. Her work is widely published and highly regarded.

Karen Smith Rotabi-Casares is a Professor in social work with a background in child protection and family support. Her work is international and she has been engaged in child rights and health promotion projects in a number of countries, to include Belize, Guatemala, Bosnia-Herzegovina, Malawi, the United Arab Emirates and Somalia. Focused on child rights, Rotabi-Casares is most interested in prevention with an orientation to the development of programs that engage the community and human service organizations in social change.

SOCIAL WORK IN HEALTH EMERGENCIES

Global Perspectives

Edited by Patricia Fronek and
Karen Smith Rotabi-Casares

Routledge
Taylor & Francis Group
LONDON AND NEW YORK

Cover image: © Getty Images
First published 2022
by Routledge
2 Park Square, Milton Park, Abingdon, Oxon OX14 4RN

and by Routledge
605 Third Avenue, New York, NY 10158

Routledge is an imprint of the Taylor & Francis Group, an informa business

British Library Cataloguing-in-Publication Data
A catalogue record for this book is available from the British Library

Library of Congress Cataloging-in-Publication Data
A catalog record has been requested for this book

ISBN: 978-0-367-62874-1 (hbk)
ISBN: 978-0-367-62873-4 (pbk)
ISBN: 978-1-003-11121-4 (ebk)

DOI: 10.4324/9781003111214

Typeset in Bembo
by KnowledgeWorks Global Ltd.

This book is dedicated to the frontline workers who worked tirelessly during the COVID-19 pandemic to care for others, especially medical and human services professionals as well as those in the service industry. Also, in remembrance of the people we lost and those they left behind.

CONTENTS

FIGURES

TABLES

BOXES

CONTRIBUTORS

Nadia C. Badran, President of the Social Workers Syndicate Lebanon, has a B.S. in Social Work, Master's in Counselling, and is a current PhD student researching ethics in social work. She has worked for the past 25 years in a civil society organization in Lebanon and in the MENA region as a consultant.

Elizabeth Bowen is an Associate Professor at the University at Buffalo School of Social Work, State University of New York, USA. Her research focuses on housing as a social determinant of health, health disparities affecting homeless populations, and social policy analysis.

Lynne Briggs is Associate Professor and Academic Lead of Field Education and Clinical Practice at Griffith University, Australia, and was at the University of Otago, Christchurch, New Zealand. Her research interests include national and international mixed-method studies, mental health outcomes for refugees, women, and the impact of child sexual abuse, demoralization, interventions in disasters, social work and field education.

Kelley Bunkers has spent close to three decades working in child protection in Eastern Europe, Africa, the Middle East and Latin America. Her work encompasses policy and programming, workforce strengthening and alternative care. She has a Master's in Child Rights and frequently contributes to articles, book chapters and webinars on the topics of child protection, alternative care and intercountry adoption.

Nicole Capozziello is a doctoral candidate at the University at Buffalo School of Social Work. Her research focuses on how nature-based interventions can impact people involved in the criminal justice system.

Ching-Wen Chang is Assistant Professor, Graduate Institute of Social Work, National Taiwan Normal University. Her current research interests are recovery for people with mental illness, youth mental health and mental health service utilization.

Marcus Chiu is Associate Professor at the Department of Social and Behavioural Sciences, City University of Hong Kong, Hong Kong. He received his postgraduate training and education from the School of Behavioural Science and Psychiatry, University of Manchester, UK. His research interest is mental health and carer advocacy.

Robert Common is a Child Protection Social Worker and psychologist. He is currently Managing Partner of The Beekeeper Practice, Cambodia. Current research interests include Buddhist approaches to trauma recovery and developmental trauma, the institutionalisation of children and LGBT advocacy.

Shelley Craig is Professor of Social Work at the Factor-Inwentash Faculty of Social Work, University of Toronto and Canada Research Chair in Sexual and Gender Minority Youth (SGMY). Her research and practice interests are cultivating the resilience of SGMY through technology and evidence-informed interventions, exploring social work in healthcare settings and developing competence in social work education.

Eliza Crossley is currently studying for a Master's in Social Work at the University of Melbourne, Australia, where she previously completed a Bachelor of Arts. Her research interests include lifespan development, family violence, mental illness and healthcare.

Roberta Di Rosa is Professor of Sociology of Migration and Social Work at University of Palermo. Her current research interests are international social work and intercultural competences, community mediation and social cohesion.

Jonathan Dickens is Professor of Social Work at the University of East Anglia, Norwich, UK. He is also Director of the UEA Centre for Research on Children and Families. His research interests focus on child protection court proceedings and children in care.

Peter C. Doherty AC FAA FRS Laureate Professor and Patron of the Doherty Institute at the University of Melbourne and Michael F Tamer Chair of Biomedical Research, St. Jude Children's Research Hospital, Memphis, TN, USA. Research interests, viral pathogenesis and immunity, particularly the "killer" T cell response. 1996 Nobel Laureate for Medicine and 1997 Australian of the year.

Claudia Fonseca is Professor in the Program of Post-Graduate Studies of Social Anthropology at the Federal University of Rio Grande do Sul, Brazil. Her research interests include anthropology of science and technology, technologies of government, health, family organization, and working-class culture.

Alan B. Franklin is a supervisory research biologist and Project Leader for the Wildlife-Borne Pathogens Affecting Food Safety and Security Research Project at the USDA National Wildlife Research Center, CO, USA. His current research interests include the ecology and dynamics of wildlife populations, integrating wildlife population ecology with wildlife disease ecology, pathogen surveillance and monitoring in wildlife, and the ecology of pathogens in wildlife populations at the wildlife-agricultural and wildlife-human interfaces.

Corlie Giliomee is Lecturer at the Department of Social Work and Criminology, University of Pretoria, South Africa, and serves as the Treasurer of the Association of Schools of Social Work in Africa. Her research interests centre around human rights, social justice, human rights education, social work education, social development and homelessness.

Louise Harms is Chair and Head of the Department of Social Work, The University of Melbourne, Australia. Her research interests are trauma and resilience, particularly as they relate to health and post-disaster experiences.

Kathryn Hay is Associate Professor at Massey University, New Zealand. Her current research interests are related to work-integrated learning, graduate readiness for practice, and social workers engagement in disaster management.

Mădălina Hideg is an instructor in the Master's Program in Social Services Management, Faculty of Sociology and Social Work at Babeş-Bolyai University of Cluj-Napoca, Romania, and Scientific Director at ARGUMENT, Social Research Institute, DC News Research & Development, Romania. Her current research interests are effectiveness and efficiency in the social work field, public opinion and public consent, and new social trends in the pandemic context.

Dorothee Hölscher is Lecturer in the School of Health Sciences and Social Work, Griffith University, Australia, and a research associate with the Department of Social Work, University of Johannesburg, South Africa. Her research interests are in anti-oppressive theory and applied ethics, with a focus on questions of social justice within the fields of social work education and practice with cross-border migrants.

Elyssa Hudson is currently a Master of Social Work student at The University of Melbourne, Australia, and an English/Humanities Teacher (BA, GradDipEd, GradDipPsych). Her research interests include family violence, natural disasters, as well as mental health issues and their presentation within young people.

Joel Izlar is a PhD candidate of Social Work at the University of Georgia, USA. His current work focuses on how functional communities operate as forms of community work, social welfare, organizing, protest and direct action that meet human needs while challenging the ecological crises of our time.

Connie Kellett is Senior Family Violence Leader in Victoria, and is part of designing, implementing and evaluating new processes following the 2016 Victorian Royal Commission into Family Violence. She is also a member of the Beyond Bushfires Research Team at the University of Melbourne, VIC, Australia. Her areas of interest are family violence, disaster and trauma.

Sungmin Kim is a social worker in Australia working at the Prince Charles Hospital. His current research interests are brain–computer interface and neuroimaging studies.

Myung Hun Kim is a social worker in Gangnam Severance Hospital, Yonsei University, South Korea. His current research interests are health technology assessment and medical social work.

Alexa Kirkland is a research assistant with the Affirmative Research Collaborative at the Factor-Inwentash Faculty of Social Work, University of Toronto, Canada.

Yoko Kobayashi currently works as Child Protection Specialist in UNICEF Kenya. She worked in Zimbabwe, Uganda, Sri Lanka, Nepal and Japan in areas of child protection, focusing on various initiatives ranging from national-level policy development to humanitarian response.

Lauren Kosta is Lecturer in Social Work at the University of Melbourne, Australia. Her research interests are parenting and family adjustment following adversity, including paediatric critical illness and post-disaster recovery.

Justin S. Lee is Assistant Professor, Department of Social work and Gerontology, Weber University, United States. Lee's practice and research focus on forced migration, health disparities, and mental health access across cultures. He has written on refugee resettlement, volunteerism, and health access among immigrant populations.

Jianqiang Liang is Lecturer and Program Advisor (International) in the School of Health Sciences and Social Work, Griffith University, Australia. His current research interests are international social work and field education, program development, and enhancing the health and psychosocial well-being of vulnerable children, women and older persons in developing countries.

Siân Long is a senior associate with Maestral International and has spent close to three decades working on child protection and HIV responses for children in Africa, Asia, the Middle East and Latin America. Her work encompasses community to national policy and programming and social service workforce strengthening.

Antonio López Peláez is Professor of Social Work and Social Services at the National Distance Education University (UNED), Madrid, Spain. His current research interests are digital social work, and youth and social work with groups.

Jane Maidment is Professor from the University of Canterbury, New Zealand, and has a long history of research and practice within field education. Edited book titles have included *Practice Skills for Social Work and Welfare* (2016); *Social Policy for Social Work and Human Services in Aotearoa New Zealand* (2016); and *Supervision in Social Work: Contemporary Issues* (2015). Jane has also researched and published widely on the influence of handcrafting for individual and community wellbeing.

Gokul Mandayam is Assistant Professor of Social Work at Rhode Island College. His 2020 co-edited book is entitled *Social Entrepreneurship, Intrapreneurship, and Social Value Creation Relevance for Contemporary Social Work Practice.* His current research interests are the practical application of creative solutions for social problems.

Donna McAuliffe is Professor of Social Work in the School of Health Sciences and Social Work, Griffith University, Australia. Her field of practice and academic expertise is professional and applied ethics, with a focus on ethical decision making, moral philosophy and interprofessional ethics education.

Kai Medina-Martinez is Assistant Professor of Social Work at California State University Monterey Bay, USA. Her research interests include social work field education, social work clinical practices with diverse communities and social work development.

Gabriela Misca is Senior Lecturer in Psychology at the University of Worcester, UK, and her research portfolio addresses diverse and/or adverse family dynamics across the life course, including families formed through (intercountry) adoption and (global) surrogacy; same-gender parenting; and military and veteran families. She is leading the ongoing international study *Families Un-Locked.*

Carmen Monico is Associate Professor in the Joint Master and PhD Social Work Programs of the North Carolina Agricultural and Technical State University and the University of North Carolina Greensboro. Her research is on intercountry adoption, global migration and human trafficking, and she has written extensively on civic engagement and social accountability.

Sharon E. Moore is Full Professor of Social Work at the Raymond A. Kent School of Social Work at the University of Louisville, USA. Dr. Moore was awarded the 8th Annual Florence W. Vigilante Award for Scholarly Excellence. She and several of her previous doctoral mentees co-authored in the *Journal of Teaching in Social Work*, "The Dehumanization of Black Males by Police: Teaching Social Justice—Black Life Really Does Matter."

Barbara Muskat is Adjunct Professor at the Factor Inwentash Faculty of Social Work, University of Toronto. Her current research interests include social group work, clinical approaches for neurodiverse populations and social work in health care.

Nicoleta Neamțu is Associate Professor of Social Work and Director of the Master Program in Social Services Management at Babeş-Bolyai University of Cluj-Napoca, Romania, and has contributed to the development of the social work profession in Romania. Her current professional interests are in the areas of effectiveness of social programs, social intervention methods, innovation in social services and change management.

Samuel Ochieng has spent close to three decades working in child protection in Kenya and social protection in Africa, the Middle East and Latin America. His work covers policy and programming, social protection strengthening and child protection system development and programming.

Malcolm Payne holds professorial roles at Manchester Metropolitan University and Kingston University, London, UK. His current research interests are social work theory, end-of-life care and social work with older people, including citizenship practice and safeguarding.

Renie Rondon-Jackson, Ph.D., LCSW, is the Field Education Coordinator and Lecturer at California State University Monterey Bay, USA. Her research interests include women experiencing homelessness, global mental/physical health, and social work field education. She has more than 25 years of working marginalised under or inappropriately served individuals and families.

Sareh Rotabi is Executive Manager of Investor Relations and Development at Humansoft Holding Company, Kuwait. She is an Experienced Economist with a demonstrated history of working in higher education, management and financial services. Her research interests are macroeconomics and macroeconomic policies, entrepreneurship and happiness.

Wanchai Roujanavong is Thailand's Representative to ACWC - ASEAN Commission on the Promotion and Protection of the Rights of Women and

Children and a Senior Consultant Public Prosecutor who has held led public service positions as Director General of several departments. He has a long history of national and international work with NGOs for the promotion and protection of child and human rights and has received two prestigious national awards for this advocacy work.

Thabile A. Samboma is a researcher under the Governance & Administration Unit at the Botswana Institute for Development Policy Analysis (BIDPA), Botswana. Her research interests are on child protection, gender development and governance.

Taghreed Abu Sarhan is Assistant Professor of Social Work at United Arab Emirates University, UAE. Her research interests are women's and child protection from a legal perspective, women and children in the criminal justice system, women killings, sexual & physical assaults against women and children, law enforcement and human rights, forensic social work, and police investigating domestic violence and child abuse, and human rights.

Deepy Sur is the CEO at the Ontario Association of Social Workers in Ontario, Canada. Her current research interests are empathy-centred care in interprofessional teams and advancing innovative models of social work practice.

Gemma Thornton is a doctoral researcher at the University of Worcester, UK, with researching interests in family psychology. Her doctoral research is focusing on the impact of COVID-19 bereavement on families from a family resilience perspective.

Ariel Kwegyir Tsiboe is a graduate from the University of Southampton's M.Sc. Global Ageing and Policy Program (UK). He is currently a Ph.D. candidate at McMaster University – Ph.D. Social Gerontology. His research interests are aged care research, relationships and social networks among older people in rural areas.

Janestic Mwende Twikirize is Senior Lecturer at the Department of Social Work, Makerere University, Uganda. Her research interests are developmental social work, indigenisation and decoloniality, child protection, and gender.

Gidraph G. Wairire is Associate Professor in the Department of Sociology and Social Work, University of Nairobi, Kenya. His main interests include social work theory and practice, community organisation, international social work, developmental social work, social work with minorities, social action for social change and interdisciplinary research. He is the immediate past President of the Association for Schools of Social Work in Africa (ASSWA).

Janet Walker is Emeritus Professor of Family Policy at Newcastle University, England. Having directed over 50 multidisciplinary studies relating to family life and relationships, she is currently a research consultant to an evaluation of support for naval families; a co-investigator of the Anglo-Australian "*Families Un-locked*" study; and Chair of the Archbishops of Canterbury and York's Commission on Families and Households.

Matthew C. Ward is Senior Lecturer in History at the School of Humanities in the University of Dundee, Scotland. His research interests are in early American history and he is currently working on a project on Native American demography.

Hilary N. Weaver is Professor and Associate Dean for Diversity, Equity and Inclusion in the School of Social Work, Buffalo State University. She currently serves as President of the Indigenous and Tribal Social Work Educators' Association, is the global Commissioner of the Indigenous Commission, IFSW, and Chair-Elect of the Council on Social Work Education Board of Directors. Her research, teaching and service focus on cultural issues in the helping process with an emphasis on indigenous populations and well-being.

Yanuar Farida Wismayanti is a researcher in the Ministry of Social Affairs of Republic Indonesia. Her current research interests are child protection, social protection, and poverty.

Tarek Zidan is Assistant Professor of Social Work at Indiana University's School of Social Work in South Bend, Indiana, USA. His research interests are Muslim/ Arab Americans and Disability.

FOREWORD BY RICHARD HUGMAN

When in late 2019, it became apparent that the world was on the brink of a global pandemic, it also became very clear that social workers and the organisations within which they work were unprepared for the extent of the impact on all aspects of practice. Although prior to this point social work has increasingly responded in the development of new practices, knowledge and theories in the field of disaster response, the emerging realities of a global pandemic have forced the profession to go further and to rethink how every aspect of social work simultaneously must be questioned in the face of such a previously unencountered challenge. At the time of the last health emergency that is recognised as a *global* pandemic, the "Spanish Flu" of 1918 to 1920, social work was in its infancy relative to today. So, in many ways, recent experience is unique.

One of the strategies used by political leaders in many countries to attempt to shape the discourse around COVID-19 is through the rhetorical device of assertions that "we're all in this together." This is true in the sense that no one is unaffected at least in some way; public health measures, in principle, apply to everyone in a given community. Yet, as we know from critical social work theory and practice, the circumstances in which people experience these supposed similarities are very often unequal in various ways (Maglajlic, 2019). Given that pandemic response measures affect all aspects of society, the impacts of such policies are felt in employment, education, health, justice, as well as in day-to-day life in families and communities. As social work knowledge and theory tell us, these are all aspects of society that are shaped by considerable inequalities, whether of access or outcome.

How people have experienced the pandemic has varied greatly, according to sex and gender, sexuality, culture and ethnicity, age, dis/ability, and geographical location. In particular, the intersection of each of these factors with socio-economic class and status has amplified the extent to which it is more true to say that "we are not all in this together," even if we are all in this in some way. The importance of addressing structural inequalities can be seen at all levels of social work, from micro-practices with families, in communities, hospitals and clinics, schools and so on, through to the macro-practice involvement that social workers undertake in research, policy formation and advocacy. Furthermore, inequalities occur not only between individuals and families, and between specific groups within societies but also between entire countries and global regions. For example, just as access to vaccines is differentially available according to income, age, ethnicity and locality within any country, there is a comparable global inequality between countries that is structured along the well-recognised divide between the global North and South. So at an institutional level, social work associations and unions can engage with the "no one left behind" advocacy of the responsibility of the OECD countries towards the rest of humanity in this regard (as in so many others). Social workers must both be prepared individually to practice in ways that address the new context of such challenges, but also collectively to act so that the contexts themselves are addressed.

In addition to the requirement for new practices and knowledge, social work also finds its core values of social justice and human rights are confronted. A recent analysis (Banks et al., 2020) indicates that in broad terms what is necessary is to use these core values integrated purposively with new knowledge in order to address the changed circumstances of practice. If we focus on the particular example of vaccines, which are a key element in overcoming the pandemic condition, social justice may require that those who are most vulnerable get first access, but in most countries so far we have seen that political leaders and other privileged groups have often been at the front of the queue. How social workers can engage with this reality in policy advocacy, while also seeking to help individuals and families whose lives are affected by lack of access, is an ethical struggle with which we are only too familiar. Similarly, access to vaccines is also a right, given that they are already available in many countries (and potentially could be in *all* countries). Where this right is denied through factors such as costs, a lack of engagement with minority groups and of practical support measures (such as income replacement for those who are unable to work while receiving treatment or getting vaccinated), social workers can act to pursue or to develop ways that will assist people to overcome these barriers.

Throughout this volume, the authors address these important differences in their careful analyses. Such an approach is, in itself, a major strength of the way Patricia Fronek and Karen Smith Rotabi-Casares have brought together authors who reflect these differences through their considerable collective diversity. Although, in each case, the authors write about their own contexts, the collection as a whole is genuinely international: in addition to global Northern views, some chapters focus on global Southern contexts and others are comparative discussions across countries and regions. This provides an important corrective emphasis to the tendency to model social work overwhelmingly on the traditions and insights of the global North. We are only able to be "all in it together" if we are "*all* in it," in social work as well as in social policy.

One of the themes that occurs in discussions of social work in emergency and disaster situations is that of preparing for the next time. Yet, although it has been 100 years since the previous occasion of a global pandemic, whether this is now a "next time" depends on the point of view we might have about regional or national health epidemic emergencies such as SARS, Avian Flu, Ebola, Zita and other viruses. In these situations, strong public health measures have been a major dimension of ending epidemics. In many parts of the world social work plays an important role in public health, usually working in collaboration with other professional groups. The North-South divide has masked the extent to which practice knowledge about such matters has already been developed through the work of colleagues in Africa, Asia and South America. The current crisis is an opportunity for the global North to learn from the global South and must be grasped as such.

Social work is as affected by the disruptions the pandemic has caused as any other part of a society, especially including those more disadvantaged groups with whom social work tends to be engaged. This places a responsibility on the profession to contribute to thinking about the future, as well as having to take sides in current debates. For example, arguments that emphasis should be placed on limiting disruption to economic activity will disproportionately place the lives of those who experience disadvantage in greater risk than those who enjoy advantage. This not only creates an ethical obligation for social workers to be involved in thinking about "next time" but also to be working (together with colleagues in related fields and beyond) towards policy and practice that values all lives in a practical sense. The health impacts of the rapidly growing climate emergency demand the same attention. For example, diseases that result from a polluted environment do not affect populations equally, either in geographical or social structural terms. Here too the global North has much to learn from the South.

The editors of this book are to be congratulated on bringing together such a diverse range of authors and to ensuring that a critical approach is taken in relation to all the different areas of social work that are addressed. In the same way that all discussions about the future raise questions about a "new normal," one that is not simply a return to how things were in 2019, social work will need to develop a new vision in practice and theory that learns from the experience of this global health emergency. This volume will contribute to that task, both in the ideas that are shared about particular aspects of social issues but also in the approach that is evident throughout.

Richard Hugman
Emeritus Professor of Social Work
University of New South Wales, Australia

References

Banks, S., Cai, T., de Jonge, E., Shears, J., Shum, M., Sobocan, A. M., Strom, K., Truell, R., Uriz, M. J., & Weinberg, M. (2020). Practising ethically during COVID-19: social work challenges and responses, *International Social Work*, 63(5), 569-583.

Maglajlic, R. A. (2019). Organisation and delivery of social services in extreme events: lessons from social work research on natural disasters, *International Social Work*, 62(3), 1146-1.

PREFACE

When the news of the novel virus broke in December 2019, we were travelling the world, Karen visiting places that quickly became hotspots including China and Patricia working in Cambodia. On return to our respective countries, Australia and the United States, Skype conversations between us, friends and colleagues, about the state of affairs sparked the idea for this book. We explored the many ideas that were predictive of human behaviour and the future of global health in the context of COVID-19. Unfortunately, many of our forecasts have materialised especially the human pain, suffering and loss of dignity experienced. Due to our experience in health care including during SARS and H1N1, we watched events unfold with some clarity as to our future and alarm at how quickly the health response was captured by politics in many jurisdictions. As social workers who have worked in many practice settings as well as global policy analysts, we were more than worried about the ineptitude of many governments to respond proactively. We also recognised the many bright spots that would be found in communities. Our considerable trust in the social work profession was not misplaced. During the pandemic social workers engaged with people in need with ingenuity and a depth of persistence while collaborating across disciplines in ways rarely seen before in the history of social work. As we learn from our past, we are reminded that *the best predictor of our future is the past.* Learning the lessons of COVID-19 is critically important, particularly as the field of public health social work unfolds with new dimensions. COVID-19 will become our past and the lessons learned that we hope will feature when we are faced with the next pandemic. It was our intent to capture the evidence and stories of the very good work carried out by our colleagues. We think that we have reached that goal and we are deeply appreciative of everyone who rapidly came together to make this book happen – from our earliest work with Claire Jarvis and her team at Routledge to the authors who have contributed critical knowledge so that we may be better prepared for present and future health emergencies, the next perhaps closer than we expect.

Patricia Fronek and Karen Smith Rotabi-Casares

1

INTRODUCING SOCIAL WORK IN HEALTH EMERGENCIES

Patricia Fronek and Karen Smith Rotabi-Casares with Jonathan Dickens

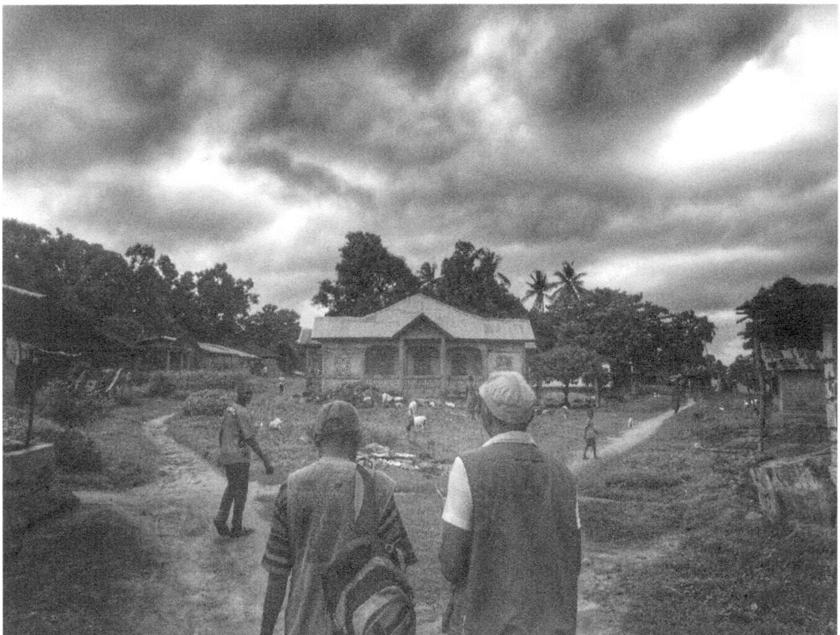

FIGURE 1.0 Surveillance officers of the Mambolo Chiefdom walking towards a clinic in the village of Tongo Walla, Sierra Leone in 2016

Source: Photographer: Louise Eduardo Torrens. Courtesy of CDC/CDC Connects

DOI: 10.4324/9781003111214-1

This book, for social workers, is about how the profession as a helping discipline has responded to *health emergencies* (see Box 1.1), in particular the COVID-19 pandemic, and how crisis response capacity has developed from these experiences. Threaded through our collection of 20 chapters, a compelling global story about practice and innovation in both resource-rich and resource-poor environments is told, firmly situating social work's place in public health practice across all social work fields. The value social work brings to the table in meeting the needs of people, especially the vulnerable, and the potential to bring expertise to future pandemic planning deserves recognition.

The COVID-19 pandemic, identified as a new contagion in December 2019, presented an opportunity to explore how a deadly, global disease has impacted all people, interrupted *normal* life, and disrupted the practice and education of social workers. This exploration presents opportunities to critique whether lessons have been learned from previous health emergencies, how governments, social workers, the general population and others responded, how new disadvantage, vulnerabilities and opportunities were created in uncertainty, and how science literacy has become an imperative for social work knowledge, practice and leadership. These understandings inform how social workers intervene during *health emergencies*, how they respond in the aftermath and how the profession should plan for the future.

BOX 1.1

WHAT IS A HEALTH EMERGENCY?

Health emergencies are threats or actual outbreaks of disease, natural and human-induced disasters, and any event that causes physical or mental illness, death or widespread injury or property destruction. A disease that escalates to epidemic or pandemic status is a health emergency that requires global cooperation and coordination. The World Health Organization (WHO) and national governments play key roles in preparing and planning for these emergencies. The International Health Regulations Monitoring Framework (WHO, 2005) requires State Parties "to have or to develop minimum health capacities to implement" the Regulations for health emergencies. Coordinated responses from all sectors, cooperation between disciplines and science literacy are necessary to address human and material need in these contexts.

In this book, we critically unpack unfolding events during the COVID-19 pandemic, explore how social workers met challenges and opportunities head-on in tragedy and hardship and how the profession has moved forward with new knowledge. As the human experience has always been shaped by its context, we explore how social workers have supported people to recognise and build resilience in the face of uncertainty and adversity and to understand human behaviour in pandemic conditions. To fully engage with health emergencies requires many ways of thinking. An ecological view helps make sense of the perfect storm of *pandemic*, *politics* and the *planet* that has led to this health emergency, shaped its management and the consequences for all people. An *ecological perspective* (see Box 1.2) provides a framework that helps us understand the complexity of multiple, systemic interactions while human dignity inclusive of human rights and the ethics and values of the profession provides the lens through which to interpret the impact of health emergencies, critique responses to it and shape social work practice.

BOX 1.2

AN ECOLOGICAL PERSPECTIVE

An *ecological perspective* focuses on the mutual interactions between multiple elements of a system, which impact a person's daily existence and social reality. Elements of a system can be identified by starting at the micro level with the individual (the body being a system in itself) as the central element in the wider system, their relationships with significant others and their community, service providers and macro elements such as legal, educational and welfare systems, culture, relationships with the natural environment and the time in which people live. All these elements interact and influence each other, impacting on the individual.

Where individuals are in their life course affects their vulnerability to particular diseases; for example, older people and people with comorbidities are more vulnerable to death from COVID-19. Exchanges between elements of the system are affected by the presence of poverty or family violence, unhygienic or overcrowded living and work conditions, the preparedness of the health system, the person's access to health care and income support, the type of political regime and even specific policies that affect groups such as the aged, prisoners or refugees, and access to food and income during quarantine and lockdowns. The *natural* and *social* are each part of human existence and are not mutually exclusive elements of an ecological system. Examples that complicate health emergencies include risks from other infectious diseases, the impact of the looming climate emergency on zoonosis (transmission of viruses from other mammals to humans) and concurrent disasters. Hundreds of thousands of naturally occurring viruses can potentially infect humans, which emphasise the necessary reduction of anthropogenic (caused by humans) climate change and threats to biodiversity to reduce these risks (IPBES, 2020).

Chronology (the time in which we live), the temporal factors such as globalisation (trade, travel and the movement of people) or political climates of economic austerity or persecution are the elements that are interconnected influencing the human condition and the well-being of people. Social workers intervene at various points within a system to improve relationships between elements of that system to improve health and overall quality of life in *micro, mezzo* and *macro* practice. Figure 1.1 depicts an ecological framework that helps understand the interrelationships of all the factors at play in health emergencies.

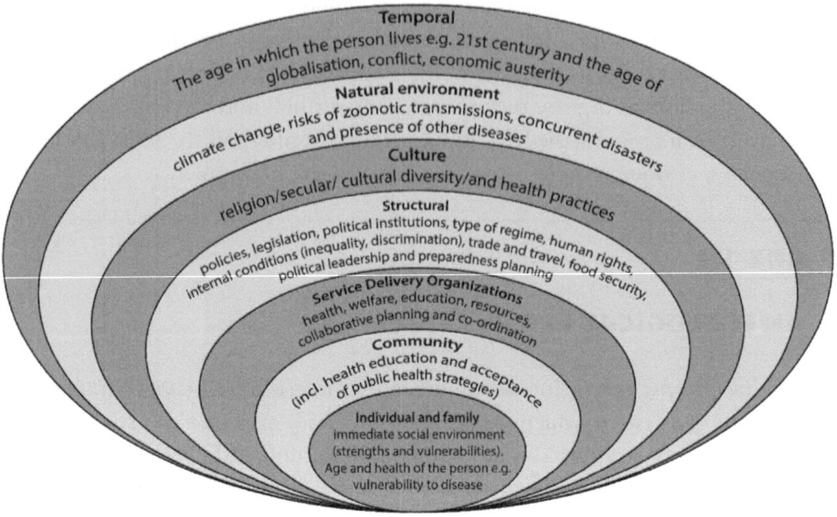

FIGURE 1.1 An ecological framework for health emergencies

Health social work

The field of health social work began mid-last century when the focus of professional practice shifted from community work to institutional social work in hospitals, thus gaining professional recognition in those settings. Critiques suggest that striving for professional status and ultimately funded services, particularly in the US, led to an overemphasis on micro practice (e.g. interpersonal work, therapy and counselling) and the foray of the medical model into social work education. Nonetheless, macro practice, orientated to structural change and organisational and community practice, has remained as vibrant and responsive to human need as it has always been.

Starting with one of the earliest documentation of community practice with the Settlement House movement, the health and safety of urban communities were core concerns in London, Chicago and elsewhere. For example, in the late 1800s, Jane Addams and the women of Hull House tackled social problems and infectious disease in the Chicago neighbourhood. They were particularly concerned with immigrant health in the context of poverty and inequality and understood social welfare as inclusive of systems of care and a government responsibility (Addams, 1910). Counting latrines among other health focused activities were included in their community assessment work and problem-solving strategies. This work is one of the earliest recorded that included an ecological understanding of social care and community development with related practices for response and reform. Addams went on to win a Nobel Prize for her ideas of peace work and obligations of society to meet the needs of vulnerable people (Farrell, 1967).

The social determinants of health

Preferencing micro practice over macro or vice versa creates a false dichotomy that quickly disappears when responses to complex health and social problems and the breadth and scope of social work practice are considered in the context of health emergencies. In these crises, the interrelationship between macro and micro are particularly clear. This leads us to the realisation that social work is a good fit with the *social*, firmly located in the *social determinants of health* (see Box 1.3) paradigm. Understanding the effects of inequalities have led to the profession's advance into public health social work (Friedman & Merrick, 2015; Moniz, 2010). The biopsychosocial and ecological understandings of health in social work practice, how social work responds to man-made and natural disasters and more recently to new health emergencies has hastened the need for skilled and knowledgeable social work practice in this emergent field (Alston et al, 2019; Walter-McCabe, 2020).

BOX 1.3

THE SOCIAL DETERMINANTS OF HEALTH

> The *social determinants of health* are the conditions in which people are born, grow, live, work and age. These circumstances are shaped by the distribution of money, power and resources at global, national and local levels. The social determinants of health are mostly responsible for health inequities – the unfair and avoidable differences in health status seen within and between countries.
>
> (*WHO, n.d.*)

Key concepts addressed are employment conditions, social exclusion, public health programs, women and gender equality, early child development, globalisation, health systems, measurement and evidence, and urbanisation.

Critical questions

With the advent of the global COVID-19 pandemic, the world changed quickly and dramatically. A paradigm shift from practice in relatively predictable circumstances to uncertainty and imminent personal risk affected social workers everywhere, requiring creative responses to continue to serve others. As a profession, social work has been propelled, regardless of fields of practice, into the public health arena, entwining understandings of micro, mezzo and macro practices into an integrated whole.

A critical approach insists on challenging beliefs, questioning assumptions and seeking disconfirming information while evaluating them against evidence, particularly when rapidly circulating misinformation or the *infodemic* is rife (WHO, 2018, p. 26). Key questions must be asked, and assumptions challenged – *How do we know this is true or false? If this is true or false, then what else is true or false?* And, *how can we, as social workers, take this knowledge and engage effectively with local and global dimensions to adequately address the needs of vulnerable people during a health crisis?* We set forth to answer these questions, while also learning from previous health emergencies such as the 1918 Influenza, SARS, H1N1, Ebola and HIV-AIDS, and the rapidly evolving science about COVID-19.

The COVID-19 pandemic

The spread of the new virus precipitated one of the most extensive health emergencies faced by the modern global population, a circumstance magnified by living in a globalised, interconnected world and the rapidly evolving climate emergency. The movement of people meant the virus travelled the world long before it was identified. The WHO upgraded COVID-19 from an outbreak to an epidemic and finally to a pandemic on March 11, 2020 (WHO, 2020), following at least three months of warnings about the potential for the disease to infect the global population when it was probable that it had already spread. As we proceed with this discussion, it is important to clarify the terms – *outbreak*, *epidemic*, *pandemic* and *endemic* – as they are often confused and incorrectly used interchangeably (see Box 1.4).

BOX 1.4

DEFINITION OF TERMS

- An *outbreak* is localised where the disease is contained to a specific community or geographical area.
- An *epidemic* is where the disease has spread, and outbreaks occur elsewhere.
- A *pandemic* has spread to many countries. The WHO defines a pandemic as "the worldwide spread of a new disease" (WHO, 2010).
- *Endemic* describes a disease that stays in the population in a particular geographical area and people learn to live with a low level of the disease. Examples are chicken pox or malaria in particular regions of the world. COVID-19 holds a strong possibility of becoming endemic in the global population.

The novel coronavirus that causes COVID-19 is *novel* because it was new and *corona* because it belongs to a family of viruses called corona that have crown-like formations when viewed through an electron microscope. Figure 1.2 shows the first photograph taken of the virus.

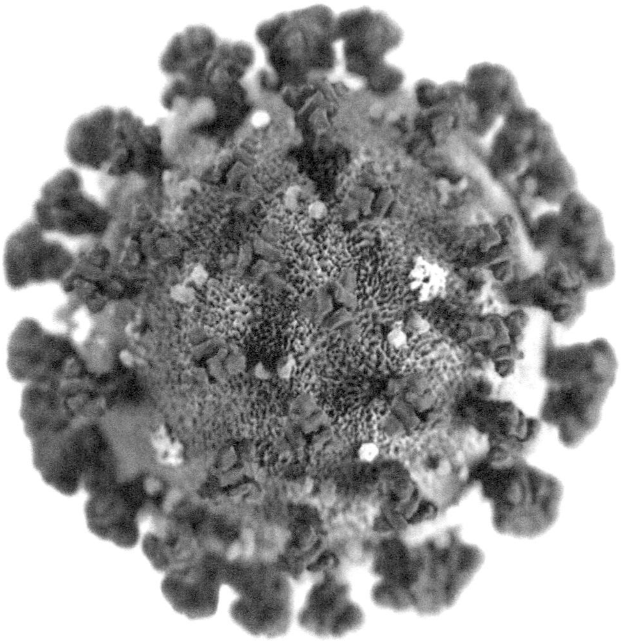

FIGURE 1.2 SARS-CoV-2

Source: Photograph by Alissa Eckert MSMI; Dan Higgins, MAMS (to check out a rotating 3-D image of the virus taken by scientists, go to https://nanographics.at/projects/sars-cov-2/360.html)

As knowledge of the novel coronavirus developed, scientists renamed the virus and the disease.

- The virus is called SARS-CoV-2.
- The disease that results from SARS-CoV-2 infection is *COVID-19*, short for Corona Virus Disease 2019.
- Variants that evolve from the original virus are named differently (e.g. B117 and B1351) eventually named according to the Greek alphabet, e.g., Delta.

Information that the virus was man-made circulated globally, and the lab-leak theory gained traction in speculative, popular discourse (Maxmen & Mallapaty, 2021). Although scientist agree all possibilities must be explored, natural origins of the virus were confirmed through genome sequencing (Ren et al., 2020). The corona family of viruses is transmitted from other mammals to humans in a process called *zoonosis*, often called *a jump* in the mass media (Franklin & Bevins, 2020).

Evolutionary studies identified that the ancestors of SARS-CoV-2 have been circulating in bats for decades and are transmitted to people via intermediary host mammals such as pangolins, a situation worsened by anthropogenic (human-induced) climate change (Boni et al., 2020). The exact transmission path of SARS-CoV-2 from other species to humans had not been conclusively determined by the time this book was completed and may take years to determine. In the Q&A of Chapter 19, we ask questions of Alan B. Franklin from the National Wildlife Centre, US Department of Agriculture, about the natural environment and the spread of infectious disease in the context of climate change, in particular, the interdependent relationships between humans, the natural environment and the spread of disease.

Although studies indicate the virus emerged earlier than December and had spread across the globe soon after, the first identified outbreak of SARS-CoV-2 was connected to the Huanan Seafood Wholesale Market in Wuhan, China. *Case Zero* (the first case) has not been identified. Confusion exists around *zero* terms such as *patient zero* as many similar terms tend to be used interchangeably to describe the first case noticed (*index case*), the first case in an outbreak (*primary case*), and the very first person to catch the virus from zoonotic transmission (*case zero*). It may be impossible to locate the first case involved in zoonosis given the nature of global travel and delays in recognising and diagnosing the disease. Matters are further complicated because people infected with SARS-CoV-2 can spread the virus even when asymptomatic and others who do become symptomatic can spread the virus for at least two days before showing symptoms.

Who is vulnerable to COVID-19?

Related viruses include multiple strains of influenza, Severe Acute Respiratory Syndrome (SARS) which infected people in China, Hong Kong and other countries in 2003, and the Middle East Respiratory Syndrome (MERS), also called Camel flu, which appeared in Saudi Arabia in 2012 and spread to 27 countries (Allimuddin et al., 2015). All coronaviruses act somewhat differently and have a death toll which varies with the virus characteristics, severity and spread, and the particular vulnerabilities within the human population. For SARS-CoV-2, older people and those with comorbidities are at most risk of complications and death, yet there is no international convention to protect the rights of older people, only principles which do not obligate signatory countries to comply. Globally, aged care facilities have been hotspots of infection and death, and alarmingly, the well-being of older people and people with disabilities were not included in many national preparedness plans, their survival given less priority, and judgements made by others about the quality of life according to life years remaining. Privatisation of aged care came with neoliberalism in many countries, precipitating a decline in quality services and conflicts between profit and serving the needs of older people. For example, Australia still had no federal pandemic plan for aged care as late as September 2020. Health vulnerabilities and other factors including inadequate preparedness and training, profit-driven models, and judgements about human dignity and ageism contributed to an unacceptable global mortality rate. Malcom Payne tackles the issue of ageism in Chapter 10.

Eight out of ten people with COVID-19 have mild or no symptoms while still infectious. The virus is transmitted primarily through the air in droplets and aerosols. Early reports suggested that the virus can remain on surfaces for extended periods. Plastic, vinyl, cloth, metal, paper and glass can become *fomites*, meaning carriers of infection. However, it has been suggested that risks of surface transmission have been exaggerated (Goldman, 2020). Children can spread disease for weeks after being infected, are more likely to be asymptomatic and the incidence of infection in children is under-reported (DeBiasi & Delaney, 2020; Grijalva et al., 2020; Hippich et al., 2020). By April 2021, the rising number of deaths of very young children from COVID-19 in Brazil became a grave concern in a country badly affected by the pandemic and the development of new variants (see Chapter 2). The Brazilian Ministry of Health reported 852 children under nine years died of COVID-19 between February 2020 and mid-March 2021 (Brazilian Ministry of Health, 2021; Passarinho & Barrucho, 2021). At the same time, a dramatic increase in the number of children presenting with COVID-19 in US hospitals was being attributed to the UK variant and spring break.

Younger people were also generally less affected by SARS-CoV-2, and outbreaks of infection have been associated with young people and adolescents who may take more risks such as participating in large gatherings. An early study in Japan found that asymptomatic or pre-symptomatic young people aged between 20 and 29 years were responsible for clusters of infections where crowds gathered, for example, bars and clubs, a pattern confirmed by other studies around the world (Furuse et al., 2020). Some people of all ages experienced negative long-term effects on the immune system, cardiovascular, neurological and respiratory systems and damage to the brain and other organs. A few cases of psychosis have been reported but causation is not determined and, for some children, the development of multisystem inflammatory disease (MiS-C) (Ahmed et al., 2020; Paterson et al., 2020). The lingering effects of COVID-19 that can last for months are commonly called *Long Covid*, affecting between 60% and 90% of people (Carfì et al., 2020; Davis et al., 2020; Huang et al., 2021; Nalbandian et al., 2021).

For people who become ill, symptoms are mild in the first week and worsen by the second week. Most deaths occur in the second and third weeks. The course of the disease for UK Prime Minister, Boris Johnson, followed this pattern (Lewin et al., 2020). Donald Trump, the ex-President of the US, and other world leaders who failed to protect their population also fell victim to COVID-19. President Jair Bolsonaro of Brazil who described COVID-19 as a *gripezinha* (little flu) tested positive and later claimed to be cured by a disproven drug also promoted by Trump. Status did little to protect people from becoming infected, given politicians, celebrities and royalty were infected and some died. However, status did ensure access to the best health care, new treatments and vaccination as they became available. By August 2020, one person in the world was dying every fifteen seconds, and by June 2021, 180 million people globally had contracted COVID-19 and four million people were known to have died from the disease (Johns Hopkins Corona Virus Resource Centre).

We consider the science further in Chapter 20 where Laureate Professor and Nobel Prize winner, Peter C. Doherty, answers questions about COVID-19 and other health emergencies. Understanding the science behind health emergencies and relevant health information empowers and equips social workers to provide accurate, life-saving information to our clients, protect ourselves on the front line, mitigate false misinformation and to respond and prepare for future health emergencies.

How the world responded

This brings us to how the world has responded. COVID-19 is simply the latest in a long line of health emergencies. Historically, knowledge gained from each health emergency has informed preparedness for the next one. For example, isolation and quarantine as public health measures can be traced back to the Black Death in the 1300s which killed one-third of the European population and are still vital strategies in containing infectious diseases today. Scientists have long predicted the inevitability of future pandemics, a circumstance worsened by the climate emergency (CDC, 2017; Doherty, 2013; Jones et al., 2008; WHO, 2017). Likewise, economic consequences were forecast in hypothetical pandemic scenarios (Rockefeller Foundation & Global Business Network, 2010). Lessons learned from past pandemics should have informed a unified global response. Unfortunately, this did not eventuate with COVID-19 for many reasons which are explored in Chapter 2.

The initial approach to COVID-19 was marred by the political opportunism of too many world leaders avoiding responsibility or finding scapegoats to deflect from the emerging disaster. For example, China was accused of secrecy and delayed reporting in the early stages of the pandemic. Indeed, a failure to report within 24 hours was a violation of international health regulation. The Chinese laboratory that submitted an article to *Nature* on 7 January 2020 about the novel coronavirus was shut down soon after (Chan & Lee, 2020; Wu et al., 2020). In response to international pressure and on the tail end of a complex geopolitical history, China admitted to weaknesses in its public health system while also exerting political muscle in Hong Kong and the South China Sea. China did share scientific findings, provided practical supplies and expertise with other nations such as Cambodia where it had heavily invested. Given global travel, it is likely the virus that had spread long before the first case was identified in China as new disease.

Conspiracy theories and political blame-shifting emanating from countries like Australia and the US proliferated. Diplomacy was not the language spoken with inevitable results. For example, the Australian Prime Minister, Scott Morrison, repeatedly demanded an investigation that focused on blaming China, not investigating COVID-19. Unsurprisingly, consequences were trade restriction against Australia and deteriorating relationships. Morrison, according to media reports is influenced by friends in QAnon and Hillsong church (Hardaker, 2019), has a reputation for admiring the ex-President Trump and also refused to reign in federal Ministers spreading false information about COVID-19.

On 19 May 2020, a more rational, apolitical approach, which focused on the virus as a critical incident rather than political blame-shifting, was presented to the 73rd World Health Assembly in Geneva. The draft resolution for an evaluation of the *international response to COVID-19* was passed, a vote which China supported (WHO, 2020). A joint investigation with China to explore the origins of the virus for future global health was conducted between 14 January and 19 February 2021, highlighting the emergence of SARS-CoV-19 as a zoonotic process. An intermediary animal and the site of origin were not able to be identified. Some early cases were linked to the outbreak in the Wuhan market, whereas other cases were not (WHO, 2021). The international team is open to further investigations and new information which could take years to reach any further conclusions, if at all. See Chapter 19 for a further explanation by Franklin.

Harvard researchers analysed satellite data about increased traffic around the five Wuhan hospitals and data on internet searches about coughs and diarrhoea which suggested that cases of COVID-19 may have appeared as early as November 2019 in China (Nsoesie et al., 2020). A recent study in conservation science confirms this, suggesting that zoonotic transfer occurred as early as October or November 2019 and had spread globally soon after (Roberts et al., 2021). Sewage analysis is being used to identify COVID-19 hotspots, a method of detection that has been used for other diseases such as polio (Hovi et al., 2001). In interesting developments, scientists have reported detecting the virus in wastewater in Brazil and Italy in November 2019, and according to a contested preprint article, traces were found in March 2019 in Spain (Chavarria-Miró et al., 2020). Other circulating illnesses such as that noted during the World Military Games held in Wuhan in October were also considered. The possibility that some studies of early detection could be a case of mistaken viral identity due to partial sequencing has been suggested (Maxmen, 2021). For a worldview of sewage monitoring, see the COVID-19 Poops dashboard (https://www.covid19wbec.org/covidpoops19).

The first response of scientists internationally was to leap into action, ultimately producing a range of effective and safe vaccinations in less than a year, a ground-breaking record, followed by work on booster vaccines. The challenges were for governments to purchase and roll out the vaccine, ensure their populations were vaccinated quickly and address inequitable distribution across the globe. Vaccination is discussed further in Chapters 16 and 18. At the time of writing this book, effective COVID-19 treatments were still being investigated.

Government and policy responses

The delivery of health and welfare were vital components of pandemic responses. Policy and the ideological positions of governments have always determined how social welfare is delivered. COVID-19 offers a good example of how the responses of governments illuminated underlying values and political ideologies that determined approaches to the economy and the social welfare and health systems of their respective societies. Governments placed different emphases on science influenced by personal beliefs and interests, the role of business and individual responsibility, and commitments to communities, social justice, human rights and equality. The responses around the world were consequently quite different.

Trust in science, as a starting point for policy making, has been underscored once again as a critical element in the equation of sound and rational social planning and policy response. We only need to look at the current climate emergency as a prime example of the choices leaders make between beliefs (which are claimed as truths) and political expediency versus scientific evidence and knowledge (Driscoll et al., 2020). The choices of governments have determined the mix of state and private enterprise and related service capacities of health and welfare. How social workers can practise within these contexts and the resources available to them has been a consistent focus of discussion during COVID-19, which highlights critical questions for public health social work. Jonathan Dickens explores the concept of welfare regimes and offers eight dimensions to evaluate how well the State might manage a health emergency using COVID-19 as an example (see Box 1.5).

BOX 1.5

WELFARE REGIMES

Jonathan Dickens

Welfare regimes offers a fertile framework for describing, evaluating and comparing national welfare systems. Esping-Andersen's (1990) *The Three Worlds of Welfare Capitalism* brought to prominence three broad approaches in capitalist economies to understand how citizens should be supported in times of hardship. He called these:

- *liberal or neo-liberal* – People should support themselves and their families, with a sparse state *safety net;*
- *conservative corporatist* – the state partners with business and voluntary sectors to provide adequate security, the aim being social stability, not change;
- *social democratic* – Taxation and state services redistribute wealth, ensuring equality and quality of treatment for all citizens.

The model, based on empirical work, also drew on centuries-old political thinking, the core approaches of *libertarianism, utilitarianism* and *egalitarianism.* Gough and Wood (2004) adapted the model for countries with different income levels and cultures, notably developing countries. They observed that Esping-Andersen's *ideal-types* were premised on wealthy states with well-functioning systems of government, which they called *security regimes,* because in different ways, they all ensured a degree of social and economic security for citizens. They expanded the model by introducing the concept of

(Continued)

BOX 1.5 (*Continued*)

WELFARE REGIMES

informal security regimes, working as a continuum. As states move along the continuum, they become increasingly weak, unable to collect taxes, deliver services and maintain order. Citizens become less able to rely on formal social policy, legislation and state-supported services. Instead, citizens rely on extended families (including remittances sent from abroad), their communities, non-state agencies and, increasingly, clientelism and corruption. At the far end, *insecurity regimes* are at risk of war, ethnic rivalries, epidemics or natural disaster. The state is ineffective and international agencies may have to step in to ensure citizens' survival and safety.

Building on these ideas, the following model describes eight dimensions to analyse and compare states and their responses to COVID-19. Like all models in social policy, it is a simplification, not a prescription – a tool for understanding and a springboard for more detailed analysis, and in this way, it could also be useful for evaluating responses to other pandemics, past and future.

Eight Dimensions of State Responses to COVID-19

1. *National wealth* – Overall wealth indicates access to housing, healthy diets, good wages, and well-funded, high-quality services for citizens therefore protecting the country from the worst effects of COVID-19. However, challenges in other dimensions will weaken these benefits – say, overall wealth disguises social inequalities or no coverage for non-citizens living in the country.
2. *Well-resourced public health* – Additional to well-resourced medical systems that respond to health emergencies, well-supported public health measures are vital for prevention such as physical distancing campaigns, and test and trace schemes. Respect for such measures will be influenced by levels of science and health literacy in the country.
3. *Secure borders* – Geography contributes to the ease of securing and maintaining borders. For example, the island nations of New Zealand and Australia can more easily respond to border security than countries that allow freedom of travel or are unable to restrict border crossings.
4. *Effective government* – All tiers of government are involved (national, federal or regional, and local). Countries that can effectively promote and enforce lockdowns and other protective measures and deliver the necessary services to support those worst affected will do better. In the absence of effective government, international agencies such as the World Bank may provide funds (which can drive poorer countries into further debt), and aid agencies may have to deliver practical and material support. But

(*Continued*)

BOX 1.5 (*Continued*)

WELFARE REGIMES

diverse political ideologies mean one person's *effective government* could be another person's authoritarianism.

5. *Economic and social equality* – Disparities in wealth, employment opportunities and living conditions increase the risk of coronavirus spread, applied to citizens and non-citizens living in the country.
6. *Access to financial and practical support* – Wealthier countries are more able to provide financial and practical support to people whose jobs are suspended or lost, making it easier to comply with lockdowns. Risks are increased when political decision-makers hold ideologies of non-intervention by the state and the prioritisation of individual responsibility. Poorer countries face practical challenges of ensuring food and income security for those who must work in order to eat, making adherence to protective measures more difficult.
7. *Favourable age profile* – Demography contributes to COVID-19 risk, that is, older people and those with pre-existing health conditions at greater risk of serious complications. Countries with a younger population may have less people seriously affected. Other countries such as Japan with a high older population did not initially experience a higher death rate, influenced by other dimensions such as economic and social equality.
8. *Collectivism* – A strong sense of wider community responsibility underpins adherence to protective measures necessary to contain the pandemic, more so than individualism, for example, certain Asian countries.

How these dimensions work together can be visualised as a radar graph (or spider graph), as shown below. A country which scores highly on each dimension should theoretically respond swiftly and effectively to the pandemic, controlling the incidence and supporting the population. A lower-scoring country would be less likely to do so. But it is a dynamic model, and strengths in some dimensions can compensate for weaknesses in others.

Figure 1.3 offers an imagined example of a relatively wealthy country with good public health services, secure borders and effective government, but with counterpoints of high inequality, limited financial supports, an older population and a culture of individualism. Despite initial advantages, one might expect challenges in managing the pandemic.

In contrast, Country 2 depicted in Figure 1.4 is relatively poor, has reasonable public health services, but has difficulties regulating cross-border movement, the government is weak, and it is not able to offer much support for citizens (support may be available from other sources). But because Country 2 does not have pronounced social divisions and inequality, has a younger population and is collectivist, the worst effects of COVID-19 might be avoided.

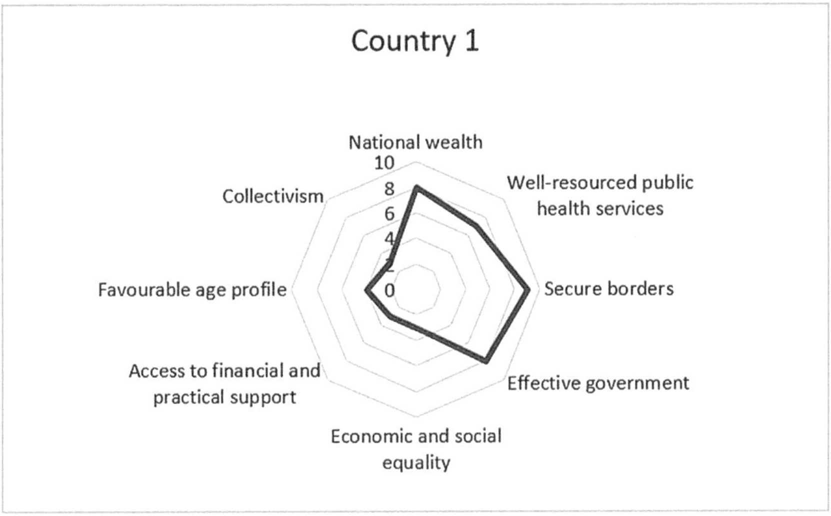

FIGURE 1.3 Hypothetical example of eight-dimension analysis, Country 1

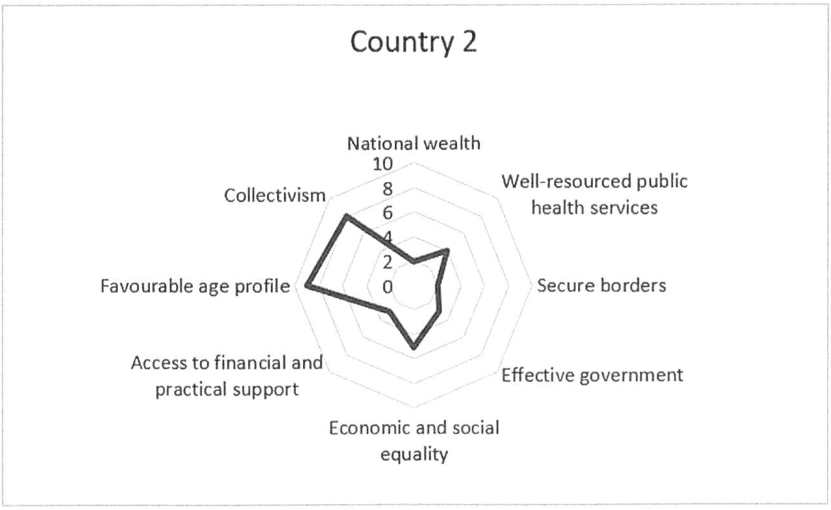

FIGURE 1.4 Hypothetical example of eight-dimension analysis, Country 2

Chapter 2 provides country examples of how Dickens' dimensions played out during the first six months of the pandemic. The marked differences in how governments first responded to COVID-19 and in subsequent decisions about mitigation, suppression or elimination, easing restrictions, and how they responded to second and third waves of infection, had significant effects on the spread of the disease and loss of life as well as on economies.

There is no standard definition of *waves*. Certainly, numbers of cases ebb and flow, and pandemics usually have two or more peaks. Some national governments, for example, the UK, Australia, and the US, prioritised saving the economy over lives before acting with variation within countries between jurisdictions depending on political flavour. In principle, such a position accepts a certain number of deaths as inevitable, whereas other regimes such as New Zealand, Iceland, Taiwan, and Vietnam prioritised lives with an elimination approach, acted quickly and recognised that a healthy population supports the economy, health and societal functioning overall. New Zealand, for example, quickly responded to subsequent outbreaks introduced by returned travellers and continued to contain the virus with strict and functional border protections and other strenuous measures which were coordinated nationally.

Governments that did not introduce protective measures such as hard lockdowns, physical distancing, handwashing, rigorous quarantine and contact tracing early enough either did not perform well from the beginning or struggled with subsequent waves. Some countries such as South Korea relied on extensive testing and tracing avoiding lockdowns which was initially an extremely promising approach but ultimately was insufficient. In many countries, borders remained porous, screening was inadequate, and testing was not available or only limited to people who met restrictive criteria. Also, of interest was how much emphasis countries gave to personal freedoms, for example, leaving mask-wearing to individual decisions or to businesses to make their own decisions, compared to prioritising the health of the community and collective responsibility. Where well-resourced countries delayed action and limited testing, the delays often related to a lack of preparedness and allocated resources, a belief that risk was not as great as forecast, a reliance on herd immunity or the prioritisation of business interests. Once vaccines became available, countries that did not focus on vaccinating their population and sharing with poorer neighbours threatened global capacity to manage the virus and its variants no matter how well they did initially.

Many governments relied on assumptions about the *R number* (the reproductive number of the virus) which is a calculation of how many people one ill person might infect. The aim is to keep the R number at one so as not to overwhelm the health system. An R number of 2.5 was estimated for SARS-CoV-2 which meant people including asymptomatic individuals could spread the virus to 2.5 others every 15 days (Sanche et al., 2020). By January 2021, the R number had risen to 3.28 and the variant first identified in South Africa had an estimated R number between 4 and 7, and later variants as high as 8. *Variants* arise as the virus mutates, a natural evolutionary process. The longer a virus is allowed to freely circulate among humans, the more *mutations* will occur creating new variants which are potentially more or less dangerous. SARS-CoV-2 and its resultant variants are deadly and highly infectious. The predictive nature of the R number is often overstated due to these changes (Shaw & Kennedy, 2021). It is important to remember that the R number is simply an average and does nothing to inform individual risks.

Superspreader refers to events where the virus spreads to a lot of people. A superspreading event relies on multiple factors – the variant, the amount of virus an infectious person emits (virus shedding), the environment (e.g. crowds, poor ventilation) and the vulnerability of others. Commonly sporting matches, political and religious gatherings were allowed to proceed by some national leaders despite limiting other large gatherings. Reasons ranged from prioritising economic benefits to awareness of religious traditions to ensuring popular votes. Schools and universities have also triggered such events. Prior to the US 2020 federal election, Trump and other Republicans who tested positive triggered a Whitehouse superspreader event which resulted in 30,000 new cases and 700 connected deaths, a situation exacerbated by Trump's self-aggrandizement, disregard for the health and lives of others and divisive politics (Bernheim et al., 2020).

The virus can be transmitted within short time frames and through cumulative short contacts (CDC, 2020; Jones et al., 2020). Calculating risk or ignoring that risk where eight out of ten people are estimated to be asymptomatic does not necessarily provide an accurate prediction of how the virus is spreading in the community at the onset of an outbreak or during the easing of restrictions, nor does it help the health system. The wider a virus spreads, the more people vulnerable to the disease will become ill, thus overwhelming even well-resourced health systems. Universal early containment and elimination strategies are the best defence. The longer the wait, the greater the spread of disease and the development of variants (Binny et al., 2020).

Sweden chose a different path, trusting citizens to do the right thing, maintaining life as usual and only recommending basic preventative measures. Sweden relied on *herd immunity* (see Box 1.6) which resulted in significant numbers of lives lost in the country, especially vulnerable elders, delivering a devasting outcome for the country.

BOX 1.6

WHAT IS HERD IMMUNITY?

The term *herd immunity*, community immunity or herd protection is an epidemiological concept that relies on a whole of community protection by either a large proportion of the population being vaccinated against a disease (e.g. measles or pertussis) or that the spread of the disease has been so extensive that a sufficient number of the population have developed antibodies preventing further spread of the disease. The problem with relying on herd immunity for new viruses in the absence of a vaccine is that a greater number of deaths are inevitable and expected.

For example, to reach heard immunity in the US without a vaccine, 70% of the population or 200 million people would need to be infected, inevitably leading to many unnecessary deaths (Dowdy & D'Souza, 2020). Early studies of countries with widespread infection showed only 2%–3% of the Wuhan

(Continued)

BOX 1.6 (*Continued*)

WHAT IS HERD IMMUNITY?

population had developed antibodies to COVID-19, 5% in Spain and 21.2% in New York, far below what is needed for herd immunity (Chow, 2020). The question of antibodies continued to undergo scientific investigation. However, by November 2020, new research (in preprint) suggested there was an adaptive immune response –in other words, the body remembers the virus and thus continues to fight it – which can last for eight to nine months or longer (Hartley et al., 2020).

There are other dangers with the unfettered spread of the virus which led to the emergence of new variants like those originating in Brazil, South Africa, India, California, New York, the UK and Peru which potentially posed greater risks.

Localised low-tech innovations emerged in different countries. For example, the city of Lund in Sweden took a unique position surrounding its parks with chicken manure to deter gatherings (Rahim et al., 2020). One Indonesian village engaged volunteers to patrol the streets. The volunteers wore ghost costumes believing people's superstitious beliefs would scare them into compliance (BBC, 2020). Unfortunately, it had the opposite effect with people seeking them out for entertainment. Many countries used actors, singers and song and dance videos to promote *physical distancing* (see Box 1.7), which could easily be accessed on mobile phones, for example, the Bangkok Train Service sang "Dance against the virus". Mexico used Susana Distancia, a cartoon superhero, to promote physical distancing and graffiti artists around the world painted public health messages (Sheridan, 2020). In Guatemala, public health messages asked people to imagine a tapir (a large animal with an extended snout) between people. See Chapter 16 for more on low-tech innovations.

BOX 1.7

PHYSICAL DISTANCING

Physical distancing (or *social distancing* which is the public health term) is used to help people keep a safe distance from each other to prevent the spread of infectious disease. The origins of the practice can be traced back to the Influenza Pandemic of 1918 (Spanish Flu). During the COVID-19 pandemic, the US Center for Disease Control and Prevention recommended that people keep a 6-foot (approximately 1.8 metres) distance from others when making essential

(*Continued*)

BOX 1.7 (*Continued*)

PHYSICAL DISTANCING

trips into the community for grocery shopping and other critical needs. The Australian government promoted 1.5-metre (approximately 4.9 feet) distance from others which demonstrates how public health information differed from country to country.

The term *social distancing* was first used in the 1950s to describe people who were socially or emotionally detached and is associated with *othering*. The term social distancing has been critiqued as being harmful for First Peoples, in Roma and other cultures, and for people with mental health conditions because it implies a cultural and social disconnection from others that goes beyond the physical. Social and cultural connections are important for holistic well-being and for others to maintain their mental and physical health. For this reason, the term *physical distancing* is purposely used throughout this book.

Flattening the curve

Many governments relied on mathematical predictive modelling based on the *Susceptible-Infectious-Recovered Model*, first written down over a century ago, which provides an equation used to calculate the spread of infectious disease (Magal & Ruan, 2014). The idea is to *flatten the curve* by reducing new daily infections. *Flattening the curve* means instigating strategies that interfere with the rate of rising infection (e.g. physical distancing and mask-wearing) rather than allowing the curve to continue an upward trend as it would without such interference. Graphical representations of the curve can show two things – bars which represent the daily number of infections and a cumulative curve, depicted by a solid line, that adds the daily totals represented by bars. The example shown in Figure 1.5 depicts how bars and lines are usually presented in these types of graphs.

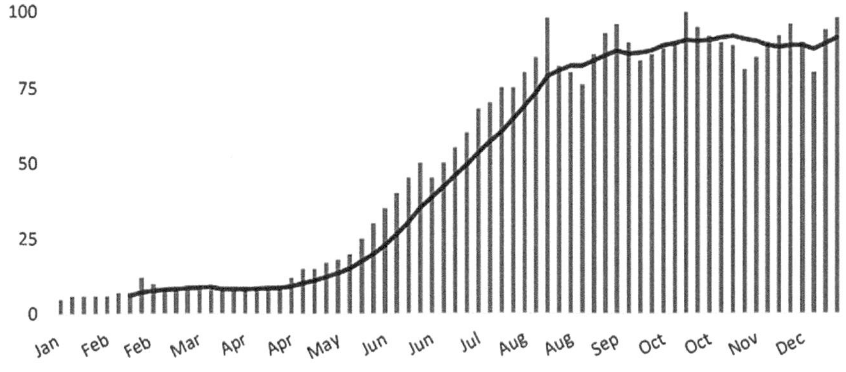

FIGURE 1.5 Example of graph showing cumulative curve and daily total cases

If a curve is high, the disease is spreading from infectious people to susceptible people quickly. If the curve is low, infectious disease is spreading more slowly (Lewin et al., 2020). Different graphic representations depict this spread. For example, the graph below shows an outbreak which has a very high, sharp curve and a lower curve achieved with some mitigation measures (see Figure 1.6). The lower the curve, the less stress on health systems. Of course, the ideal interference to a curve are the combination of measures that dramatically arrest the curve's progress and ideally includes widespread vaccination (Lewin et al., 2020).

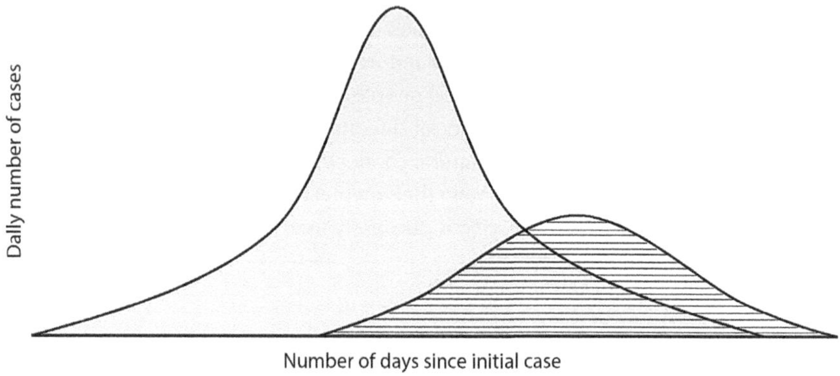

FIGURE 1.6 Example of graph showing high and low curve

In relation to COVID-19, some governments waited until the curve began to rise quickly before acting or meted out measures in increments in attempts to keep economies active and not overwhelm under-resourced health systems. To flatten the curve, individual US States eventually moved forward with critical decisions to control the spread of the virus due to the inaction of federal and many state governments, a similar experience to Australia and other parts of the world where responsibilities were left to the states (Adeel et al., 2020). In the US, extensive social marketing to flatten the curve came first from the private sector rather than the Trump administration. The federal Australian government had good scientific information from the start but chose to delay actions as long as possible, left decisions to businesses and meted out restrictions in a slow and piecemeal fashion.

The idea of flattening the curve became *real* to many ordinary people who were coming to terms with how they could personally participate in controlling the spread of disease while others denied its existence, which in turn affected individual collective behaviour. For the US, realisation came too late as it became the most affected country in the world with New York the first epicentre of disease in the US, discussed further in Chapter 2. Although Australia also delayed actions, it fared better due to a good universal public health system, geographical advantage enabling strict border closures, and the eventual introduction of more stringent strategies to flatten the curve instigated by state governments, not due to coordinated national governance and planning.

Subsequent outbreaks came with poor quarantine oversight, premature opening of borders, allowing large gatherings, and poor coordination. The federal government ultimately failed to protect the population, provide safe quarantine facilities, purchase sufficient vaccines and efficient rollout, bring citizens home from overseas and provide income support for individuals.

Each government's level of denial, preparedness or their priorities determined when they introduced proactive measures and which measures they adopted. For example, Italy, one of the most heavily affected countries in Europe only introduced lockdown 27 days after the 100th case. Multiple factors led to Italy's crisis and response, including an overwhelmed health system. The initial outbreaks in Italy and Spain were traced to trade, international travel and large sporting matches. Concepts related to pandemic approaches (see Box 1.8) are *mitigation, suppression, controlled suppression, elimination, controlled adaptation and eradication* (Ferguson et al., 2020; Group of Eight, 2020).

BOX 1.8

CONCEPTS RELATED TO PANDEMIC APPROACHES

Mitigation "focuses on slowing but not necessarily stopping epidemic spread – reducing peak healthcare demand while protecting those most at risk of severe disease from infection".

Suppression "aims to reverse epidemic growth, reducing case numbers to low levels and maintaining that situation indefinitely" (Ferguson et al., 2020, p. 1).

Controlled suppression is about using mitigating strategies to keep the rate of infection as low as possible.

According to Ferguson and colleagues (2020), both mitigation and suppression have challenges. Even the best-managed mitigation would still result in hundreds of thousands of deaths globally and overwhelmed health systems. The length of time needed to maintain strict measures until a vaccine is available brings other problems. For example, in many countries where poverty is rife, food security is an issue and people must work and travel to be able to eat on a daily basis in the absence of government assistance. For other countries which prioritise the economy, suppression is considered undesirable due to the perceived impact on globalised and local business.

Elimination is about defeating the disease in a jurisdiction, for example, New Zealand's and Vietnam's response to COVID-19. The challenge here is about protecting the country from the disease re-entering. For example, after being virus-free for 100 days, travellers brought the virus

(*Continued*)

BOX 1.8 (*Continued*)

CONCEPTS RELATED TO PANDEMIC APPROACHES

back into New Zealand and a localised 3-day shutdown was instigated in Auckland when four cases were identified.

Controlled adaptation concerns a phased easing of lockdown conditions. This approach accepts further incidents of illness and death and is claimed to be better for the economy.

Eradication completely defeats the disease. Smallpox is the only disease affecting humans ever eradicated globally. Eradication is unlikely for COVID-19.

Country outcomes concerning the spread of COVID-19 and resultant *mortality* (deaths) in accrued numbers and per population are mixed highlighting varying approaches to health emergencies as well as contributing conditions, data recording and collection. The influencing factors are diverse and variable, rooted in the social and political context of each country and their concepts of freedom, the role of government and its reach into the sphere of family and community-life, efforts to support uninterrupted economic functioning, and trust in leaders to respond in the interests of the people. As such, responses in countries with a strong orientation to *individualism* versus *collectivism* and *repressive* versus *liberal societies* have generally been quite different.

When examining the whole picture, the lack of a coordinated global approach to pandemic management is a standout, even with concerted efforts by the WHO to warn, advise and share the reality of a rapidly spreading infectious disease. Countries and regions chose their own policy and social planning pathways, often with little recognition of *how* their policy affected neighbouring countries, entire regions and beyond. The hope is that one outcome of the COVID-19 pandemic will be the universal adoption of a global rapid response system informed by common values and the lessons learned worldwide to avoid the ongoing consequences beginning in 2020 and to ensure that future pandemics are not used as opportunities to advance political agendas to the detriment of world health.

Human behaviour

Beginning as a political concept in the UK, *behavioural fatigue* or the idea that people will only tolerate restrictions for a limited period of time gained traction. The inherent assumptions were not critiqued nor supported by research. The concept was adopted by politicians in other countries as a justification for delayed actions and premature opening. Whereas countries and communities with previous epidemic and pandemic experiences, for example, in Asia, were notable at the level of community behavioural responses that interfaced with their governments' rapid public health policy rollouts such as the early adoption of multiple strategies. It could be argued that the problem of fatigue that did emerge is more related to the yoyo effect evident in those countries where the pandemic was not managed strictly in the beginning or where governments and the business sector pushed for premature openings causing people to move in and out of *lockdown* (see Box 1.9) situations creating considerable uncertainty and hardships related to financial resources.

It has been suggested that fatigue is strongly related to social context in terms of perceived vulnerability and severity or how a person perceives their chances of catching the disease and how sick they expect to become if they do, making leadership messages that downplay the effects of the disease particularly dangerous (Joseph et al., 2009). New Zealand Prime Minister, Jacinda Adern, showed how trust, empathy and clear evidence-informed messaging positively influenced behaviour even during strict lockdown (Mazey & Richardson, 2020). An issue that further affects behaviour is *proof of no appearance* (Naumova, 2020). In other words, when the disease is effectively controlled, people do not personally see the impact of disease and therefore some people conclude that the risk was overblown or non-existent (especially if this coincides with pre-existing beliefs). The focus then shifts to individual hardships experienced during lockdowns rather than disease prevention.

BOX 1.9

LOCKDOWN

Lockdown (or *Shelter-in-Place*) is the term used when people are required to stay at home to stem the spread of disease, except for workers providing essential services and activities such as caring for others and grocery shopping. The term lockdown originates in prisons where inmates are confined for extended periods following incidents such as riots. Lockdown is usually instigated in stages of severity where complete lockdown is the highest stage of restrictions.

A survey of 2,250 people aged between 18 and 75 years of age in the UK conducted by Kings College London during lockdown found three clusters of people who behaved and responded differently (Duffy & Allington, 2020). They named these groups – *the accepting*, *the suffering* and *the resisting*. The accepting group (48%), nearly always followed lockdown rules and tended to be in the older age group. The majority coped well despite concerns about future financial problems. The suffering group which had more women, thought about COVID-19 all the time, checked social media often and were worried, anxious and depressed. Those who were suffering also followed the rules and, like the accepting group, supported police action to keep people in check. The majority in the resisting group (9%) held false beliefs about COVID-19 (i.e. the virus was manufactured in a laboratory) and used homeopathic remedies for prevention; they also felt the pandemic was overblown and resisted official advice or external intervention. They followed the rules less, visiting others or working instead of following requirements. More people in this group expected financial distress and were mostly in the youngest age group. However, they were also more optimistic than the other groups.

As the pandemic progressed and exit strategies from lockdown scenarios were developed, some countries (New Zealand being the first) adopted a *bubble* or *pod* approach in an attempt to balance emotional, social and cultural needs with protective health measures, and to contain risky behaviours (Leng et al., 2020). A bubble or pod could constitute a single, family unit or an extended bubble where others could be nominated to join the bubble, an approach suitable for non-traditional family units and cultural practices. Within the bubble, individuals would not physically distance nor wear masks but were to remain faithful to only indulging these behaviours within the social bubble. Later, bubbles between safe countries were employed to stimulate economies as well as connecting people.

During initial response periods, messaging from world leaders also influenced the positive or negative behaviour of people. Denial, misinformation, violence and racism proliferated in some countries, while, in others, leaders supported community cohesion encouraging communities to rally together and help others. We consider these issues in Chapter 2 when we explore these factors and the human and material costs in different societies during the first six months of the pandemic. In addition to policy, politics and welfare regimes, influences include the level of pandemic preparedness; geographical advantage; resources including the health system, population density, pandemic measures (quarantine, lockdowns, extensive tracing and testing), access to the manufacture and supply of masks, sanitisers and soap, and treatment equipment (ventilators) and later access to vaccines and the vaccine rollout. The provision of income support, access to food and factors such as culture and health beliefs combined with educating the population are further influences. The pandemic bought untold suffering to many people who faced loss of roles and income, illness and death, and uncertain futures.

The position of social workers

Experience in responses to COVID-19 has improved our understanding of the psychological, social and behavioural impact of pandemics in the modern world which, in turn, has expanded social work practice to include how to best support people during a pandemic, help them deal with failing systems and the aftermath of widespread disease on families and communities as well as working to change systems at the macro level and to value social work as an essential contributor to health emergency planning. Social workers are on the front line whether that be in institutional or community care. Social workers have a core commitment to preventive practices and interventions at *primary*, *secondary* and *tertiary* levels (see Box 1.10).

BOX 1.10

STAGES OF PREVENTION

Primary prevention aims to prevent a disease developing in the first place. Promoting vaccination and scientific information through health education is an example.

Secondary prevention aims to prevent at-risk groups who may be susceptible to disease or at risk of exposure and becoming ill. For example, providing education specifically to immunosuppressed people on physical distancing, handwashing and wearing masks, or working with people to address anxieties and distress about COVID-19 or supporting people in lockdown to ultimately prevent the further spread of the infectious disease.

Tertiary prevention is rehabilitative and responds to disease in its fullest manifestation. In other words, maximising psychosocial and health outcomes during and after serious illness to improve survival chances, prevent further complications and promote well-being. For example, educative, practical, psychosocial or supportive interventions for people in recovery.

Professional practice includes interactions with vulnerable populations, addressing needs from a social justice and human rights–based value alongside preventative and responsive practices which shape programs and services. This lens combined with our professional commitment to human dignity are threads woven throughout this book. Rights, values and ethics also extend to the profession itself and *how* we practise in the context of health emergencies. These major concepts come to life in the chapters that tackle particular fields of practice with vulnerable groups and settings that either promote or infringe upon human dignity and well-being. We build upon dignity with our shared moral and ethical imperatives related to life and health as explored throughout the collection.

During the COVID-19 pandemic, social workers were faced with preserving their own health, safety and well-being while maintaining services, particularly to those people made more vulnerable in *lockdown* situations or unprotected in under-resourced and unprepared contexts. In many countries, there was little readily available guidance on personal protection for social workers to safely do their job due to a lack of personal protective equipment (PPE) and even access to soap in many places. Social workers have not always been included in planning for essential frontline workforces as PPE such as masks, where available, were reserved for medical professionals with an emphasis on the front line in hospitals rather than in the community or other types of institutions such as aged care facilities. Of course, there are many complications inhibiting resources locally, and within and between countries. Professional social work associations and organisations did develop guidelines and social workers turned to electronic communications and social media as a means of sharing information and disseminating guidance for safe practice and innovative interventions (Jiang, 2020; López Peláez et al., 2020).

Developing response systems had significant limitations as social workers were literally placed in a position of responding respectfully to human need while keeping physical distance and dealing with their own personal trauma and that of their families. The challenges were immense and at times overwhelming. Social workers had to find novel methods of engagement including using technological tools. The nature of work changed for the social work profession across all fields. Adapting to the pandemic accelerated changes previously progressing more slowly such as social work practices using tele-health and online counselling, online teaching, supervision, professional development and going about organisational business. The COVID-19 pandemic threw a spotlight on both the resourcefulness and resilience of the profession as well as how unprepared social work was for a global health emergency. Social work as a profession has adapted and continues to evolve.

The structure of the book

The book is constructed in three sections which tell a cogent story of social work innovation in health emergencies across world regions. Sections 1 and 2 of the book focus primarily on COVID-19 with reference to other historical and contemporary health emergencies while Section 3 looks to the future. The book concludes with two Q&A bonus chapters in conversation with eminent scientists.

In the first section of the book, *Regional, historical and social work perspectives*, we explore pandemic and public health concepts with a specific focus on understanding the COVID-19 pandemic and the perfect storm of pandemic, politics and the planet. Then, in Chapter 2, our international authors take us on a journey through the diverse regions of the world in an exploration of the different approaches to COVID-19 in its first six months, each influenced by unique histories, the actions of leaders, the preparedness of health systems and the capacity of countries to manage disease alongside the global movements of people, goods and services. Compounding the health emergency, some regions experienced concurrent disasters, for example, locust plagues in East Africa, tornadoes and fires in the US, a massive explosion in Lebanon, the devastation of the Amazonian environment, floods in Japan, the Nangka storm that devastated South East Asia and Cyclone Harold in Fiji and Vanuatu, and the re-emergence of Ebola in Guinea, to name only a few. We then turn to the long history of health emergencies for clues about challenges and human behaviour, authored by Matthew Ward. The section finishes with human dignity which underscores and contextualises pandemic social work practice in Chapter 4 by Donna McAuliffe with case studies by Hilary N. Weaver on First Nations, Sharon E. Moore on Black Lives Matter and Robert Common on LGBTQIA issues.

The middle section of this book, *Social work practice issues and responses*, presents issues, challenges and responses pertaining to 11 fields of social work practice.

Throughout the ensuing chapters, protection for social workers is considered alongside novel adaptions and experiences.

Barbara Muskat and colleagues unpack the social work experience and practice from research conducted in Canadian hospitals at the height of their second wave. Social workers across fields identified new or intensified risks such as those for older people, children, family violence as well as other forms of abuse and neglect within families and wider communities. Children living on the streets or in residential childcare institutions in low-resource countries experienced heightened risks. Child protection in Botswana is explored by Thabile Samboma in Chapter 6. Louise Harms and colleagues address family violence in the Australian state of Victoria. Gabriela Misca and colleagues present their research on the experiences of UK families in lockdown which created extraordinary stress and the need to adapt. In Chapters 9 and 10, Tarek Zidan discusses the immense challenges for people with disabilities and Malcolm Payne tackles the issue of ageism which became terribly apparent in pandemic conditions.

The chapter on global challenges and the terrible plight of people on the move is presented by Justin Lee and Carmen Monico. Ching-Wen Chang and Marcus Chiu address issues of mental health in Hong Kong in a politically charged pandemic environment in Chapter 12. Elizabeth Bowen and Nicole Capozziello tackle urban homelessness in the US, highlighting how these problems also exist in high-resourced countries. Joel Izlar explores the innovations found in community organising, proposed as the New Social Service. The final field of social work practice addressed in Chapter 15 discusses the disruption to higher education specifically field placement in Australia, New Zealand and California, authored by Lynne Briggs and colleagues.

Preparing for the Future, the final section of the book, returns to broader concepts of public health social work concerned with innovation, living in the world with coronaviruses, preparedness and future practices as social work enters a new era of service delivery. Gokul Mandayam and colleagues examine low- and high-tech innovations further in Chapter 16 on social innovation with case studies from India and Kenya. In Chapter 17, we challenge the profession to consider how we can prepare for the next pandemic which is predicted to occur much sooner than we think. We conclude the section with a precis of our journey through the COVID-19 health emergency bringing us not to the end of the pandemic rather up to has happened to the world since the first six months of the pandemic to June 2021 and continuing our gaze into the future.

The final two bonus chapters bring ecological and scientific understandings by contributing scientists. We ask questions of Dr Franklin about the links between humans, animals and the environment. Dr Franklin is a leading research biologist who specialises in ecology and the dynamics of wildlife populations, pathogen surveillance and monitoring in wildlife, and the wildlife-agricultural and wildlife-human interfaces. In our final bonus chapter, Laureate Professor and Nobel Prize winner, Peter Doherty, whose special interests are viral pathogenesis and immunity, answers our questions about COVID-19, new variants, immunity, vaccines and much more. To reflect on issues raised in this chapter go to Box 1.11

BOX 1.11

REFLECTION

1. Consider the ecological model. How do the relationships between micro, mezzo and macro work together to shape the impact of a pandemic on individuals?
2. Reflect and discuss the kind of welfare regime in your country and analyse the response according to Jonathan Dicken's Eight Dimensions of State Responses
3. COVID-19 is expected to become endemic. What might be the implications of this?
4. What was your key learning in this chapter? Did anything surprise you?

References

Addams, J. (1910). *Twenty years at Hull-House.* The McMillan Company.

Adeel, A. B., Catalano, M., Catalano, O., Gibson, G., Muftuoglu, E., Riggs, T., … Zhirnov, A. (2020). COVID-19 policy response and the rise of the sub-national governments. *Canadian Public Policy*, 46(4), 565–584.

Ahmed, M., Advani, S., Moreira, A., Zoretic, S., Martinez, J., Chorath, K., … Moreira, A. (2020). Multisystem inflammatory syndrome in children: A systematic review. *EClinical Medicine*. https://doi.org/10.1016/j.eclinm.2020.100527

Allimuddin, Z., Hui, D. S., & Pearlman, S. (2015). Middle East respiratory syndrome. *The Lancet*, 386(9997), 995–1007.

Alston, M., Hazeleger, T., & Hargreaves, D. (2019). *Social work and disasters: A handbook for practice*. Routledge.

BBC. (2020, April 14). Coronavirus: Indonesian Village Uses 'Ghosts' for Distancing Patrols. *BBC News*. https://www.bbc.com/news/world-asia-52269607

Bernheim, B. D., Buchmann, N., Freitas-Groff, Z., & Otero, S. (2020). *The effects of large group meetings on the spread of COVID-19: The case of Trump rallies*. Department of Economics, Stanford University. https://sebotero.github.io/papers/COVIDrallies_10_30_2000.pdf

Binny, R. N., Hendy, S. C., James, A., Lustig, A., Plank, M. J., & Steyn, N. (2020). *Effect of alert level 4 on R_{eff}: Review of international COVID-19 cases*. https://www.tepunahamatatini.ac.nz/2020/04/22/effect-of-alert-level-4-measures-on-covid-19-transmission/

Boni, M. F., Lemey, P., Jiang, X., Lam, T. T.-Y., Perry, B. W., Castoe, T. A., … Robertson, D. L. (2020). Evolutionary origins of the SARS-CoV-2 sarbecovirus lineage responsible for the COVID-19 pandemic. *Nature Microbiology*, 5(11), 1408–1417.

Brazilian Ministry of Health. (2021). *Special Epidemiological Report. Disease from Coronavirus COVID-19. No. 52 [Boletim epidemiológico especial: Doença pelo coronavirus COVID-19]*. https://www.gov.br/saude/pt-br/media/pdf/2021/marco/05/boletim_epidemiologico_covid_52_final2.pdf

Carfì, A., Bernabei, R., Landi, F., & Covid-Post-Acute Care Study Group. (2020). Persistent symptoms in patients after acute COVID-19. *JAMA*, 324(6), 603–605.

CDC. (2017). *National pandemic strategy*. Centers for Disease Control and Prevention. https://www.cdc.gov/flu/pandemic-resources/national-strategy/index.html

CDC. (2020, October 21). *Contact Tracing. Case Investigation and Contact Tracing Guidance. Appendices*. https://www.cdc.gov/coronavirus/2019-ncov/php/contact-tracing/contact-tracing-plan/appendix.html#contact

Chan, L.-H., & Lee, P. K. (2020, May 20). The World Health Organization must answer these hard questions in its coronavirus inquiry. *The Conversation*. https://theconversation.com/the-world-health-organization-must-answer-these-hard-questions-in-its-coronavirus-inquiry-138959

Chavarria-Miró, G., Anfruns-Estrada, E., Guix, S., Paraira, M., Galofré, B., Sáanchez, G., … Bosch, A. (2020). Sentinel surveillance of SARS-CoV-2 in wastewater anticipates the occurrence of COVID-19 cases. *medRxiv*. https://doi.org/10.1101/2020.06.13.20129627

Chow, D. (2020, May 15). Can Herd Immunity Help Stop the Coronavirus? Experts Warn It's Not That Easy. *NBC News*. https://www.nbcnews.com/science/science-news/can-herd-immunity-help-stop-coronavirus-experts-warn-it-s-n1207351

Davis, H. E., Assaf, G. S., McCorkell, L., Wei, H., Low, R. J., Re'em, Y., … Akrami, A. (2020). Characterizing long COVID in an international cohort: 7 months of symptoms and their impact. *medRxiv*. https://doi.org/10.1101/2020.12.24.20248802

DeBiasi, R. L., & Delaney, M. (2020). Symptomatic and asymptomatic viral shedding in pediatric patients infected with Severe Acute Respiratory Syndrome Coronavirus 2 (SARS-CoV-2): Under the surface. *JAMA Pediatrics*. https://doi.org/10.1001/jamapediatrics.2020.3996

Doherty, P. C. (2013). *Pandemics: What everyone needs to know*. Oxford University Press.

Dowdy, D., & D'Souza, G. (2020). *Early Herd Immunity against COVID-19: A Dangerous Misconception*. https://coronavirus.jhu.edu/from-our-experts/early-herd-immunity-against-covid-19-a-dangerous-misconception

Driscoll, D. A., Garrard, G. E., Kusmanoff, A. M., Dovers, S., Maron, M., Preece, N., … Ritchie, E. G. (2020). Consequences of information suppression in ecological and conservation sciences. *Conservation Letters*. https://doi.org/10.1111/conl.12757

Duffy, B., & Allington, D. (2020). *The Accepting, the Suffering and the Resisting: The Different Reactions to Life under Lockdown*. https://www.kcl.ac.uk/policy-institute/assets/Coronavirus-in-the-UK-cluster-analysis.pdf

Esping-Andersen, G. (1990). *The three worlds of welfare capitalism*. Polity Press.

Farrell, J. C. (1967). *Beloved lady: A history of Jane Addams' ideas on reform and peace*. Johns Hopkins University.

Ferguson, N. M., Laydon, D., Nedjati-Gilani, G., Imai, N., Ainslie, K., Baguelin, M., … Ghani, A. C. (2020). *Impact of Non-Pharmaceutical Interventions (NPIs) to Reduce COVID-19 Mortality and Healthcare Demand*. https://www.imperial.ac.uk/media/imperial-college/medicine/sph/ide/gida-fellowships/Imperial-College-COVID19-NPI-modelling-16-03-2020.pdf

Franklin, A. B., & Bevins, S. N. (2020). Spillover of SARS-CoV-2 into novel wild hosts in North America: A conceptual model for perpetuation of the pathogen. *Science of The Total Environment, 733*. https://doi.org/10.1016/j.scitotenv.2020.139358

Friedman, B. D., & Merrick, J. (2015). *Public health, social work and health inequalities*. Nova Science Publishers.

Furuse, Y., Sando, E., Tsuchiya, N., Miyahara, R., Yasuda, I., Ko, Y. K., … Oshitani, H. (2020). Clusters of coronavirus disease in communities, Japan, January–April 2020. *Emerging Infectious Diseases*, 26(9). https://doi.org/10.3201/eid2609.202272

Goldman, E. (2020). Exaggerated risk of transmission of COVID-19 by fomites. *The Lancet Infectious Diseases,* 20(8), 892–893.

Gough, I., & Wood, G. (2004). *Insecurity and welfare regimes in Asia, Africa and Latin America: Social policy in development contexts*. Cambridge University Press.

Grijalva, C. G., Rolfes, M. A., Zhu, Y., McLean, H. Q., Hanson, K. E., Belongia, E. A., … Talbot, H. K. (2020). *Transmission of SARS-COV-2 Infections in Households — Tennessee and Wisconsin, April–September 2020.* https://www.cdc.gov/mmwr/volumes/69/wr/mm6944e1.htm?s_cid=mm6944e1_w#suggestedcitation

Group of Eight. (2020). *COVID-19 Roadmap to Recovery – A Report for the Nation.* Australia. https://go8.edu.au/research/roadmap-to-recovery

Hardaker, D. (2019, October 31). Scott Morrison's conspiracy-theorist friend claims he has the PM's ear – and can influence what he says. *Crikey.* https://www.crikey.com.au/2019/10/31/scott-morrison-qanon/?utm_campaign=SundayRead&utm_medium=email&utm_source=newsletter

Hartley, G. E., Edwards, E. S. J., Aui, P. M., Varese, N., Stojanovic, S., McMahon, J., … van Zelm, M. C. (2020). Rapid and lasting generation of B-cell memory to SARS-CoV-2 spike and nucleocapsid proteins in COVID-19 disease and convalescence. *medRxiv.* https://doi.org/10.1101/2020.11.17.20233544

Hippich, M., Holthaus, L., Assfalg, R., Zapardiel-Gonzalo, J., Kapfelsperger, H., Heigermoser, M., … Ziegler, A.-G. (2020). A public health antibody screening indicates a 6-fold higher SARS-CoV-2 exposure rate than reported cases in children. *Med.* https://doi.org/10.1016/j.medj.2020.10.003

Hovi, T., Stenvik, M., Partanen, H., Kangas, A. (2001). Poliovirus surveillance by examining sewage specimens. Quantitative recovery of virus after introduction into sewerage at remote upstream location. *Epidemiology and Infection,* 127(1), 101–106.

Huang, C., Huang, L., Wang, Y., Li, X., Ren, L., Gu, X., … Cao, B. (2021). 6-month consequences of COVID-19 in patients discharged from hospital: A cohort study. *The Lancet,* 397(10270), 220–232.

IPBES. (2020). *Escaping the 'Era of Pandemics': Experts Warn Worse Crises to Come Options Offered to Reduce Risk.* https://ipbes.net/pandemics

Jiang, Q. (2020). What small NGOs can deliver: A case study of a Canadian community-based project making fabric scrub caps for healthcare workers during the COVID-19 pandemic. *International Social Work.* https://doi.org/10.1177/0020872820959374

Johns Hopkins Corona Virus Resource Centre. Johns Hopkins University. https://coronavirus.jhu.edu/

Jones, K. E., Patel, N. G., Levy, M. A., Storeygard, A., Balk, D., Gittleman, J. L., Daszak, P. (2008). Global trends in emerging infectious diseases. *Nature,* 451(7181), 990–993.

Jones, N. R., Qureshi, Z. U., Temple, R. J., Larwood, J. P. J., Greenhalgh, T., & Bourouiba, L. (2020). Two metres or one: What is the evidence for physical distancing in covid-19? *British Medical Journal,* 370. https://doi.org/10.1136/bmj.m3223

Joseph, G., Burke, N. J., Tuason, N., Barker, J. C., Pasick, R. J. (2009). Perceived susceptibility to illness and perceived benefits of preventive care: An exploration of behavioral theory constructs in a transcultural context. *Health Education & Behavior,* 36(5_suppl), 71S–90S.

Leng, T., White, C., Hilton, J., Kucharski, A. J., Pellis, L., Stage, H., … Flasche, S. (2020). The effectiveness of social bubbles as part of a Covid-19 lockdown exit strategy, a modelling study. *medRxiv.* https://doi.org/10.1101/2020.06.05.20123448

Lewin, S., McCaw, J., Harper, I., Damousi, J., & Kapur, S. (2020, April 16). Life beyond coronavirus: The expert view. In *Pursuit.* University of Melbourne. https://pursuit.unimelb.edu.au/articles/watch-episode-1-life-beyond-coronavirus-the-expert-view

López Peláez, A., Marcuello-Servós, C., Castillo de Mesa, J., & Almaguer Kalixto, P. (2020). The more you know, the less you fear: Reflexive social work practices in times of COVID-19. *International Social Work.* https://doi.org/10.1177/0020872820959365

Magal, P., & Ruan, S. (2014). Susceptible-infectious-recovered models revisited: From the individual level to the population level. *Mathematical Biosciences*, 250, 26–40.

Maxmen, A. (2021, March 30). WHO report into COVID pandemic origins zeroes in on animal markets, not labs. *Nature Briefing*. https://doi.org/10.1038/d41586-021-00865-8

Maxmen, A., & Mallapaty, S. (2021, June 8). The COVID lab-leak hypothesis: What scientists do and don't know. *Nature*. https://www.nature.com/articles/d41586-021-01529-3

Mazey, S., & Richardson, J. (2020). Lesson-drawing from New Zealand and COVID-19: The need for anticipatory policy making. *The Political Quarterly*, 91(3), 561–570.

Moniz, C. (2010). Social work and the social determinants of health perspective: A good fit. *Health and Social Work*, 35, 310–313.

Nalbandian, A., Sehgal, K., Gupta, A., Madhavan, M. V., McGroder, C., Stevens, J. S., … Wan, E. Y. (2021). Post-acute COVID-19 syndrome. *Nature Medicine*. doi:10.1038/s41591-021-01283-z

Naumova, E. N. (2020). Public health response to COVID-19: The forecaster's dilemma. *Journal of Public Health Policy*, 41(4), 395–398.

Nsoesie, E. O., Rader, B., Barnoon, Y. L., Goodwin, L., & Brownstien, J. S. (2020). Analysis of hospital traffic and search engine data in Wuhan China indicates early disease activity in the Fall of 2019. *Digital Access to Scholarship at Harvard*. http://nrs.harvard.edu/urn-3:HUL.InstRepos:42669767

Passarinho, N., & Barrucho, L. (2021, March 16). Why Are So Many Babies Dying of Covid-19 in Brazil? *BBC News*. https://www.bbc.com/news/world-latin-america-56696907

Paterson, R. W., Brown, R. L., Benjamin, L., Nortley, R., Wiethoff, S., Bharucha, T., … Neurosurgery, C.-S. G. (2020). The emerging spectrum of COVID-19 neurology: Clinical, radiological and laboratory findings. *Brain*. https://doi.org/10.1093/brain/awaa240

Rahim, Z., Mahmood, Z., & Pettersson, H. (2020, May 1). Swedish City Uses Chicken Manure to Encourage Social Distancing. *CNN*. https://edition.cnn.com/travel/article/sweden-lund-chicken-manure-scli-intl/index.html

Ren, L.-L., Wang, Y.-M., Wu, Z.-Q., Xiang, Z.-C., Guo, L., Xu, T., … Wang, J.-W. (2020). Identification of a novel coronavirus causing severe pneumonia in human: A descriptive study. *Chinese Medical Journal*, 133(9), 1015–1024.

Roberts, D. L., Rossman, J. S., & Jarić, I. (2021). Dating first cases of COVID-19. *PLoS Pathogens*. https://doi.org/10.1371/journal.ppat.1009620

Rockefeller Foundation & Global Business Network. (2010). *Scenarios for the Future of Technology and International Development*. https://www.nommeraadio.ee/meedia/pdf/RRS/Rockefeller%20Foundation.pdf

Sanche, S., Lin, Y. T., Xu, C., Romero-Severson, E., Hengartner, N., & Ke, R. (2020). High contagiousness and rapid spread of severe acute respiratory syndrome coronavirus 2. *Emerging Infectious Disease journal*, 26(7), 1470.

Shaw, C. L., & Kennedy, D. A. (2021). What the reproductive number R0 can and cannot tell us about COVID-19 dynamics. *Theoretical Population Biology*. https://doi.org/10.1016/j.tpb.2020.12.003

Sheridan, M. B. (2020, March 26). From Mexico's Newest Superhero to Iran's Most Elegant Hand-Washer: Watch How Countries Are Promoting Coronavirus Safety. *The Washington Post*. https://www.washingtonpost.com/graphics/world/2020/03/26/watch-how-countries-are-promoting-coronavirus-safety/

Walter-McCabe, H. A. (2020). Coronavirus pandemic calls for an immediate social work response. *Social Work in Public Health*, 35(3), 69–72.

WHO. (n.d). *Social determinants of health*. World Health Organization. https://www.who.int/social_determinants/sdh_definition/en/

WHO. (2005). *International Health Regulations Monitoring Framwork*. World Health Organization. https://www.who.int/data/gho/data/themes/international-health-regulations-(2005)-monitoring-framework

WHO. (2010, February 24). *What is a pandemic?* World Health Organization. https://www.who.int/csr/disease/swineflu/frequently_asked_questions/pandemic/en/

WHO. (2017, May). *Pandemic influenza risk management: A WHO guide to inform & harmonize national & international pandemic preparedness and response*. World Health Organization. https://www.who.int/influenza/preparedness/pandemic/influenza_risk_management/en/

WHO. (2018). *Managing epidemics: Key facts about major deadly diseases*. World Health Organization. https://apps.who.int/iris/handle/10665/272442

WHO. (2020, March 11). *WHO Director-General's Opening Remarks at the Media Briefing on COVID-19 – 11 March 2020*. https://www.who.int/dg/speeches/detail/who-director-general-s-opening-remarks-at-the-media-briefing-on-covid-19—11-march-2020

WHO. (2020, May 19). *Historic Health Assembly Ends with Global Commitment to COVID-19 Response* [Press release]. World Health Organization. https://www.who.int/news-room/detail/19-05-2020-historic-health-assembly-ends-with-global-commitment-to-covid-19-response

WHO. (2021). *WHO-Convened Global Study of Origins of SARS-CoV-2: China Part*. https://www.who.int/publications/i/item/who-convened-global-study-of-origins-of-sars-cov-2-china-part

Wu, F., Zhao, S., Yu, B., Chen, Y.-M., Wang, W., Song, Z.-G., … Zhang, Y.-Z. (2020). A new coronavirus associated with human respiratory disease in China. *Nature*, 579(7798), 265–269.

PART I

Regional, historical and social work perspectives

2

REGIONS OF THE WORLD AND THE COVID-19 HEALTH EMERGENCY

Patricia Fronek and Karen Smith Rotabi-Casares with Jianqiang Liang, Wanchai Roujanavong, Myung Hun Kim, Sungmin Kim, Yanuar Farida Wismayanti, Gokul Mandayam, Antonio López Peláez, Roberta Di Rosa, Jonathan Dickens, Nicoleta Neamțu, Mădălina Hideg, Claudia Fonseca, Carmen Monico, Renie Rondon-Jackson, Gidraph G. Wairire, Janestic Mwende Twikirize, Dorothee Hölscher, Corlie Giliomee, Taghreed Abu Sarhan, Nadia C. Badran, Tarek Zidan, Sareh Rotabi and Lynne Briggs

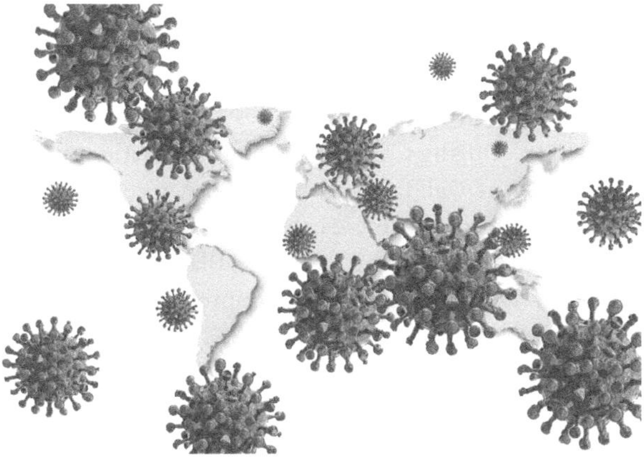

FIGURE 2.0 COVID-19: a global pandemic

DOI: 10.4324/9781003111214-3

How governments first responded to the COVID-19 pandemic provide insights into how the virus was able to spread, how subsequent outbreaks and new variants were managed and the long-term consequences for people. Importantly, these actions underscore the importance of leadership, clear and truthful messaging and the values that shape them. To this end, this chapter explores the populated regions of the world – Asia, Europe, the Americas (north, south and the Caribbean), Africa, Middle East and North Africa (MENA) and Oceania – examining government responses to the COVID-19 pandemic and the key issues affecting people in these regions during the first six months of the global health emergency, from December 2019 to 31 May 2020. Antarctica remained the only unaffected continent in this period but by December 2020, it too was affected by COVID-19, raising further ecological concerns about its impact. As we traverse the globe, the focus is on major hotspots and contrasting approaches to managing the pandemic rather than attempting to represent every world nation.

Public health is not simply about managing disease, it is political. Understanding the first actions and non-actions tells us much about the key role of leaders, their priorities and whether they heeded the science. The World Health Organisation's Director General, Dr Tedros Adhanom Ghebreyesus, declared a pandemic on 11 March 2020, and said:

> If countries detect, test, treat, isolate, trace, and mobilize their people in the response, those with a handful of cases can prevent those cases becoming clusters, and those clusters becoming community transmission.
>
> *(WHO, 2020, March 11)*

The health, social and economic impacts of the COVID-19 pandemic will last well beyond its immediate impact, through second and third waves. While the aftermath will adversely affect people for many years to come, new opportunities have also arisen. A study conducted on the 1918 Influenza pandemic in the US found that where actions were taken swiftly and aggressively, negative impacts on economies and people were fewer and less extreme (Correia et al., 2020). Importantly, they found lower mortality rates and quicker economic recovery with aggressive action. During COVID-19, many US cities that did not manage the COVID-19 pandemic well faced bankruptcy. A recent interrogation of data from 45 countries found governments that swiftly contained COVID-19 had less economic damage (Smithson, 2020). The Blavatnik School, University of Oxford, developed a tracking tool to collect prospective data on government policy responses internationally (Hale et al., 2021). Consider these findings in conjunction with pre-existing inequalities and the social consequences of death and disease as we journey through world regions comparing responses to managing this latest pandemic.

COVID-19 was first identified in Asia in December 2019, followed closely by Europe, the Americas, Oceania, MENA and Africa. By the end of May 2020, the most affected countries in the world by the number of cases were the US,

Russia, Brazil and the UK followed by Spain and Italy. Other countries such as India rose higher in the list of the most affected countries after May. During the first six months, countries had variable success in containment, some were successful, others reported widespread infections and an upward trend, while others were dealing with isolated clusters of infection. A true gauge of circumstances was difficult to determine in under-resourced and many well-resourced countries during those first few months due to testing limitations and, in some cases, lack of transparent reporting. Overall, countries that heeded the science, acted early and decisively with lockdown, quarantine, widespread testing and contact tracing alongside other measures such as physical distancing and mask-wearing, did better in the short and longer term. Those countries that only put a selection of these measures in place, ignored the science, had weak or corrupt leadership, intervened late or introduced measures in reluctant stages, prioritised the economy over health, relied on herd immunity, or had under-resourced health systems did worse with higher human costs in the first six months.

Understanding how governments protected the most vulnerable people in society is of particular importance to social workers. Certainly, as restrictions began to ease around the world, countries faced second and third waves of infections especially when attempts to reboot economies meant premature easing of restrictions. The global numbers of cases and deaths continued to rise with a total of almost six million cases and 369,254 deaths recorded on 31st May and continued to rise rapidly forecasting the devastation to come (Johns Hopkins Coronavirus Resource Center). Total number of cases should be considered proportional to the populations of each country.

Asia

Because COVID-19 was first identified in China, it is therefore useful to start our journey through world regions by exploring China's response as the first known epicentre of the virus (see Box 2.1).

BOX 2.1

CHINA

Jianqiang Liang

Cases of pneumonia with unknown *aetiology* (cause) were first reported in Wuhan, China, in early December 2019. However, the disease is believed to have emerged as early as November (Chen et al., 2020). The outbreak in China began under the shadow of global controversy. Dr Li Wenliang, an ophthalmologist, initiated a WeChat group discussion with other Wuhan

(*Continued*)

BOX 2.1 (*Continued*)

CHINA

doctors on 30th December about the cluster of SARS-like pneumonia cases. Similar to actions in other oppressive regimes where citizen and professional journalism is tightly controlled, the Wuhan Public Security Bureau detained eight people including Dr Li and Dr Ai Fen, a prominent doctor in Wuhan for spreading rumours and censored journalists. Their detainment resulted in a public outcry including an open letter by academics from Wuhan's Central China Normal University about China's constitutional protection of free speech. Dr Li died on 7th February from COVID-19. An official Chinese Inquiry later exonerated him and formally apologised (Investigation Committee of the State Supervisory Commission, 2020). Deaths of frontline health workers were many and the disease spread quickly through the population.

On the 31st of December, an epidemiological alert was sent out by the local authority and an expert response team was formed (Huang et al., 2020). The seafood market, considered the source of the outbreak, closed on January 1st and the WHO prepared for further outbreaks. On January 8th, the National Health Committee declared a new virus was the cause and on January 12th, a virologist leaked the virus genome sequence confirming a coronavirus which pushed the government to act. China was criticised for not then providing a biological sample. On January 20, human-to-human transmission was confirmed. Eighty Chinese cities including Wuhan went into lockdown on 23rd January.

China chose strategies to eliminate the disease, a monumental task given the size and density of the population. By February, a 1,000-bed hospital in Wuhan had been built in 10 days with a second almost completed. By March 10th, less than 20 new cases a day were being reported in China (Johns Hopkins Coronavirus Resource Center). The country's success in managing the pandemic included government-imposed lockdown, restricting the movement of people and intensive cleaning of cities alongside, widespread testing, monitoring temperatures, isolation, quarantine, contact tracing, mask-wearing, handwashing, and physical distancing. The onset of COVID-19 in a country where people rely heavily on traditional medicines coincided with the influenza season and the upcoming Lunar New year presenting further challenges across Asia because many people cross the globe to celebrate with families. Unfortunately, for a range of reasons including the training of those policing and enforcing, and diverse local governance, breaches of human rights came to the fore in China. People were forcibly removed from their homes and others were locked inside their homes with supplies of rice. Some older people and people with disabilities died as a result. Suppression of citizen reporting was heavy handed.

(*Continued*)

BOX 2.1 **(*Continued*)**

CHINA

Some might argue that suppression and population compliance is only possible in authoritarian regimes using coercive control. Yet, the Chinese private sector was also involved in supporting these measures and China had early success in flattening its curve. Once numbers reduced and the 11 million Wuhan residents tested, Wuhan began a staged easing of restrictions on April 8th. In May, new clusters were identified in the north eastern province of Jilin (four cases) and in Shulan city (11 cases). Smart phone applications were used for monitoring and tracing with a colour coded system – green for healthy people allowed to work and travel. China had not experienced a significant second wave by the end of May and had low numbers of new infections. A chartered flight arranged by the German Chamber of Commerce flew into China on 31st May to progress business. Despite rigid screening and monitoring before the flight, one passenger landed in China with COVID-19.

Hong Kong acted quickly due to previous experience of SARS in 2003 and H1N1 in 2009 and the tough social and economic consequences experienced. Responding to events in Wuhan on January 2nd, the Hong Kong government held a cross-departmental meeting to heighten alert and strengthen surveillance, prevention and control measures (Government of the Hong Kong Special Administrative Region, 2020a). Hong Kong's close linkages to authorities and health institutes in mainland China enabled the sharing of information and border control. On January 9th, legislation was amended to include mandatory reporting of pneumonia cases with unknown aetiology and a travel history from Wuhan (Government of the Hong Kong Special Administrative Region, 2020b). From the outset, the public had high awareness of hygiene measures embracing hand washing and wearing masks.

By 30th May, health workers were protesting to close borders. Enabled by press freedom, Hong Kong media criticised the lack of transparency and the effectiveness of public health actions by the Chinese central and local governments. On May 21st, mainland China announced new security laws for Hong Kong which would override press and assembly freedoms reigniting public protests. Social workers were already serving prison sentences for participating in public protests against the Extradition Bill. In Hong Kong, the number of new daily cases were significantly reduced by the 12th of April. Due to early action including the cooperation of health workers and communities, there were only four deaths reported including *no deaths in Hong Kong care homes*. No new cases were reported in the last week of May.

As of May 31st, 4,555 deaths and over 84,128 confirmed cases had been reported in China (Johns Hopkins Coronavirus Resource Center).

Taiwan also acted quickly. As soon as the novel coronavirus in Wuhan became known, Taiwan imposed border controls and a 14-day isolation period for international arrivals, banned gatherings and the export of supplies such as masks to ensure local supply. Taiwan had only seven deaths and 442 confirmed cases by 31 May 2020.

The first case outside China was diagnosed in Thailand (see Box 2.2). Although Thailand has a relatively good health system, there are marked health and wealth disparities. COVID-19 devastated the poor and the tourism industry on which many were dependent. Thailand already had one of the highest suicide rates in South East Asia, followed by Myanmar (WHO, 2016). Increases in suicide were reported in the media in many countries attributed to loss of employment and lockdowns (Salvá, 2020; Wang et al., 2020). However, a later study found little basis to support an increase in suicides attributable to COVID-19 in most countries (Pirkis et al., 2021).

BOX 2.2

THAILAND

Wanchai Roujanavong

After receiving reports of an epidemic in China, the Ministry of Public Health established Emergency Operation Centres at airports on the 4th of January to screen arrivals from China. On January 8th, a Chinese tourist was confirmed as the first case of COVID-19 outside of China. The first Thai citizen, returning from China, was diagnosed on January 15th. On March 12th, the National Centre for COVIID-19 Situation Administration (CCSA) was established with full powers to deal with the virus. The strength of the CCSA was that it was administered and led by doctors and other health experts not politicians. Two superspreader events, one in a boxing stadium and the other in a bar in Bangkok, were identified. The Government ordered partial lockdown on April 2nd and closed all airports to foreigners while allowing Thai citizens to return with a strict compulsory 14-day quarantine. All new cases were identified in returning travellers while in quarantine. No new cases of COVID-19 were found in Thailand between 26th and 31st of May.

A key prevention mechanism involved the Village Health Volunteer (VHV) teams established more than a decade ago by the Government under the Ministry of Public Health. The VHV teams are local people trained to work in every rural village on all aspects of health promotion and disease prevention. Thai people were cooperative with lockdown, wore masks, washed hands and physically distanced. When no new cases were identified for 28 days within territories, lockdown measures were revoked step by step. Plans to open schools and to gradually reopen activities and businesses proceeded from the 1st of July. The CCSA was not complacent, planning concurrently for a second wave when

(Continued)

BOX 2.2 (*Continued*)

THAILAND

tourism would reopen. Tourism, key to the Thai economy, held little hope of early recovery as global numbers were still rising and as yet, there was no vaccine.

Because the economic impact was dire with millions of workers forecast to lose their jobs, the Government provided financial assistance of US $500 to approximately 30 million people, nearly half the Thai population. The problem was how long before life returned to where it was before COVID-19. As of 31st May, there was 3,081 total cases and 53 deaths in Thailand (Johns Hopkins Coronavirus Resource Center).

The next stop on our journey takes us to Korea. It was difficult to determine the situation in North Korea due to the nature of the political regime. Reports included allegations that suspected cases were imported from South Korea to Kim Jong-un claiming the country was virus-free. However, propaganda was strongly suspected especially as borders between North Korea and China were open until the end of January. In South Korea, the first case was confirmed on January 19th, soon after Thailand. Although South Korea has experienced high economic growth from the 1960s, nonetheless, health and wealth inequalities existed in the country with health and social services unequally distributed.

BOX 2.3

SOUTH KOREA

Myung Hun Kim and Sungmin Kim

Hard lessons learned from MERS in 2015 paved the way for South Korea's approach to COVID-19. Korea took decisive and rapid action and carefully managed subsequent clusters. Korea's primary focus was on widespread testing and tenacious tracing while aiming to minimise restrictions on daily life. Immediately after the first confirmed case, the Korean government issued the highest level of National Crisis Alert and established the Central Disaster and Safety Countermeasures Headquarters in the Korean Centers for Disease Control & Prevention. Local infectious disease prevention and control teams worked closely with the central government. Local quarantine authorities were responsible for tracing, monitoring quarantine, supervising facilities, and allocating confirmed cases to shelters or hospitals. Drive-through testing centres, selective screening infirmaries for symptomatic people, and secure outpatient dispensaries in 91

(*Continued*)

BOX 2.3 (*Continued*)

SOUTH KOREA

designated hospitals were established. Existing technological competence from previous pandemics allowed for the rapid development and manufacture of testing kits by biomedical companies enabling widespread testing. Rapid tracing was possible via the collection of data from mobile phones, credit cards and CCTVs. A Smart City Data Hub Platform could identify hotspots of infections in ten minutes. While transmission paths were widely publicised through SMS messaging and on government websites, the National Human Rights Commission of Korea ensured the protection of personal information.

In ordinary times, access to healthcare is not the same for all Koreans. During the pandemic, the government met all costs of testing, living in treatment shelters and inpatient treatment. Paid sick leave allowance for salaried employees based on their wages and a living allowance for others were provided. These strategies ensured the basic needs of the disadvantaged were met, avoided the early spread of disease for those people who could not afford healthcare and who may otherwise have hidden in the community. Government leadership was critical to central and local coordination, the rapid development, testing and approving of testing kits and other supplies, and supporting the health and livelihoods of the community. The cooperative and adaptive characteristics of the Korean people inspired social solidarity during the crisis demonstrated by following advice and volunteering, characteristics important to successfully manage the pandemic. Notably, there was no panic buying and people remained calm during the pandemic. Korea's early success was also attributed to quick public health action, high quality healthcare, income protection, strong leadership, responsibility and prior experiences.

As of 31st May, there was 11,468 total cases and 262 deaths in South Korea (Johns Hopkins Coronavirus Resource Center).

Travelling west to Japan, we find a century-long tradition of wearing masks dating back to the 1918 Influenza (Horii, 2014). Although Japan initially did relatively well compared to countries in Europe and the US and was reported to have flattened the curve with fewer deaths reported by the end of May, a second lockdown was instigated after easing restrictions too soon in response to industry and business pressure (Tashiro & Shaw, 2020). Both South Korea and Japan experienced an escalation of cases in the second half of 2020. Korea adjusted and tightened their approaches in response, while the Prime Minister of Japan, Yoshihide Suga, was strongly criticised for encouraging tourism. Both countries had not implemented nationwide hard lockdowns at the onset of the virus.

Heading south to Malaysia, the first case was confirmed on 25th February. The Tabligh Akbar, an annual Islamic celebration held in Malaysia, attracts people from around the world – Thailand, Singapore, Cambodia, Vietnam, Brunei, the Philippines, Australia and Indonesia, to name a few. This mass event, held in February 2020, included 2,000 Rohingya attendees and is thought to have contributed to the further spread of SARS-CoV-2 to other countries. Strict lockdown measures were put in place on March 18 after a sharp increase of cases and, of concern, these measures were eased in early May to stimulate the economy. Spikes in numbers of infections in Malaysia triggered discrimination towards refugees, particularly in Rohingya communities. Malaysia is just one example where true numbers were difficult to determine due to limited testing. The number of cases and deaths officially reported in Malaysia were relatively low. The total number of cases recorded by the end of May was 7,762 with 110 deaths (Johns Hopkins Coronavirus Resource Center).

Major international airports posed high risks of imported infections. For example, Singapore's Changi airport served 68.3 million passengers in 2019. Singapore only put restrictions in place once numbers began to escalate. Its approach was also to control and contain not to impose strict lockdown. On 24th May, a surge of 600 new infections were reported attributed to migrant workers and associated with poverty, crowded conditions, and limited access to health-care and social services. Official statistics in Singapore do not necessarily include immigrant workers and when masks were distributed to the population, migrant workers were excluded. Singapore, relying on contact tracing apps, experienced the beginnings of a second wave by the end of May. Singapore had a total of 34,366 cases and only 22 deaths reported on May 31st.

The next Asian destination is Indonesia (see Box 2.4) which became the worst affected country with the highest death rate in Asia during the first six months.

BOX 2.4

INDONESIA

Yanuar Farida Wismayanti

Indonesia is the largest Muslim-majority country outside the Arab world. Many Indonesians live in poverty in a country with nascent health and welfare systems and with social problems similar to many other low- and middle-income countries. The people are all too familiar with the impact of natural disasters such as volcanic eruptions, earthquakes and tsunamis. According to the Joint United Nations Programme on HIV/AIDS (UNAIDS), 640,000 people were living with HIV in 2018 as well as outbreaks of measles, malaria, cholera and other infectious diseases.

The first documented case of COVID-19 was on 2nd March and by early April, the disease had spread to all 34 provinces. Jakarta, Banten and West

(Continued)

BOX 2.4 (*Continued*)

INDONESIA

Java were the worst affected regions. Timor-Leste (East Timor), an outlier, imposed severe restrictions from its first case on March 21st with no new reported cases since 24th April. By May 21st, Indonesia had 19,189 confirmed cases and 1,242 deaths reported despite limited testing capacity and personal protective equipment (PPE). To further complicate the situation, many Indonesians rely on traditional medicines which can give a false sense of protection. President Joko Widodo declared on a government website that he drank a tea made of red ginger, lemongrass, turmeric and curcuma to defend against the coronavirus. The health system was unable to deal with the pandemic with only 309,100 hospital beds for a population of over 270 million people and only 2.7 intensive care beds for every 100,000 people, most on the island of Java and the lowest number in Asia (Setiati & Azwar, 2020).

Internal movement of people was difficult to control. As well as the unique sociopolitical context of Indonesia, Islam, like other religions, played a role in COVID-19 paradoxically providing faith and comfort for people while at the same time contributing to its spread. From the beginning, mass gatherings posed problems. *Ramadan* (a sacred month of fasting and prayer) which fell on 23 April 2020 was followed by *Lebaran*, a major national holiday. *Mudik*, a tradition where Muslims leave cities to return to their villages to participate in a celebration called *Idul Fitri* which occurs towards the end of *Ramadan*. Mudik was banned in 2020 (Spagnoletti, 2020). Provincial leaders held different opinions about management. Instructions to stay-at-home were openly ignored in Aceh, a conservative province. Mixed messages at political levels caused confusion and lockdown continued to be avoided for some time including closing mosques for Ramadan, ultimately only partially implemented. Although physical distancing was encouraged, it was almost impossible to achieve due to the living conditions of many Indonesians. In effect, it was not until May 18 that Widodo extended physical distancing rules, travel bans and ruled out easing restrictions as Indonesia faced continuing and rapidly escalating numbers of infected.

Widodo's lack of action is attributed to early denial and the country's unique sociopolitical context. As he explained to Aljazeera, Widodo opted for a patchwork solution, not herd immunity, as total lockdown would only drive people further into poverty, an approach he claimed was consistent with Taiwan, Vietnam and Japan (Aljazeera, 2020). Overall, a lack of transparency, under-reporting and under-diagnosing cases also impeded an adequate response (Djalante et al., 2020). It became clear that Indonesia was ill-prepared to address the needs of vulnerable groups and the health and economic challenges of the pandemic. As of 31st May, there was 25,773 total confirmed cases and 1,483 deaths in Indonesia (Johns Hopkins Coronavirus Resource Center).

Moving on to Pakistan, Bangladesh and India, we find these are also countries familiar with natural disasters and communicable disease. Cyclone Amphan hit West Bengal and Bangladesh in May 2020 adding to existing vulnerabilities and compounding risks of virus spread as the 2.5 million people evacuated were relocated to crowded emergency shelters. Rohingya refugees were already in an extremely vulnerable position in Bangladesh. Pakistan allowed prayers in mosques where worshippers were provided with sanitiser and instructed to remain six feet apart. Many markets closed worsening the situation for Pakistan's poor. From April 18th, 35 repatriation flights brought thousands of Pakistanis home from places like Dubai and Abu Dhabi. The under-resourced and unprepared health system in Pakistan triggered strikes and protests from health workers. Concerns escalated over time about the extent of the SARS-CoV-2 spread in Pakistan and India. Pakistani-administered Kashmir made their own decisions and fared better with stricter measures implementing lockdown after its first case in mid-March resulting in only 5,000 reported cases and 59 deaths by the end of May.

Meanwhile across India (see Box 2.5), 1.3 billion people were in lockdown. The poor everywhere bore the brunt of COVID-19 and none more so than in India where for many people it was once again deciding between eating or protecting themselves from COVID-19. India's population (1.3 billion) has 176 million people living on less than $1.90 a day. Many had no option but to risk the disease.

BOX 2.5

INDIA

Gokul Mandayam

On 30 January 2020, the first case of COVID-19, a student returning from Wuhan, was confirmed in Kerala (Sharma & Paul, 2020). By March, the number of cases had increased rapidly linked to travellers and religious and public gatherings (Lingam & Sapkal, 2020). In the months ahead, case numbers surged in Delhi, Mumbai and Chennai. On the 25th of March, a national lockdown was announced almost two months after the first case. Migrant workers in metropolitan areas had to leave with only four-hours of notice. Many were left stranded without shelter, food or transportation resulting in deaths due to hunger and exhaustion as people walked home to their villages. After the national lockdown, states enacted various lockdown mandates based on the spread of the virus within each state.

The Ministry of Health and Family Welfare operates countrywide, grassroots public health initiatives and services executed by Accredited Social Health Activist (ASHA) workers, predominantly women. Their responsibilities came to include monitoring and counselling COVID-19 cases in communities

(*Continued*)

BOX 2.5 (*Continued*)

INDIA

including returning migrant workers. ASHA workers carried the burden in semi-urban and rural areas while at personal risk due to scarce PPE. The lack of a robust health system, high population density and the caste system posed immense challenges. The Dalit population or India's *untouchables* who work menial jobs in construction, tannery or janitorial work, and scavenging, were severely impacted with limited access to healthcare and other social protections. With few options, many poor households were forced to send their children to work. School closures added to increased risks of child labour. Orphaned and separated children were particularly vulnerable to trafficking, forced begging, or death due to starvation. Non-government and community-based organisations distributed food grains, ran community kitchens and helplines for counselling support (Lingam & Sapkal, 2020). Cases of mental health concerns and alcohol misuse increased. The COVID-19 Innovation Challenge, a government initiative, was launched on March 16th, bringing together wisdom from universities, industry and government. Multiple strategies resulted including technologies (drones, robots, cell phone applications), and education on community radio and the government television channel. Alternative medicine options such as Ayurveda, an ancient holistic approach to wellness was important to the people. While the Prime Minister, Narendra Modi, claimed India's recovery rate outperformed other countries, this did not ultimately play out and the pandemic exposed grave deficits in social and economic policies. After lockdown was eased, cases dramatically increased and India eventually became the second most affected country in the world.

As of 31st May, there was 182,490 total confirmed cases and 4,638 deaths in India (Johns Hopkins Coronavirus Resource Center).

The true rate of infection can be difficult to ascertain in many regions, especially in low-resource countries due to health infrastructure, testing rates and access to free testing, transparent reporting and other health, political and economic factors. In Afghanistan, for example, doubts have been raised about official figures as the country had the lowest testing rates in the world. While saying that, people listen to governments' directions in many Asian countries and many governments heeded the advice and support from China as well as from international organisations. Importantly many countries acted early due to prior experience with SARS and H1N1. The Association of Southeast Asian Nations (ASEAN) had been working on an agreement for the prevention, control and eradication of zoonotic diseases since 2012, and for the rapid sharing of information with members when outbreaks occur.

Geography also played a role in Asia. Cambodia has a dense population in Phnom Penh and a significant amount of internal movement as people return to villages at weekends and national holidays, similar to Indonesia. Many older people live in villages and elders return to them to live out their old age. These rural areas are not densely populated which was somewhat protective against the pandemic. As with much of Asia, tourism is the economic lifeblood for Cambodia particularly in the casino region, Sihanoukville, where regular flights arrive direct from Wuhan. China suspended these flights on 23 January 2020 (Pech, 2020). Prior to the suspension, 1,539 people had flown into Sihanouk and 1,539 to Siem Reap from Wuhan. Following three false alarms, the first reported case of COVID-19 was a Chinese tourist in Sihanoukville, diagnosed in late January. From early January, many Cambodians were acutely aware of COVID-19, sanitiser was used in tourist hotels and many staff wore masks. As the world locked down, hotels closed as tourists stopped coming and many people lost their livelihoods. As of 31 May 2020, only 125 cases were reported in Cambodia with no available mortality data.

Other countries with low reported numbers were Brunei (141 cases, 2 deaths), Myanmar (224 cases, 6 deaths) and Bhutan (43 cases and no reported deaths). Despite Nepal's strict lockdown, its borders are porous. Nepal had 1,401 confirmed cases with only five deaths. During lockdown, Nepal took no action to increase tracing and testing. Common to many developing countries, the Nepalese government relied on non-government and international organisations to supply the country with the equipment and PPE, and corruption was a concern. Later reports from Nepal indicated coronavirus patients suffered discrimination and vilification on social media. According to ASEAN, Laos also reported low numbers of cases. In the authoritarian regime of the Philippines, President Rodrigo Duterte authorised the police and military to shoot if there was any resistance to lockdown and warned the 110 million Filipinos "Instead of causing trouble, I'll send you to your grave" (Cook, 2020). Disturbing examples of children being punished have been reported. Two children were locked in a coffin and five children were locked in a dog cage for violating curfew. Further examples included children being arrested, cutting hair as punishment and a child stripped naked and forced to walk home for resisting (Cook, 2020, citing Human Rights Watch).

Moving south again, we explore Vietnam (see Box 2.6), a country that successfully managed the pandemic attracting criticism for breaching human rights while doing so.

BOX 2.6

VIETNAM

As with all countries that fared well in containing the disease, Vietnam acted early and hard. After the first case on 23rd January, urgent and clear information was distributed by government and health departments (Dinh et al., 2020). Similar to Cambodia and Thailand, many people live in village and commune settings which required community-based strategies. The army

(*Continued*)

BOX 2.6 (*Continued*)

VIETNAM

was mobilised, health measures were compulsory and state-run quarantine centres were established alongside mass surveillance using both technology and traditional methods to ensure the population complied (Klinger-Vidra et al., 2020). More than 100,000 people were quarantined.

As early as February, targeted testing and compulsory temperature screening at airports were in place and schools and other gathering places closed prior to the Lunar New year. People were criminally charged if they gave false declarations. Testing stations were established, and lockdowns were immediately imposed wherever the disease was detected. Like China, the private sector cooperated implementing hygiene and testing strategies which included apartment buildings. As reported by Klinger-Vidra et al. (2020), the most significant aspect of Vietnam's success was the development of three brands of cheap and effective testing kits by 5th March. Vietnam also donated kits and masks to neighbouring Laos, Cambodia and countries outside Asia badly affected by the pandemic. The authors attributed the fast development of testing equipment to government as a convening and mobilising agent, innovation and collaboration, and the shared mission between government, the private sector and Vietnamese society. ASEAN also played a key role in sharing information with Vietnam and other member countries and partners.

Vietnam has been hailed as a prime example of elimination. No deaths and only 328 cases were reported by 31st May in a population of 97 million. Fast forwarding to August, Vietnam had 99 days with no new infections, achieving elimination, until a later outbreak in a tourist region in early August.

Europe

The global pattern of vastly different approaches to pandemic management in the first few months is well demonstrated in the European context. A study of 25 European countries, explored differences focusing on three main factors – social relations, restrictions and institutional trust (Oksanen et al., 2020). Societal and psychosocial factors were influential in how the pandemic spread. The researchers hypothesised that there would be differences between southern versus northern Europe. Low institutional trust had been a crucial issue in the spread of Ebola in Liberia and the Congo as people were more likely to not comply with the advice of governments. The researchers were therefore interested in how distrust in governments, for example, in eastern Europe affected people's responses to COVID-19. After grouping European countries according to their characteristics, the researchers found little statistical difference between low and high institutional trust. However, it was a protective factor. They also found early action was the most important factor in managing the pandemic. Late action resulted in a significantly 2.5 higher mortality rate. Not surprisingly, sociability with closer physical contact was associated with a higher mortality rate.

As well as restrictions already imposed in most countries by mid-March, the European Commission announced on 17th March that borders would close to all non-essential travel for at least 30 days, a plan approved by *Schengen* area members (see Box 2.7).

BOX 2.7

WHAT IS THE SCHENGEN AGREEMENT?

The Schengen Agreement began as a treaty signed in the village of Schengen in Luxemburg on 14 June 1985. The Treaty outlined a commitment to the free movement of people, goods and services by abolishing European border visa requirements. Initially only five countries signed the Treaty – France, Germany, Belgium, Luxemburg and The Netherlands. On 19 June 1990, a Convention was signed for its implementation which began in 1995. Twenty-six member states, associate members, soon-to-be members (Bulgaria, Croatia and Romania) and non-member states (Monaco, San Marino, Vatican City, Norway, Iceland, Switzerland and Liechtenstein) opened their borders. The exceptions are Ireland and Cyprus. The UK never became a member and it is unlikely with Brexit.

As the pandemic spread across Europe, seasonal workers across the continent returned to home countries leaving a shortage of farm and other workers. Across Europe, xenophobia and discrimination against refugees and asylum seekers increased as conditions worsened. The protection of refugees and asylum seekers already displaced and vulnerable was of great concern. Italy, Spain and Greece are on the *Central Mediterranean Migration Route*, an extremely dangerous route taken by many thousands of people including unaccompanied children. The largest refugee camp, Moria, on the Greek island of Lesbos, held particular pandemic risks due to the size of the camp. The fate of Moria is discussed further in Chapter 11. Fast forward to May, groups were protesting in parts of Europe demanding the right to not wear masks and to return to normal activities while business interests pushed for open borders. These protests highlighted problems with the influence of the far right, the economic impact of the pandemic, and individualistic schema that claimed rights to individual freedoms rather than responsibility to society as a whole which was concerning as the pandemic was far from over. France, Italy and Spain (see Box 2.8), the next destinations in our itinerary, became the first and worst affected European countries in the early weeks of the pandemic.

BOX 2.8

ITALY, FRANCE AND SPAIN

Antonio López Peláez and Roberta Di Rosa

Years of austerity and outsourcing services weakened response capacities in Italy, France and Spain (López Peláez & Gómez Ciriano, 2019). Intergenerational solidarity is strong in in these countries and provide the welfare safety net (Moreno Mínguez et al., 2012). Coping fell heavily on families during lockdowns and the subsequent economic crises (di Ateneo Studi & sulla Famiglia, 2020).

In 2019, France received the most tourists worldwide, Spain second and Italy fifth. The economic impact on tourism, leisure and hospitality was weighty and the initial lack of coordination between countries combined with global tourism highlighted underestimated risk. Debates about the how to proceed raised questions of herd immunity versus confinement, whether to make masks mandatory, to prioritise health or economic activity, and the shortage of PPE.

The first confirmed case in France was on January 24th. The first death occurred in Spain on February 13th and the second in France on February 14th. In mid-March, President Macron instigated an eight-week lockdown and mandatory mask-wearing. On April 22nd, cases rose to nearly 160,000, bringing the overall death toll to 21,000 (Andolfatto & Labbé, 2020). In some districts, video cameras were used to monitor mask-wearing and physical distancing. On May 12th, people could return to work and shop, but restaurants and cafes remained closed in Paris, and religious services were allowed from May 24th.

In Italy, a nationwide health alert and state of alarm were activated on January 31st. The Codogno area locked down on 23rd February, followed by the northern region on March 8th, and nationwide on March 9th. Lockdown was strict and fines were heavy. Only hospitals, food, and other essential services such as the public bus services were operating.

In Spain, the central government encouraged people to attend the International Women's Day demonstrations on March 8 and imposed lockdown one week later. Construction and factory workers returned to work in mid-April, followed ten days later by non-essential workers in Madrid. After six weeks of lockdown, children under 13 years were allowed outside for one hour from April 26th. After a spike in numbers, lockdown was extended to May 9th. On May 20th, when 67,000 cases were recorded in Madrid, city authorities canvassed the Supreme Court to ease restrictions. On May 21st, Spain passed legislation to make mask-wearing and physical distancing of one metre compulsory.

(*Continued*)

BOX 2.8 ***(Continued)***

ITALY, FRANCE AND SPAIN

The scarcity of PPE and ventilators overwhelmed hospitals amplifying the impact of COVID-19 in these countries. Triage decisions about which patients should be admitted produced terrible situations, particularly for the elderly (Allegri & Di Rosa, 2020). By May 10th, there were 16,678 COVID-19 deaths in Spanish care homes (Comas-Herrara et al., 2020). In France, the Conseil National Professionnel de Gériatrie which represents nursing homes wrote to the Minister of Health, Olivier Véran, on March 26th highlighting the drastic need to provide workers with PPE (CNP, 2020).

Throughout lockdowns, social workers developed rapid responses including providing virtual services. Spanish practitioners launched initiatives to disseminate good practices and combat misinformation (López Peláez et al., 2020). The General Council of Social Work in Spain developed several projects to support social workers in their day-to-day work, providing a toll-free hotline to provide health and social service professionals with emotional support (www.cgtrabajosocial.es). Under Order SND/295/2020 of March 26th, the Spanish government declared social services to be essential services. In Italy, social workers developed strategies that guaranteed essential services, strengthened internal cohesion and spread safety information (Sanfelici et al., 2020). Among other strategies, French social workers in the Reception and Social Reintegration Centres (CHRS) reorganised their working days to accompany people in fragile psychological states.

Lockdown compounded the refugee situation and lack of access to the same services as citizens. NGOs in Italy reported that in many cases lockdown was implemented in prison-like environments and uncertain futures worsened psychological problems. Asylum seekers in France staged a hunger strike due to no PPE, poor living conditions and fear of illness. Undocumented refugees continued to be arrested and detained, and flights were unavailable for deportation (Yang & Castanier, 2020).

As of May 31st, Italy had confirmed 232,664 cases and 28,834 deaths, France 188,752 cases and 27,125 deaths and Spain 239,228 cases and 27,134 deaths (Johns Hopkins Coronavirus Resource Center).

In Germany where strong leadership was shown, large numbers of infection still plagued the country. Germany took the approach of attempting to balance health and the economy by taking the least restrictive approaches possible. A preprint publication presented an epidemiological study that examined the change points aimed at flattening the curve in Germany and the effectiveness of these interventions (Dehning et al., 2020). Although, the first case of COVID-19 was detected on 27th January in Bavaria, Germany, and like many countries,

Germany's three-step strategy was only implemented in early March. The first phase involved cancelling large events such as football matches. Schools, child-care and non-essential stores were closed on March 16th and March 23rd, the third step, *Kontaktsperre,* involved banning small public gatherings and closuring restaurants and more stores. A significant reduction in new cases occurred between March 9 and March 15, but new cases were still exponential suggesting strong weaknesses in the incremental approach. Kontaktsperre was most effective, reducing new cases over the subsequent two weeks. Individual actions, such as physical distancing, were not included in the modelling. On May 31st, there were 183,189 confirmed cases in Germany and 7,734 deaths.

Our next destination, the UK (see Box 2.9), was criticised for weak leadership and lack of action leading to the UK becoming among the worst affected and least effective in flattening the curve in the world.

BOX 2.9

UNITED KINGDOM

Jonathan Dickens

Political leadership lends insight into the UK response to COVID-19. There was no uniform *UK response* as the overall Conservative government is responsible for immigration, taxation and welfare benefits, while health and social policy is devolved to England, Scotland, Wales and Northern Ireland. Mixed messages from the Prime Minister, Boris Johnson, about the seriousness of the virus and how best to respond were compounded by notable country differences to lockdown and other measures as governments sought to balance public health, economic stability and individual liberties.

The first documented case was on 31 January 2020 in England. As numbers rose, Johnson's messages were to keep calm and carry on as normal. A major horseracing event, the Cheltenham Festival, attended by 60,000 people daily for four days, proceeded in mid-March. A national lockdown was announced on 23rd March. Soon after, Johnson became seriously unwell with COVID-19. A UK-wide scheme to financially support workers on *furlough* and small businesses temporarily closed was a remarkable step for Conservatives who espoused non-interventionist economics and low public expenditure.

The daily rate of infections started to fall from early May. Alongside assurances that the virus was under control came advice that a *world beating* test and trace system was underway, claims disconfirmed by facts. Guidance became more ambiguous, creating widespread confusion about what was required. Leading government adviser, Dominic Cummings, was reported to

(Continued)

BOX 2.9 (*Continued*)

UNITED KINGDOM

have broken lockdown in the first few weeks adding to this confusion. Despite a public outcry, no action was taken, and his excuses became a national joke, contributing to further resentments (Mason, 2020).

COVID-19 exposed and exacerbated existing inequalities and health disparities (Public Health England, 2020). Mortality rates in the most deprived areas were more than double those in the least deprived areas. The highest death rates were for people from Black, Asian and Minorities Ethnic (BAME) groups who were more likely to be working on the front line as consultants, nurses, social care workers and cleaners, and in public-facing jobs such as bus and taxi drivers, shop workers and catering. By May, 200 health care workers had died from COVID-19. Six in ten were from BAME backgrounds (Marsh & McIntyre, 2020).

As of 31 May 2020, there were 274,219 reported cases and 38,458 deaths, the highest numbers of cases and deaths in Europe, and fourth in the world at that time (Johns Hopkins Coronavirus Resource Center).

Our journey through Europe continues to central and eastern Europe and Russia. These countries have long and complicated political, economic and social histories. Human rights violations have been reported during this pandemic particularly related to discrimination against minorities such as Roma communities. Poverty, inequality and lack of social services were issues prior to the COVID-19 pandemic. Belarus, like Sweden, did not instigate lockdown nor put adequate health measures in place resulting in over 40,000 confirmed cases and 131 reported COVID-19 deaths by the end of May 2020. A lack of trust in government, and escalating health consequences were reported. In April, the BBC highlighted the plight of the vulnerable, in particular, those children in institutions which were bereft of funds due to the cessation of donations (BBC News, 2020). In the same period, the Ukraine reported 23,204 confirmed cases and 668 deaths and at least one hundred stranded babies born to cross-border commercial surrogacy (Fronek & Rotabi, 2020). Russia reported 396,575 cases and 4,515 deaths, an unusually small number of deaths given the reported infection numbers. Russian health workers lacked PPE and there were reports of abuse as people feared health workers would spread the disease. Domestic violence was a significant pre-existing problem in Russia, and common to experiences in all countries, the incidence of violence increased during the pandemic. The Czech Republic was slow to respond prioritising business interests, resulting in the upward trend of identified cases. Next, we turn to events in Romania, Bulgaria, Hungary and Poland (see Box 2.10) during the first six months.

BOX 2.10

ROMANIA, HUNGARY AND POLAND

Nicoleta Neamțu and Mădălina Hideg

A minority, centre-right, neoliberal National Liberal Party government took the leadership of Romania in November 2019. From January and prior to the state of emergency, public perceptions of SARS-CoV-2 were divided between trust in science and the proliferation of conspiracy theories often due to economic interests. The majority of political decision makers were perceived by ordinary people as incompetent and not meeting real needs during the pandemic. Health spending in Romania, historically the lowest in the European Union, meant access to health care posed barriers, especially for people in rural areas where distribution of health services is unequal. Health workforce shortages were critical, with the number of doctors and nurses among the lowest in Europe because of the emigration of medical professionals (European Commission, 2019).

Following WHO recommendations, Romania authorised COVID-19 emergency plans in January (CNSCBT, 2020a). Challenges were faced at different stages of epidemic control, including large numbers of Romanian diaspora returning from highly affected European countries, inadequate healthcare system infrastructure, mismanagement of human resources and sociocultural determinants. The first case of COVID-19 was confirmed in Gorj county in south-western Romania on the 26th of February. The infected person had been in close contact with an Italian national who had visited Romania (Digi24, 2020). By 14th March, Romania exceeded 100 confirmed cases, mostly citizens returning from abroad, followed by local spread (CNSCBT, 2020b; Schitea, 2020). A state of emergency was declared on the 16th of March 2020 for 30 days, limiting freedom of movement and closing non-essential businesses (Romanian Government, 2020a).

On 25th March, a military curfew was imposed (Romanian Ministry of Internal Affairs, 2020). New measures included confining citizens over the age of 65 to their homes, reducing outings to essential shopping and visiting pharmacies or hospitals. On 26th March, the total number of confirmed cases of infection exceeded 1,000. By 15th May, the national state of emergency was lifted, and replaced with state of alert measures relaxing most restrictions. Romanian social workers were already integrated into Emergency Reception Units and in hospitals from 2008 (Romanian Ministry of Public Health, 2020). Recognizing the vital role of health professionals including

(*Continued*)

BOX 2.10 (*Continued*)

ROMANIA, HUNGARY AND POLAND

social work, the government did not allow them to work abroad from April (Romanian Government, 2020b).

The political regimes of Hungary (KNDP) and Poland (PiS) were characterised as autocratic and populist. Hungary seemed to fare well until 31st May. Hungary's health system was weak, underfinanced, and had a deficit of health professionals as about 5,500 doctors had left Hungary between 2010 and 2016 (Karáth, 2020). During the first waves, Poland and Hungary also began with imported cases, then shifted to local transmission. Early restrictions in Hungary kept the number of cases low initially, but many were infected while hospitalised. On March 4th, Hungary registered the first case, and Poland on March 15th. After the first death, Hungary declared a 15-day state of emergency on March 11th that was extended indefinitely. On March 30th, Prime Minister Orban received the right to rule the country by decree (abolished in June). Travel was restricted and border checks at the Austrian and Slovenian borders were re-implemented. On March 16, entry was restricted to Hungarians only. Schools were closed and events with more than 500 participants were banned until the end of May. In Poland, school closed until April 26th, and offices and mass events between March 10 and 12. On March 25th, non-family gatherings were reduced to two people, and religious gatherings to six people until April 20, when 50 people could gather. On March 31st, parks, beauty salons and boulevards closed. Borders closed between March 15th and May 3rd, except for the Polish citizens. From April 16, everyone had to cover their nose and mouth in public places. A plan for public assistance to business was launched on April 1st (Anti-crisis Shield) and Poland provided medical supplies to other countries in the West and Baltic regions.

As of 31st May, Romania had 19,133 confirmed cases and 1,061 deaths, Hungary had 3,867 cases and 498 deaths and Poland 23,571 cases and 997 deaths (Johns Hopkins Coronavirus Resource Centre).

Belgium had more deaths proportional to their COVID-19 cases, 16.3%. As of May 31st, Belgium had 58,186 cases and 8,530 deaths and the Netherlands 46,460 and 5,186 deaths. Travelling north west to the Nordic countries (see Box 2.11), we explore social democracies renowned for societal obligations and well-developed health and welfare systems. Surprisingly, when it came to managing the pandemic, the response was starkly varied.

BOX 2.11

THE NORDIC COUNTRIES

The Nordic countries, usually share similarities when it comes to social policy, diverged markedly by addressing the health and safety of the population very differently. Sweden and Iceland stood out for very different reasons. The first confirmed case of COVID-19 in Sweden was on 11th March. Sweden chose a herd immunity approach led by epidemiologist, Anders Tegnell, claimed to be a common-sense approach which prioritised individual freedoms and the economy, placing trust in their citizens to do the right thing. Sweden did take some measures banning large groups, encouraging physical distancing, closing schools for older children while conversely actively discouraging mask-wearing. The approach of allowing the virus to spread freely throughout the population with minimal protective strategies and few tests was predictably risky in the absence of a vaccine. The approach was marked by inadequate protections for at-risk groups, particularly the elderly. King Carl Gustaf publicly criticised the government's approach which meant Sweden had a much higher death rate than its neighbours and the highest per capita number of deaths in the world by the end of May (over 4,000 deaths with 88% of deaths of people over 70). Sweden eventually conceded its failed experiment was a mistake. An announcement by Prime Minister Stefan Löfven of a future inquiry into the high number of nursing home deaths followed.

Early reports suggested the anticipated antibody protection did not eventuate with only 7.3% of the population developing antibodies (Folkhälsomyndigheten, 2020). Sweden's approach also did little to protect Sweden from the economic fallout and a declining gross domestic product (GDP). As with other countries, not all COVID-19-related deaths were reported as such. Migrant communities suffered a disproportionate number of deaths and foreign workers and migrants with no legal protection were threatened with deportation and loss of work visas if they became unemployed.

The contrast with Sweden was so great, Denmark and Norway opened tourism to Iceland and other countries excluding Sweden. Denmark and Norway acted early with the range of non-pharmaceutical interventions – lockdown, testing, physical distancing, hygiene, and quarantine. Denmark, similar to Iceland and New Zealand, locked down early. Interestingly, Danes have a cultural attachment to the word *hygge* related to the English word *hug*, a concept popularised in recent years (Wiking, 2016). It can be interpreted as creating a cosy, warm atmosphere at home, perhaps an attitude offering a functional adaptation to lockdown. *Hyggelige* (smiling and happy) Danes and Icelanders are renowned for having high trust in government and concern for the collective. In mid-March, Prime minister Mette Frederiksen encouraged

(*Continued*)

BOX 2.11 (*Continued*)

THE NORDIC COUNTRIES

Danes to place the well-being of the community over the individual or to show *samfundssin* (Statsministeriet, 2020).

After its first diagnosed case, Iceland aided by a small, homogenous population flattened its curve quickly instigating mask-wearing, physical distancing, extensive contact tracing, quarantine and mass screening, more testing per population than any other country. The evaluation of Finland's experiment with Basic Universal Income was released in May 2020, showing the potential utility of Universal Basic Income models during pandemic periods which ensures people do not have to make decisions been their health and starvation. As well as demonstrating positive employment results, a positive effect on physical and mental well-being was shown, results which suggests benefits for people during lockdown and unemployment scenarios (Kangas et al., 2020; Kela, 2020).

Greenland and the Faroe Islands had very few confirmed cases and deaths. As of 31st May, there was 11,833 confirmed cases and 528 deaths in Denmark, 6,826 cases and 310 deaths in Finland, Iceland had 1,806 cases and ten deaths, Norway 8,437 cases and 229 deaths and Sweden had 37,113 cases and 4,371 deaths (Johns Hopkins Coronavirus Resource Center).

During this period, conservative politicians across Europe exerted pressure to reopen European borders (where they were closed) while others expressed the importance of lives over profit. The pandemic was also far from over in Europe. We leave Europe for the Americas where the US topped the list of the worst affected countries along with Brazil among the worst performing nations globally.

The Americas

The Americas, north and south, were badly affected by COVID-19. We go first to the US and Canada. Two men returning from Wuhan were the first cases of COVID-19 in the US and Canada, confirmed on 19th January in Washington State and on 27th January in Toronto. In stark contrast to the US under the Trump administration, Canada's national government shared concerns about health as well as economic recovery. Learning from previous SARS experience, national, provincial, territorial governments and international partners cooperated with a shared pandemic preparedness and action plan. Canada imposed prison sentences (six months) and financial penalties (up to $750,000) or arrivals who breach self-isolation, and up to one million dollars for causing the death or serious bodily harm of another person under the Quarantine Act (Public Health

Agency of Canada, 2020). By 31st May, Canada had 91,681 documented cases and 5,970 deaths (Johns Hopkins Coronavirus Resource Center).

New York city became the epicentre of infection in the north. On March 20th, New York city accounted for 5% of global infections. On March 22nd, the city went into lockdown. In the midst of the crisis, hospital staff were forbidden to talk the media and the system was so overloaded that bodies were transported in refrigerated trucks. In April, police had no PPE, 20% of the police force were not working due to illness, and 2,500 people had the virus. National politics and the Trump leadership played important roles in the US shining a very bright floodlight on systemic problems – privatised health and social welfare structures – and on the performance of governments (see Box 2.12).

BOX 2.12

THE UNITED STATES OF AMERICA

Due to a very slow response, multiple strains of the virus entered the US. The nation succumbed rapidly becoming the worst affected nation in the world in the first six months of the pandemic. According to a PBS (2020) documentary, daily briefings alerted the Whitehouse throughout January and ex-President, Trump, knew personally by 18th January. Doctors and scientists became increasingly alarmed at the lack of action as Trump adopted a position of denial with no national approach to containment (PBS, 2020). One US study in preprint, conducted between March 15th and May 3rd, estimated that acting even two weeks earlier would have saved 50,000 lives (Pei et al., 2020). The lack of national leadership and presidential discourse that encouraged conspiracy theories made existing political and social cracks into chasms. Polarised positions were further cemented escalating into civil and health crises as the pandemic ravaged the country. Movements such as *Black Lives Matter* and *I can't breathe* later railed against structural racism and the deaths of African Americans at the hands of police while anti-mask protests and COVID-19 parties contributed to the curve's continued upward trajectory. African Americans, minority groups, Indigenous Peoples, the elderly and those with comorbidities were vulnerable, and people of all ages died. 1.3 million vulnerable people lived in nursing homes, 800,000 in assisted living facilities, and 75,000 in intermediate care facilities with three million workers employed in these facilities (Chidambaram, 2020). Only 23 states reported COVID-19-related deaths in these facilities. Insufficient testing suggested that there were many more deaths of older people than the reported 50% of all deaths in the country.

Three million people, mainly from Europe, entered New York State alone between January and March. The earliest superspreader events were gatherings

(Continued)

BOX 2.12 (*Continued*)

THE UNITED STATES OF AMERICA

of faith communities in New York City. Governor Andrew Cuomo responded to the federal leadership vacuum and failure to anticipate the pandemic's impact by taking control of the health emergency in the State. Cuomo and the Mayor of New York City adopted aggressive measures to contain the virus, support the overburdened health system and deal with the many deaths in the city. Physical distancing and lockdown for all but essential workers were policed by law enforcement. Testing increased from 400 daily to nearly 16,000 by the end of May. Field hospitals and temporary morgues were established and the navy assisted deploying the hospital ship *Comfort* to New York. Cuomo was later criticised for nursing home residents with COVID-19 being discharged from hospitals and the under-reporting of subsequent aged care deaths.

As numbers rose, Trump derided mask-wearing and the Surgeon-General advised the public against them. Cuomo instead advised *wear a mask, get tested, and save lives,* and in April enacted mask-wearing into law by executive order. With the Obama administration's pandemic plan disregarded, the spectacle of Trump downplaying the pandemic became a pointed focus of Cuomo's daily briefings thus becoming the go-to politician for many people around the US Cuomo called for the sharing of resources such as ventilators between States. Across the country, Governors who recognised the emergency (e.g. California and Maryland) banded together for mutual cooperation and creatively sourced equipment and PPE while guarding supplies from federal seizures. Other State Governors took variable actions including those that adopted positions of denial. Those resistant states were primarily those Red (Trump) states. Consequently, States like Georgia, Texas, Arizona, South Carolina and Florida saw exponential escalation of infections and deaths. Voices of reason constantly mitigated against the damage caused by Trump on top of the impact of COVID-19. Grassroots organisations rallied to address the health, economic and social problems in communities, while hate and divisiveness emerged.

On 31st May, the US was heading towards two million cases and over 100,000 Confirmed deaths and rising (Johns Hopkins Coronavirus Resource Center). The US was a long way from reaching its peak.

This brings our journey to South America. The first confirmed case in South America was on 26th February in São Paulo, Brazil, soon followed by other countries. The first cases were in affluent neighbourhoods where people had access to more resources than the poor in this region. By the end of May and rising, there were over 155,671 confirmed cases in Peru and 3,334 deaths, 1,459 cases and 13 deaths in Venezuela, and 16,214 cases and 524 deaths in Argentina.

Health systems in many parts of South America were under-resourced and unable to meet health needs before the pandemic, and many people had few, if any, safety nets. Peru acted early, testing and locking down the country but numbers continued to increase mainly in the labouring class blamed on the impact of neoliberalism on the Peru's social and economic structures (Lust, 2021). In Bolivia, the Health Minister, Marcelo Navajas, was arrested under suspicion of corruption due to price gouging on the purchase of ventilators. He was subsequently removed from his position.

In Columbia, cardboards beds that could be folded into coffins after death were manufactured to reduce contact between medical staff and the deceased (The New Daily, 2020). Ecuador and Panama were overwhelmed by February. Media reported corpses left in the streets of Guayaquil and people were turned away from overfull hospitals and funeral parlours. It was only after a severely strict lockdown did the rate of infections begin to slow (Altman & Valarezo, 2020). Uruguay fared well compared to most other South American countries due to experience with other infectious diseases, an attitude that considered health expenditure as a necessity not a burden, and scientists, health experts and politicians working together. Turning a critical gaze on Brazil (see Box 2.13), we come to understand how COVID-19 came to devastate this country.

BOX 2.13

BRAZIL

Claudia Fonseca

The radically-right, Jair Bolsonaro, became Brazil's president in January 2019. Institutional reforms that diminished job stability, reduced pension benefits and privatised banks, utilities, schools, health and other public services were rapidly introduced. These measures, accompanied by moral platitudes against *eroding traditional family values*, exacerbated the extreme inequality that has plagued Brazil since colonialisation.

A domestic worker infected by her employer who had returned from overseas officially became the first death to COVID-19. Within days, the Minister of Health confirmed community transmission throughout Brazil and made emergency recommendations consistent with WHO policies of physical distancing, closing borders, limiting intercity transportation, closing schools, and reducing activities of *non-essential* public and commercial services. Many state and county executives followed suit in their respective territories. Nonetheless, the President and most of his cabinet followed Donald Trump by describing COVID-19 as a *paltry flu* that did not warrant economic sacrifice. By mid-April, having failed to endorse Bolsonaro's enthusiasm for chloroquine, the Health Minister fell, replaced by yes-men who established no effective

(Continued)

BOX 2.13 (*Continued*)

BRAZIL

actions for prevention, testing or treatment. In the name of individual liberty, Bolsonaro defied physical distancing, attended national rallies where, maskless, he shook hands and embraced supporters. As the pandemic spread, it became evident that the country's run-down public health system fell far short of actual need. Especially in poorer regions, decentralised and sporadically funded health administrations faced obstacles finding test kits, PPE, functioning ventilators, and building and equipping quality field hospitals.

Manaus, the capital of the State of Amazonas and an important crossroads for many Indigenous groups, became one of the first hardest-hit cities. The elderly, black, Indigenous and poor already affected by chronic unemployment, low wages, structural racism, police violence, and others with chronic, poverty-related health conditions comprised the majority of deaths. Early on, self-help networks typical of the favelas acted quickly to address hardship. As well as the work of NGOs and community associations, impromptu soup kitchens sprung up operated by local women and reliant on donations. Although emergency benefits provided by the federal government to over 60 million lower-income citizens provided momentary respite, it did not revert the tragic long-term effects of the pandemic combined with the social and economic pandemonium caused by the far-right regime.

By 20th May, Brazil was the third worst affected country in the world following only the US and Russia. Brazil had 498,440 confirmed cases and 28,744 deaths by the end of May and rising (Johns Hopkins Coronavirus Resource Center).

The next stop is Mexico (see Box 2.14). Leading up to May 31st, Mexico had fewer confirmed cases than the US, and limited success in flattening the curve worsened by endemic poverty, resources and leadership.

BOX 2.14

MEXICO

Carmen Monico

The first case of COVID-19 was reported on 29th February and a national health emergency was declared on 30th March. Mexico's capacity to respond was severely limited due to an under-resourced health system

(*Continued*)

BOX 2.14 (*Continued*)

MEXICO

and widespread corruption. The Médecins Sans Frontières established treatment centres to meet need in borderlands and rural communities. Insufficient testing, incompetence, corruption, and nepotism contributed to escalating cases and unnecessary deaths in an already impoverished country. President Andres Manuel López Obrador was criticised for populist and confusing messaging, refusing to close borders, limit travel or promote physical distancing. Eventually the business sector frustrated with government inaction, developed their own responses (McCormick, 2020). Interestingly, despite political tensions between the US and Mexico, much of the approach to health, the economy and politics mirrored many of Trump's actions including appealing to religiosity and promoting non-scientific *protections*, and like Bolsonaro in Brazil, mingling with crowds without PPE.

By April, physical distancing and public health messaging promoted safety, alongside limiting travel, stay-at-home and quarantine were introduced. With limited access to safety nets and labour protections, the 56% of Mexican workers in the informal economy had to choose between staying home or earning a living. Eventually, the government announced social and job creation programs to respond to COVID-19. Mexico City residents rallied to support and help each other. Héroeslocales.mx (Local Heroes) distributed food aid and Ayuda Mutua CDMX, a mutual aid organisation, distributed food, masks and hand sanitiser. Reports of family violence, child abuse and sexual offences increased during stay-at-home orders (Vilar-Compte et al., 2020). As in other regions, organised crime stepped in. Drug cartels offered food relief while exerting increased control, conflict and takeovers. Migrants and people living in poverty were badly affected especially those subjected to deportation from the US and family separations. Outcomes for disadvantaged group were expected to worsen.

The death toll in Mexico including deaths along the US/Mexico border immigrant trail was considered to be underestimated. Mexico recorded 87,512 cases and 9,453 deaths on 31st May (Johns Hopkins Coronavirus Resource Center).

From Mexico, we travel south to the Central American Northern Triangle (CANT) to explore Guatemala, El Salvador and Honduras (see Box 2.15).

BOX 2.15

GUATEMALA, EL SALVADOR AND HONDURAS

Carmen Monico

COVID-19 badly affected Guatemala, El Salvador and Honduras given endemic poverty and frequent natural disasters. For example, prior to the COVID-19, over 60% of people in Honduras experienced poverty or extreme poverty, disproportionally affecting rural families. The pandemic worsened existing poverty, food security, and social and economic forecasts. In Guatemala, stay-at-home orders imposed by government further aggravated food insecurity as people were unable to work and feed their families. The social and cultural marginalisation of Indigenous people and those of African descent worsened in these countries. Over 50% of the population in Guatemala are of Mayan heritage and 1% identify with Afro-Latino culture. Seven percent of the population in Honduras and 0.2% in El Salvador are Indigenous or Afro-Latino. These communities experience higher levels of poverty, unemployment, and discrimination especially in accessing health care.

The World Bank projected a 7.2% economic decline in Latin America in 2020 due to COVID-19, deepened by the lack of governments' preparedness and failure to address long-standing social and structural inequalities in the CANT (World Bank, 2020a). With a long history of dictatorships, civil conflicts, socioeconomic disparities, corruption, insufficient social protection and a large informal sector, government responses were repressive and hard to implement. The Council on Hemispheric Affairs (COHA) condemned the heavy-handed and violent approach by police in El Salvador which included the mistreatment of prisoners and the detention of working people. Lockdowns resulted in increased incidences of sexual and gender-based violence, femicides, child abuse and hate crimes (UNHCR, 2020). Disappearances, murders, and death threats by organised criminal networks escalated during lockdown. Politicians and gangs responded to the pandemic for their own political purposes under the guise of humanitarianism. Although border closures reduced the spread of disease and death, reports by human rights entities and individuals regarding the mistreatment of immigrants and people returning home proliferated. The lack of adequate facilities for people arriving at borders and airports and subjected to 30–40 days of quarantine resulted in the death of at least two people.

A collaboration between Cuba and Guatemala previously assisted during natural disasters and health emergencies. The Cuban Medical Brigade was again invited to assist Guatemalan health workers during the pandemic. As of March 1, 302 doctors, 98 nurses, 30 technicians and 11 support workers were providing services in 16 Guatemalan departments. The UNHCR expanded

(*Continued*)

BOX 2.15 (*Continued*)

GUATEMALA, EL SALVADOR AND HONDURAS

cash transfer programs in the region and the provision of food, medicines, bedding and housing, reaching 1.2 million people. In April 2020, the Latin American chapter of the International Federation of Social Workers (IFSW), which included the Association of Social Workers of El Salvador, issued a call for action to respond to the COVID-19 crisis, condemning the impact of imposed restrictions on vulnerable, historically excluded and impoverished people, the shortage of PPE for health care and frontline workers, and the lack of universal service systems. Nonprofit organisations shifted programming to address the needs of most vulnerable. Most impressive were the acts of kindness reported across the CANT countries including bringing food to those unable to provide for themselves during lockdown.

On 31 May 2020, Guatemala recorded 4,739 cases and 83 deaths, El Salvador had 2,517 cases and 46 deaths, and Honduras 5,094 cases and 195 recorded deaths. (Johns Hopkins Coronavirus Resource Center).

Our final destination before leaving the Americas are the nations in the Caribbean Sea made up of independent nations, territories and other statuses governed by countries including Britain, the Netherlands, Venezuela, France, the US and Columbia. The independent nations of the Caribbean are Antigua and Barbuda, the Bahamas, Barbados, Cuba, Dominica, Dominican Republic, Grenada, Haiti, Jamaica, Saint Kitts and Nevis, Saint Lucia, Saint Vincent and the Grenadines, and Trinidad and Tobago (see Box 2.16).

BOX 2.16

JAMAICA, CUBA AND HAITI

Renie Rondon-Jackson

The unique sociopolitical environments of Jamaica, Cuba and Haiti demonstrate the diversity in the region. Travellers brought the SARS-CoV-2 into Jamaica by 10th March, followed by Cuba on 11th and Haiti by 19th March. Once under British colonial rule, Jamaica is a constitutional monarchy and middle-income country. Although crime and violence remain high and 19% of people live in poverty, socioeconomic inequality is much lower than most other Caribbean countries. Cuba, an independent socialist state, is

(*Continued*)

BOX 2.16 (*Continued*)

JAMAICA, CUBA AND HAITI

renowned for its free, universal health system. The health system is well resourced with the highest ratio of doctors per population in the world. By comparison, Haiti, a country still heavily dependent on US aid, faced the pandemic with weak, under-resourced health and social protection systems, and a population heavily impacted by intergenerational poverty, natural disasters and a history of colonisation and slavery. Complicating matters, the US deported Haitians diagnosed with active COVID-19, amplifying the crisis in Haiti.

The Jamaican Health and Wellness Ministry convened a COVID-19 response team that included members from the private sector, religious leaders, the Jamaica Defence Force, and the University of the West Indies. The government stressed community responsibility to stop the virus urging people to follow infection prevention and control measures. A limit of no more than 20 individuals in a public space, restricted numbers on public transport and physical distancing of one metre were introduced. In January, restrictions on people arriving from China were imposed which extended to South Korea, Iran, Singapore and Italy by February.

Due its natural disaster history and robust health system, Cuba had a well-developed disaster plan which included strategies to address the needs of the vulnerable although resources were still scarce attributed to pre-existing debt and strained relationships with the US. The Cuban government also acted swiftly introducing lockdown and travel bans and supported work from home. Free healthcare continued and social protection efforts made use of La Libreta, a pre-existing rationing system. Although expensive, there was a focus on testing and tracing. Meanwhile, foreign volunteers brought the pandemic to Haiti, already battling infectious diseases and social problems. The President banned travel, closed borders, shut down factories and schools and imposed curfews but the curve continued to climb.

Regardless of differences between countries, the poor and vulnerable bore the impact of the pandemic and rising curves. By May 31st, Jamaica had fared best with only 581 confirmed cases and nine deaths. Cuba reported 2,025 cases and 77 deaths. Numbers in Haiti were 1,865 cases and 38 deaths recorded.

Africa, next on our tour, is a vast continent with many countries and cultures, and so in this next section we will visit only a few. Countries have been colonised, often more than once. By the end of May, Africa's curve had still to peak.

Africa

Social workers in Africa, as elsewhere, were challenged with upholding human dignity which threatened to worsen pre-existing health, economic and social issues with few resources to support food and income security. African countries have histories of colonisation, often more than once, which invariably leave social and health problems in their wake. Human rights violations, inequalities, hunger, rural exclusion and inadequate healthcare were problems felt across the continent (Amadasun, 2020).

Across Africa, the spread of COVID-19 appeared to be slower than elsewhere attributable to geographical factors and a younger population (median age 19.7 years and even lower in some countries). Although comorbidities such as HIV/AIDs and other diseases added to health risks, fewer deaths were reported well into 2020 (Lone & Ahmad, 2020). Modelling predicted a quarter billion COVID-19 infections and 190,000 deaths would affect 47 countries but that the spread of the disease would be slower than other regions due to its unique socio-ecological factors such as scattered population, few linked road systems and limited travel (Global Health Now, 2020). One study reported an association between Neanderthal genes (almost completely absent in African population) and the severity of illness which suggested Africans may be less susceptible (Zeberg & Pääbo, 2020). Matthew Ward points out in Chapter 3 that in the face of risk factors such as overcrowding, African Americans had a lower mortality rate during the 1918 Influenza Pandemic which was attributed to earlier exposure. Although scientists questioned genetic advantage, African Americans and people of African-Caribbean descent in the UK were at greater risk. If the suggested genetic advantage proves true, this could possibly be due to mixed ancestry, while not dismissing the impact of the social determinants of health. The science has yet to answer this and other questions. Hypotheses also turned to environmental protective factors including exposure to other diseases in the environment such as parasites and microorganisms (Mbow et al., 2020). Others focused on the possible protective factors of previous vaccinations to account for lower rates of infection in Africa and Asia. The answers are likely to be complex.

At the onset of the pandemic, African nations responded quickly to the threat of Covid-19 within their resource capacity. Communicable diseases, the leading causes of death in Africa, include HIV/AIDS, diarrhoeal diseases, malaria and tuberculosis. Nations have dealt with these and other deadly outbreaks such as Ebola. It is these experiences with communicable diseases that prepared many nations to respond to COVID-19. However, healthcare capacity across Africa is weak and ill-equipped. Some countries lacked even the most basic provisions and had no ventilators.

Anti-vaccination beliefs fuelled by some leaders are problematic in Africa (Adepoju, 2021). Throughout Africa there are strong beliefs in traditional medicines which may have provided some comfort in the absence of well-resourced health systems but also paved the way for misinformation. For example, the Malagasy President of Madagascar, Andry Rajoelina, actively promoted a drink made from sweet wormwood (artemisia annua) as a COVID-19 cure, distributing the drink to other African countries. Because an anti-malarial drug was derived from wormwood, there were concerns that its use would fuel drug resistant malaria in Africa (Nordling, 2020). In Ghana, 33 herbalists submitted medicines to the Ghana Food and Drug Authority. These were not approved for use although these *cures* were still sold in local markets.

Full or partial lockdowns were in place in 42 of the 54 countries by May (Economic Commission for Africa, 2020). The experience of lockdown and the easing of restrictions was variable across the continent. Fifty-six percent of urban populations live in slums. A survey conducted in Nairobi slums found over 75% of people left their homes on average three times in 24 hours during lockdown, 32% could not afford extra soap, 81% lost jobs or had reduced income and 70% skipped meals (Economic Commission for Africa, 2020). Yet another example of having to choose between health and meeting daily needs. Community and reliance on others are important for survival making protections against COVID-19 difficult. Similar to many places in Africa, older people in Ghana, Eswatini and Zimbabwe were particularly vulnerable because they often live in villages without family support due to rural and urban migration with limited access to adequate healthcare (Nhapi & Dhemba, 2020; Kwegyir Tsiboe, 2020). African experiences again suggest the need to view social protection as a national investment rather than a burdensome expense.

As with other regions, groups already discriminated against were at increased risk (e.g. LGBTQIA+). People with albinism in parts of Africa, also at high risk, are victims of violence and discrimination under non-pandemic circumstances. Lockdown in communities where they were at risk meant they were unable to meet health and other needs (Amnesty International. 2020). Belief systems and organised crime that led to their murder and mutilation during past crises and elections, indicated heightened risks during the pandemic. In Mozambique, terrorist groups took advantage of the focus on the pandemic to increase their presence and influence over the people, and in the last few months of 2020, concerns about civil war, genocide and a humanitarian crisis in Ethiopia came to the fore with the escalation of internal conflict. We proceed with our journey through Africa in Kenya (see Box 2.17).

BOX 2.17

KENYA

Gidraph G. Wairire

Kenya was unprepared when first case of COVID-19 was detected in March 2020. Except for Mombasa and Kiambu, many county governments were caught flat-footed as they had not established fully functional COVID-19 control measures. The national government through the Ministry of Health provided daily updates about essential mitigation measures. The majority of people in Kenya depend on the agrarian economy and small businesses which were immediately

(Continued)

BOX 2.17 (*Continued*)

KENYA

affected. Transport, restaurants, hotels, and the education sector were particularly affected. Universities, schools, Technical and Vocational Education and Training institutions and commercial colleges closed. Learners lost an academic year with emotional and practical consequences, and teachers, particularly in private institutions, suffered salary cuts or job loss. Some institutions already had online learning while others struggled to embrace it with minimal success. This indirectly promoted socioeconomic injustice since the majority of learners could not afford the mandatory requirements for online learning including electricity, internet, smart phones and computers. Learners from middle-income families could learn digitally while those from poor, low-income groups could not. Yet, all were required to sit same institutional and national examinations.

The wearing of masks, physical distancing, hand washing with soap, and the closure of churches and mosques for a highly religious society were difficult for many people. The stigma associated with COVID-19 especially on the families of patients, those in isolation centres and those bereaved was traumatic (Wango et al., 2020). Strict burial procedures were traumatising for families, entire neighbourhoods and villages. Viewing the body was not allowed and the coffin and everywhere it passed also needed to be fumigated.

Regionally, the impact of COVID-19 also caused uneasy relationships with neighbouring countries, specifically Tanzania and Uganda, over the casual handling of COVID-19 and the status of their nationals entering Kenya. This caused a near diplomatic standoff between the three countries especially between Kenya and Tanzania to the point where Tanzania banned flights from Kenya for three months which badly affected the Kenyan economy.

Critical implications for social workers revolved around confidentiality for patients and families especially during the initial stages, contract tracing, moving to isolation centres against their wishes and burial procedures. Implications for human rights related to access to healthcare as stakeholders responsible were in most cases unable to play their roles effectively. Conversely, COVID-19 brought the nation together, people stood together in unity, and new songs that stroked feelings of national resilience that encouraged and captivated some hope were released. Many Kenyans grieved. Others laughed at it with a *never give up* attitude that did not allow COVID-19 to dampen their spirits.

As of 31st May, Kenya had 1,888 confirmed cases and 61 deaths. (Johns Hopkins Coronavirus Resource Center).

This brings us to the neighbouring country of Uganda (see Box 2.18), a country with a history of colonisation, war, and ruthless and corrupt dictatorships.

BOX 2.18

UGANDA

Janestic Mwende Twikirize

Uganda confirmed its first case of COVID-19 on 21st March and immediately implemented strict lockdown measures to stem the spread of the pandemic, including closing of borders, schools, businesses, places of worship, and transport. The President, Yoweri Museveni, promoted measures to stem the pandemic and the political leadership worked closely with the scientific committee to promote the WHO recommended measures against COVID-19. Mandatory quarantining of returning residents, strict contact tracing, isolation of those who tested positive with or without symptoms, and delayed community spread kept infection rates low for three to four months. An inevitable gap was allowing cross-border truckdrivers to enter and exit the country. Most positive cases came through this avenue as Uganda is landlocked.

Uganda's previous experience with epidemics such as HIV/AIDS, Ebola and others provided good ground for the reasonably fair handling of COVID-19. Uganda was right in the middle of fighting to prevent Ebola and had been screening travellers at all entry points to stop the importation of Ebola from neighbouring countries. A key lesson applied from past epidemics was of critical importance as was strict political leadership in rallying the masses around preventative measures. Another feature of the pandemic in Uganda was the mostly asymptomatic presentation of the infection. Given the very weak health system, one would have imagined disastrous effects as had been anticipated for the African continent. Instead, most cases were asymptomatic, and the rate of recovery was unexpectedly high.

Despite the reasonable handling of the pandemic, strict lockdown measures had far reaching social and economic effects. Available evidence suggested that Uganda was already experiencing increases in the incidence of domestic and gender-based violence, unprecedented levels of suicide, child abuse and loss of livelihoods (4Children Uganda, 2020; Byamukama, 2020). School closures affected more than 17.5 million children and young people and deprived hundreds of thousands of teachers employed in an estimated 17,859 private schools of a source of income. Closures in the tourism sector have left more than 1,000 workers unemployed (UNDP-Uganda, 2020) and affected several informal sector workers who constituted 84.9% of the urban population (Uganda Bureau of Statistics, 2017). People with COVID-19 and returning residents were quickly stigmatised and blamed for importing the virus. Meanwhile, the Government focus was on the medical aspects of the pandemic while the economic, and psychosocial effects including mental health impacts remained largely ignored potentially leading to serious problems for the population.

As of 31st May, Uganda reported 413 confirmed cases and no deaths (Johns Hopkins Coronavirus Resource Center).

Next, we explore the impact of COVID-19 in Ghana (see Box 2.19), situated on the coast of the sub-region of Western Africa.

BOX 2.19

GHANA

Ariel Kwegyir Tsiboe

The first two cases of COVID-19 were recorded on 12th March. These two individuals had returned from Norway and Turkey to Ghana and became ill a few days later. After confirmation of these first two cases in the country, the Government of Ghana (GoG) immediately began contact tracing and testing for potential cases. Although the contact tracing exercise was helpful, there were instances of undetected cases in the country. Consequently, the number of confirmed cases increased while generating fear in the country.

The emergence of COVID-19 negatively affected the economy, especially among people in small businesses. As confirmed cases increased day by day, many traders took advantage and capitalised on the sale of hand sanitisers by increasing its price. This made patronizing hand sanitisers among low-income earners problematic. Other sectors such as hospitality, transportation and education were greatly affected. The academic year came to a standstill leaving students idle and teachers in the private education sector most vulnerable. The majority suffered salary cuts and some lost their jobs.

Two regions in Ghana, Kumasi and Accra, became COVID-19 hotspots and were placed under partial lockdown for three weeks. Although this measure aimed to flatten the curve, the majority of Ghanaians reported emotional and economic hardship due to movement restrictions. Another notable challenge was the inability of the health sector to cope with surges and demand, especially those in need of respiratory support and beds. Clearly, the Ghanaian health sector faced difficulties before the emergence of the COVID-19 pandemic which made combating the disease even more challenging.

Given the heightened public health burden in Ghana, the GoG imposed lockdown protocols and placed a nationwide ban on all social gatherings. As occurred in developed countries, the GoG called on its citizens to trust the government through several televised presidential addresses. To support its people, the GoG introduced three forms of assistance. It fully financed the electricity bills of all Ghanaians who consumed 0–50 kilowatts per hour and subsidised electricity bills for the rest of the population for three months. The GoG also absorbed water bills for the entire country for three months and distributed food for 470,000 families during the three-week lockdown in Kumasi and Accra.

As of 31st May, Ghana had 7,768 confirmed cases and 35 deaths (Johns Hopkins Coronavirus Resource Center).

Before we explore MENA and North Africa, we travel to the southern most tip of the African continent to South Africa (see Box 2.20) which later became overwhelmed by COVID-19.

BOX 2.20

SOUTH AFRICA

Dorothee Hölscher and Corlie Giliomee

The first COVID-19 case was recorded in South Africa on the 5th of March. The virus affected affluent urban areas first and spread to poorer and rural areas within two weeks. By 22nd, almost 200 cases were confirmed, and the first person died on 26th (Singh 2020). The government declared a state of disaster on the 15th of March. On 25th, a multidisciplinary ministerial group was established and one of the world's tightest lockdowns was effected on 26th March, the same day as the first casualty of the pandemic was reported. Measures included the closure of workplaces and schools, strict limitations on mobility, and alcohol and tobacco bans (Ramaphosa, 2020; Singh, 2020). Incremental easing of these restrictions commenced on the 1st of May alongside provision of social relief for the vulnerable and support to key sectors in the economy, (UNDP, 2020). After decades-long neglect, homeless people received government support in the form of shelter and food during lockdown (Socio-economic Rights Institute of South Africa, 2020).

Preparing the health system was severely hampered by difficulties importing key resources. Health measures were criticised for responding to the fears and needs of the upper and middle classes at the expense of the poor who often live in overcrowded conditions with limited access to clean water and sanitation (Muller, 2020). Further criticism centred on the military and police tasked with enforcement, and on the lack of transparency surrounding mitigation decisions (Singh, 2020). The pandemic overlaid socioeconomic conditions of extreme inequality, high public debt and social problems (Eyewitness News, 2020; World Bank, 2020b). Groups already vulnerable were exposed to unintended socioeconomic effects. Widespread job losses imposed further risks in the informal economy, especially for female headed households, leading to widespread hunger being reported (UNDP, 2020). During the first three weeks of lockdown, calls to the national helpline from abused women and children doubled (Eyewitness News, 2020). Although saving lives in terms of the pandemic, hard lockdown in the absence of adequate material and psychosocial support escalated social problems and economic hardship.

By May 31, 2020, South Africa had recorded 30,967 cases with only 610 coronavirus-related deaths (Johns Hopkins Coronavirus Resource Center).

We now move on to the Middle East and North Africa (see Box 2.21)

Middle East and North Africa (MENA)

BOX 2.21

WHICH COUNTRIES ARE IN MENA?

The countries included in the MENA region often depends on who you ask. Sometimes it refers exclusively to the Arab world whereas other parameters are based on geography. According to the World Atlas, "There are 19 countries that are generally considered part of the MENA region. These are Algeria, Bahrain, Egypt, Iran, Iraq, Israel, Palestine, Jordan, Kuwait, Lebanon, Libya, Morocco, Oman, Qatar, Saudi Arabia, Syria, Tunisia, United Arab Emirates, and Yemen".

Before coronavirus, MENA was a region fraught with conflict, and political, cultural and religious diversity. Inequalities and political tensions are high in some countries. In Israel and the occupied Palestinian territory, official reports of coronavirus infections were low but widespread testing was absent. Significant spikes were later noted in Israel particularly in ultra-orthodox communities (Saban et al., 2020). Israel was one of the first countries to introduce a two-week quarantine period for overseas arrivals. People in Gaza already deprived of basic resources were reliant on NGOs. People in poor socioeconomic circumstances were 2.26 times more likely to test positive. Israel and United Arab Emirates (UAE) later led the world in vaccinating their populations, but for Israel, initially excluding Palestinians.

War-torn Syria reported its first death on the 30th of March and imposed a night-time curfew, banned gatherings, restricted internal travel, and closed borders, schools and universities. Although low numbers of infection were being reported, initially only 100 people were tested daily. The health system was unable to meet pre-existing demand especially the millions of internally displaced, vulnerable people. Turkey and Iran were badly affected with large numbers of confirmed cases and deaths. In Iran, over 5,000 people died or were left with damaged organs or were blinded after drinking methanol to cure or prevent coronavirus. Throughout MENA, there were vast disparities in wealth and health and many migrant workers were left without access to formal health and other services. COVID-19 brought significant challenges for religious practices in the region, especially for the Islamic traditions of Ramadan and pilgrimages where large groups of people gather.

The first case of COVID-19 in the Middle East was confirmed in the United Arab Emirates (UAE) on 29 January 2020 and in Jordan (see Box 2.22) where the first case was confirmed on March 2nd.

BOX 2.22

UNITED ARAB EMIRATES AND JORDAN

Taghreed Abu Sarhan

The United Arab Emirates (UAE) and Jordan are countries that took quick and decisive actions after the first confirmed cases of COVID-19. The UAE, a country with a population under 10,000,000 people, immediately closed schools and businesses. Nursery schools closed on the 1st of March and the flagship university on the 5th. Online education was rapidly developed to deliver the curriculum necessary to complete the spring semester. Other government services either closed or were severely restricted. In this constitutional monarchy, Orders were made by Royal Decree including those related to physical distancing. The government rapidly increased its COVID-19 response capacity in medical centres and people were encouraged to seek testing at centres established in easily accessible locations. Employers mandated testing, including teachers. Disinfecting activities commenced with teams of workers deployed to clean the streets and spray chemicals aimed at killing the virus. The metro in Dubai was a key area for cleaning.

Countrywide, updates on public safety interventions were clearly communicated with an influential digital communication network, daily text messages to remind people of physical distancing expectations and curfews, and television and radio broadcasts. Movement between the seven states was curtailed and only essential personnel were permitted to move around in public spaces. Drones and cell phone surveillance were used for monitoring as well as and the use of ankle monitors to specifically oversee the quarantine of those people who tested positive. The Government provided free meal delivery services to the homes of sick people. This aggressive monitoring of people with the disease were seen as necessary steps, rather than intrusive.

Faith leaders played an important role in preparation for Ramadan, establishing that the ritual of breaking fast should be undertaken in greater solitude as family groups and friends were not permitted to gather for feasts. This set a clear tone for a different atmosphere alongside the intensive social marketing campaigns which emphasised the importance of restraint and calm. Government actions were viewed by the people as supportive, as concerned for people's well-being and therefore trusted, resulting in a high level of cooperation with testing and other containment measures. The level of surveillance and aggressive measures may be interpreted as a government overreach by other regimes, but in this collectivist society with a strong sense of social solidarity, these moves were considered necessary to contain the disease. The use of ankle bracelets enabled people to quarantine at home and ensured compliance proving more effective than quarantine measures in those countries that used hotels (often making exceptions for celebrities) which became sources of

(*Continued*)

BOX 2.22 (*Continued*)

UNITED ARAB EMIRATES AND JORDAN

transmission clusters in many places much like cruise ships. Foreign workers were repatriated. Measures to curtail COVID-19 were viewed as necessary for the well-being of all and ultimately as an individual social responsibility.

The Jordanian government also took extraordinary measures, including implementing strict emergency laws. By the 14th of March, Jordan was in total lockdown and a curfew was imposed. The National Crisis Management Centre was launched, modelled after a military command centre, with video screens showing real time reporting of new infections and the direction of the curve. Every day at 6 pm across the country, a siren sounded at curfew which required people to be home and stay indoors. Sirens were previously only used in wartime. The Jordanian armed forces and police were deployed to patrol the Kingdom's streets to enforce the curfew.

By 31st May in the UAE, the curve was on a downward turn with a total of 33,896 confirmed cases and 257 deaths. In Jordan, 739 cases and 9 deaths were reported in Jordan (Johns Hopkins Coronavirus Resource Center).

The next stop is Lebanon (see Box 2.23), a post-civil war nation, experiencing political upheaval and protests in the midst of the onset of the COVID-19 pandemic. A massive, accidental blast in the city with loss of life followed in the second half of 2020 devastating the city. During the first six months of the pandemic, poverty was exacerbated for Lebanese people as well as the population of 1.6 million Syrian and Palestinian refugees.

BOX 2.23

LEBANON

Nadia C. Badran with the Social Workers Syndicate Lebanon

In January 2020, the Ministry of Interior and Municipalities requested information from governmental and non-governmental bodies about responsibilities for pandemic response and preparedness (Circular No. 8/2020). On 21st February, a returning pilgrim was the first confirmed case of COVID-19, and from that point numbers continued to rise. By the end of March, Lebanon had significantly flattened its curve through testing returning travellers, quarantine and other mitigation strategies. However, clusters and spikes continued eventually rising to a greater number of cases than the first peak, adversely affecting the poor, women, migrant workers and the 1.5 million Syrian refugees.

(*Continued*)

BOX 2.23 ***(Continued)***

LEBANON

Half of Lebanon's six million population and 75% of Syrian refugees were already living below the poverty line. The pandemic escalated the country's precarious economic position expected to be worse than the aftermath of the 15-year civil war that waged between 1975 and 1990. Prime Minister, Hassan Diab, warned that many people would be unable to afford bread.

Unlike many countries, Lebanese social workers were an integral part of the national pandemic planning and response. The Social Workers Syndicate Lebanon (SWSL) joined the coordinated response that included several ministries, disciplines and UN agencies (Badran, 2020). The focus was on public health prevention and interventions to ensure people were properly and safely confined in their homes and to oversee the management of community quarantine and isolation centres. Twenty-four social workers assumed the responsibility of coordinating 365 social workers mobilised to form 25 crisis cells at governorate and municipality levels under a NAPA COVID-19 strategy which comprised a seven-stage crisis intervention model built on three foundations. The first being a wide range of preventative strategies to address risks to health at individual and community levels; the second, to seek synergy across sectors to address inequality; and the third to ensure vulnerable communities were reached and served. Social workers assessed and responded to the needs of 2,000 families, 3,000 women and 1,000 older people affected by the coronavirus and mitigation measures. Interventions included case management; health education; assessments of residential environments, economic distress and biopsychosocial needs; initiating collective relationships and resources; and counselling which explored emotional states and coping strategies. At a community level, the distribution of information aimed to address stigma, discrimination and human rights breaches fuelled by COVID-19. In Lebanon, social workers played a vital role in responding to the public health crisis at a national level.

As of 31st May, Lebanon had 1,220 confirmed cases and only 27 deaths.

Although on the African continent, Morocco, Egypt and Algeria are considered to be in the MENA region. In Morocco, the first case of COVID-19, a person who returned from Italy, was diagnosed on the 2nd of March. Morocco immediately began screening passengers at airports. As further cases were identified, hygiene measures and physical distancing were implemented in mosques on the 12th of March. Flights from Europe ceased on the 14th. All learning institutions and cultural and arts activities were closed. Numbers of staff working in organisational offices were reduced, and large gatherings were banned on 16th March. A state of health emergency was declared on 19th March and a one-month lockdown was imposed the next day (Maneesh & El Alaoui, 2020). Morocco had 7,780 confirmed cases and 201 deaths as of 31st May. The country continued to struggle with the disease. Our attention now turns to Egypt and Algeria (see Box 2.24).

BOX 2.24

EGYPT AND ALGERIA

Tarek Zidan

The first confirm cases of COVID-19 were on the 14th of February 2020 in Egypt, closely followed by Algeria on 19th February. Egypt and Algeria are countries with significant health and wealth disparities indicating pre-existing health vulnerabilities. The Arab Spring, a series of large-scale anti-government protests fuelled by social media, had affected much of the Arab world in 2011 (Fronek, 2017). For Egypt, the promise of better living conditions sought during the Arab Spring did not eventuate as poverty is still widespread in Egypt. The economy depends heavily on tourism and the Suez Canal, industries in which 100 million Egyptians are employed. Tourism over the 2019 Christmas/New Year holiday period heightened risks which threatened the public health system, already struggling before the pandemic. With the onset of cases, the main concerns were in densely populated areas along the banks of the Nile especially in Luxor and Aswan. Some protective measures were implemented. Because cases continued to increase, the government imposed a stricter, complete lockdown and a curfew in mid-May and airports were closed. After lockdown ended, Egypt implemented a 14-day quarantine period for international arrivals. Other preventative measures such as physical distancing continued to be encouraged and several campaigns on television and other media outlets were funded. The Egyptian government allocated 125 billion pounds to the health sector and provided free testing and treatments for COVID-19 patients in hospitals specifically designated for the treatment of COVID-19 in the most affected regions. Egypt's curve did not begin to flatten until June following the stricter lockdown.

In Algeria, the health system is fully funded by government with the best medical care in the capital, Algiers. The Saharan areas have lower population density. Measures included economic stimulus (e.g. loans, a moratorium on debt repayments), tax relief measures (e.g. payment deferrals, rate reductions), employment-related measures, equipping hospitals and establishing a toll-free hotline. On May 19, the first nationwide lockdown was imposed affecting Eid Al-Fitr (Feast of Breaking the Ramadan Fast) due to begin on May 24th. Closing borders, wearing masks and banning travel were other measures. Although trust in government is reported to be low due to widespread corruption, the curve was beginning to flatten by the end of May.

On 31st May, Egypt reported 23,449 confirmed cases and 894 deaths. Algeria had a total of 9,267 confirmed cases and 643 death (Johns Hopkins Coronavirus Resource Center).

Although the response across the Arab countries varied and some countries were slow to impose strict measures, others learned lessons from the MERS experience especially for those countries that quickly imposed strict measures. For example, the UAE and Bahrain that reported 10,793 COVID-19 cases and 17 deaths. Saudi Arabia and Kuwait (see Box 2.25) are next on the tour.

BOX 2.25

SAUDI ARABIA AND KUWAIT

Sareh Rotabi

Saudi Arabia, the largest economy in MENA, is signatory to the WHO International Health Regulation, reports on pandemic preparedness, and established a national committee as early as January (Algaissi et al., 2020). In late February, travel was banned from COVID-affected regions and incoming travellers were monitored. Saudi Arabia was vulnerable to rapid spread due to high levels of tourism, business and the largest religious gatherings in the world. The first confirmed case of COVID-19 was on 2nd March. Extensive cleaning, closing educational institutions and preventing large religious gatherings followed. Lockdown and curfews were introduced at the end of March. In April, at least 150 members of the royal family were reported to have contracted COVID-19 and the Governor of Riyadh was being treated in intensive care. These high-profile cases served to caution the nation as it was clear that even the wealthiest were not immune to the virus. Although the mixed private, military and free public health system was robust, it was challenged during the pandemic. As Ramadhan began, prayer was to be practised in greater solitude and the breaking of fast in small family groups. As the Hajj approached, the Kingdom hosted a modest pilgrimage to Mecca only allowing citizens and residents to participate, limiting crowd density to a small fraction of the 2.5 million people who gathered in 2019. A virtual Hajj experience using an internet-based application was developed. This innovation was praised for enabling global participation for pilgrims who had planned their travel years in advance. Saudi Arabia relied heavily on technology for telehealth, education and health communication, especially social media.

Kuwait's first case was confirmed on 24th February and the Kuwaiti government took several initiatives to control the pandemic including establishing a high-level planning committee. A partial lockdown was imposed on 1st March closing schools, workplaces, mosques and malls. Two areas with high infections rates were quarantined. A full lockdown followed on May 10th in place until after Ramadhan on the 31st of May, and borders were locked down on March 15. Around 30,000 Kuwaitis were repatriated from abroad. Unlike many countries, the government did not charge Kuwaitis for their repatriation.

(Continued)

BOX 2.25 (*Continued*)

SAUDI ARABIA AND KUWAIT

Random testing including drive-throughs and Ministry of Health press briefings were daily events. Telecom companies offered free calls and data, banks postponed repayments, and landlords eased rents and offered premises such as hotels for government use. Importantly, the community rallied to help each other.

The number of infections continued to rise in both countries until early June. On 31st May, 83,384 confirmed cases of COVID-19 and 330 deaths were reported in Saudi Arabia (Johns Hopkins Coronavirus Resource Center). According to the Kuwait Ministry of Health, as of May 31st, there was 27,043 total cases and 212 deaths in Kuwait.

Oceania

Oceania includes island nations in Australasia, Melanesia. Micronesia and Polynesia. Every nation in Oceania has a history of European colonisation except for Tonga, the last remaining Kingdom in the region (see Box 2.26). Tonga became a British Protectorate in 1900 thereby technically avoiding German colonisation. Tonga became fully independent in 1970.

BOX 2.26

THE NATIONS OF OCEANIA

There are 14 countries in the Oceania region and 12 dependent territories and autonomous Areas of Special Sovereignty.

Countries – Australia, Fiji, Kiribati, Marshall Islands, Micronesia, Nauru, New Zealand, Palau, Papua New Guinea, Samoa, Solomon Islands, Tonga, Tuvalu, Vanuatu.

Territories – American Samoa, Cook Islands, Federated States of Micronesia (Yap, Chuuk, Pohnpei and Kosrae), French Polynesia, Guam, New Caledonia, Niue, Norfolk Island, Northern Mariana Islands, Pitcairn Islands (Pitcairn, Henderson, Ducie and Oeno Islands), Tokelau, Wallis and Futuna.

Several factors influence the vulnerabilities of the people across Oceania in health emergencies. Histories of colonisation, economic development, inequalities, geography, health systems and leadership are some of these factors. Colonisation, as with other world nations, has had detrimental effects on cultures, poverty and health outcomes. For example, First Australians, the Aboriginal and

Torres Strait Islander peoples of Australia, have significantly worse health outcomes and life expectancy compared to the rest of the population. Sixty-four percent of the disease burden is due to chronic conditions which places these people at high risk during the COVID-19 pandemic (AIHW, 2016). Further risks in communities involved safety, housing, employment and access to healthcare and education (AIHW, 2019). First Australians are over-represented in prisons and the child protection system, a circumstance with roots in colonisation and racist policies such as the Stolen Generation that devastated cultures and family life by the removal of Aboriginal children from their families and communities (Commonwealth of Australia, 1997). Health outcomes for all Australians are further complicated by natural disasters, storms, floods, droughts, and bushfires including the extensive damage caused by the Black Summer bushfires in 2019–2020.

The Māori people make up about 14% of the New Zealand population compared to 3.3% of First Australians. Although Māori people suffer similar inequalities and significant disparities in health outcomes and life expectancies compared to the non-Māori non-Pasifika population, New Zealand has fared much better than Australia in that the country is bi-cultural preserving Māori culture and language and supports Māori leadership beyond tokenism. Māori and Pasifika peoples are 50% more vulnerable to dying from COVID-19 than Pākehā (non-Māori New Zealanders) (Steyn et al., 2020). Along with other countries in the region, New Zealand was still recovering from earthquakes beginning in Christchurch in 2011. Many Pacific Islanders live in New Zealand while those New Zealanders and Pacific Islanders who live in Australia have access to far fewer safety nets than New Zealand offers.

Many nations in in Oceania are dependent on aid from international organisations, governing countries, former colonisers and Australian and New Zealand governments. Health crises involving measles, drug-resistant tuberculosis and polio outbreaks have plagued the region. In January 2020, 5,707 measle cases and 83 deaths were reported in Samoa, followed by Tonga, Fiji, American Samoa and Kiribati. Samoa was heavily impacted by the 1918 Influenza, the effects of which are still strong in the country's collective memory. Community distrust of vaccinations was heightened by the death of two children following vaccination (Craig et al., 2020). On investigation, the WHO's Global Advisory Committee on Vaccine Safety found causation was due to medical negligence in mixing the vaccine and other systemic factors, not the vaccine itself. The circulation of anti-vaccination sentiment, social media campaigns by anti-vaccination groups and particular Christian and traditional belief systems jeopardised the health of many. In 2019, 14 children were on ventilators as a result of infectious disease (Dyer, 2019).

Overall aid to the Pacific from Australia increased by AUD 214 million in 2019–2020. However, funding to health programs was reduced to Samoa by 36%, the Solomon Islands by 13%, Fiji by 22% and the Cook Islands by 75% and the funds of AUD three billion were instead for investment in infrastructure projects (Lyons, 2020). Atoll islands including Kiribati, Tuvalu, Maldives, the Marshall Islands, Tokelau and smaller islands of Papua New Guinea are the *canaries in the coalmine* for climate change bearing the brunt of sea level rise, coral reef destruction and natural disasters of greater intensity which are destroying the islands, cultures and homes (Aung et al., 2009). The majority of countries in Oceania have low resilience against infectious disease. The combination of natural disasters superimposed on existing health and social problems magnifies the vulnerabilities of many people in Oceania during health emergencies.

This leads us to the COVID-19 pandemic. The smaller Oceania countries had limited or no capacity to deal with a pandemic that reached their shores. Different sources reported that Papua New Guinea is estimated to have between 500 and 600 doctors and between 3,000 and 5,000 hospital beds for a population of eight million people (Fainu, 2020). Even with external assistance, the health system was inadequate, struggling to cope with ordinary health issues, outbreaks of dengue fever, malaria, measles, polio and drug-resistant tuberculosis. Island geography helped protect against SARS-CoV-2 while tourism did not. Two days after the first identified case, a state of emergency was announced on 20th March and people suffered food insecurity and loss of livelihoods (Lau et al., 2020). By March 2021, New Guinea was overwhelmed with disastrous consequences for its communities.

Countries adopted variable strategies against the virus once cases were identified. As with all countries, how political leaders responded to the pandemic was important. Media suppression, freedom of speech, and problems disseminating information to the public was of concern in Fiji, Papua New Guinea and Guam. For example, after battling Cyclone Harold and 18 confirmed cases of COVID-19, the military leadership of Fiji imposed strictly controlled lockdown and physical distancing while supressing media reports of COVID-19 (Anthony, 2020). New cases were reported daily in the Pacific. Few resources and limited testing meant the reported number of cases were likely to be an underestimate. Next we explore Australia and New Zealand (see Box 2.27).

BOX 2.27

AUSTRALIA AND NEW ZEALAND

Lynne Briggs

The two largest and best equipped countries in the region with good access to health care were Australia and New Zealand, each managing the COVID-19 pandemic differently. After a delayed start that prioritised the economy, the Australian federal government, philosophically committed to individual freedoms and business interests, initially took a mitigation approach to address COVID-19 and controlled suppression to closures and the premature easing

(Continued)

BOX 2.27 (*Continued*)

AUSTRALIA AND NEW ZEALAND

of restrictions. Australia missed its chance for early elimination, complicated by federal failures to properly manage international arrivals, quarantine and risks to vulnerable groups, in particular older people (Duckett & Mackey, 2020). The first known COVID-19 case, a man who had arrived from China, was admitted to hospital on 24 January 2020 (Caly et al., 2020).

It is important to note that from January, testing in Australia was only for those people with symptoms who had been in contact with a known case of COVID-19 or had arrived from specific overseas locations, and others with symptoms were denied tests. In the early months, travellers at Australian airports were merely asked if they had visited China in the last two weeks. Flights from China were stopped at the beginning of February while at the same time tourism was being encouraged. By the 12th of March, there were 140 cases and three deaths in Australia, Mitigation strategies were not seriously implemented until well into March including stopping other selected flights (Caly et al., 2020).

By 28th March, 495 new cases were identified including a senior federal politician, 14 deaths were recorded, and over 100 healthcare workers infected. Testing guidelines remained restrictive. Communication from national political and federal health leadership was vague, contradictory, and meted out in small doses. For example, seeking to delay banning large gatherings to allow sporting matches to proceed, then gatherings of no more than 500 people were permitted, and slowly reducing down to two people in public spaces by 29th March. From the start, the federal government minimised risks and COVID-19 was compared to the common cold with no risk of community transmission. At the same time, general practitioners had to source their own PPE and hospitals their own additional ventilators. The government continued to deny the need for masks. The media and opposition parties failed to provide early critique of federal government actions for the sake of a united front in the *war* against the virus.

First Australian communities previously heavily impacted by H1N1, showed strong leadership to protect their vulnerable Elders and communities achieved a remarkably good early result compared to the rest of the population, again in the face of federal government inaction (Australian Government, 2020; Eades et al., 2020). Action was immediate by Indigenous communities – restricting travel, closing communities, ensuring clear, culturally appropriate communication, stockpiling PPE, providing for basic needs, educating and supporting. Success was attributed to early action, combined Indigenous and health knowledge, and Indigenous-led and culturally appropriate responses (Eades et al, 2020; Hart, 2020).

A national plan for people with disabilities was not forthcoming until September 2020 and the fate of older people, a federal responsibility was

(*Continued*)

BOX 2.27 (*Continued*)

AUSTRALIA AND NEW ZEALAND

essentially left to the States to manage. Protecting these vulnerable groups were still not properly actioned well into 2021. The federal government failed to provide co-ordinated national planning for safe quarantine protocols for people entering the country, made many exceptions for business and celebrities, and later failed to purchase sufficient vaccinations. Services were contracted out and left to these businesses to attend to safety. Successes in Australia were due to States stepping into the leadership vacuum, science and medical commentators, health workers and to community action. States managed subsequent spikes differently depending on political flavours.

How national leaders responded to the pandemic in the first few months provided insights into the political regimes of these countries and ideological conceptualisations of how people are affected by inequality and social injustices. The first case of COVID-19 in New Zealand was identified on 28th February. In stark contrast to Australia, the New Zealand Prime Minister, Jacinda Adern, immediately prioritised the health of people and adopted a highly successful elimination strategy and unlike Australia managed outbreaks. New Zealand locked down on 23rd March when there were 102 cases and no deaths (Cousins, 2020). Adern's messages to the New Zealand public, the media and in social media chats were honest, clear and consistent. She promoted concern for the safety of others as motivators and brought the public with her. In contrast to Morrison, the Australian Prime Minister, she did not make grand statements of success, acknowledged the limitations of testing and how true numbers of cases were difficult to determine at that stage.

By 31st May, both countries were doing well comparative to other world regions, especially New Zealand where no new cases had been reported for 16 days. Meanwhile, Australia was still dealing with new clusters which led to second waves in Victoria and New South Wales while at the same time easing internal movement and business restrictions, state by state. The approach by New South Wales, later threatened the entire country. Australia's approach, disproportionally influenced by the business sector, has been severely critiqued in terms of welfare and economic costs (Kompas et al., 2020). New Zealand had 1,504 diagnosed cases and 22 associated deaths and Australia, 7,195 diagnosed cases and 103 deaths at the end of May (Johns Hopkins Corona Virus Resource Centre).

Trusting the numbers

Because numbers can be confusing, it is important to understand the numbers being reported here. The cases and deaths in countries reported in this chapter are simply the total numbers reported from the first confirmed case to

31st May. It is useful to further consider the numbers proportional to the population of each country to gauge the full impact of COVID-19 in particular countries.

Speculation about the reliability of lower mortality rates in many countries compared to richer countries proliferated during the first six months of the pandemic. The answer is complex and includes factors such as the type of regime, exposure to previous pandemics, decisive action, clear public health campaigns and the priorities of leaders, philosophies of community responsibility verses individualism, and the availability of widespread testing. Generally, the spread of COVID-19 was underestimated due to poor data collection or when hospital care was scarce or inaccessible. Older people in many countries were not prioritised for hospital care nor included in death counts. This included older people and younger people with disabilities living in care homes. Furthermore, due to ageism, being assigned a different cause of death or as a consequence of limited access to healthcare or its rationalisation, many people died without a diagnosis of COVID-19 including in developed countries. Under-reporting was common in developed and developing countries.

The reliability of data from countries that reported low infection and death rates were questioned but determinations of the reliability of reported rates are often supported by interrogating other data such as the number of funerals held, *excess deaths* (the number of deaths above what is usual), traffic flow, air pollution levels, and how the economy performed. For example, excess deaths of older people and people with disabilities identified in domiciliary and institutional care are good indicators (Burki, 2020; Glynn et al., 2020). A statistical analysis of the death rate in Australia found 800 excess deaths from January to March indicating the number of deaths due to COVID-19 was likely underestimated (ABS, 2020). The reality is that it may take years to know the true number of cases and deaths from COVID-19, if we ever do.

Concluding remarks

Some countries took their first actions when the first case was identified in the country, others as cases began to mount. However, given the rapid movement of millions of people across the world, and as reported in Chapter 1, the virus was already circulating the globe as early as December 2019. One thing is true across all regions, countries, states within countries, that jurisdictions universally *did their own thing*, at least at the start despite WHO advice on collective global action and, in some cases, inconsistent with national health emergency plans. The WHO has also been criticised for delays in announcing a pandemic and late advice on mask-wearing. Some national governments relied primarily on select health advice, others on epidemiological modelling, others like the Czech Republic and Australian governments preferred the business sector to make decisions while others drew on multidisciplinary health expertise and prior planning to respond. Even where the same strategies were adopted, such as lockdown, implementation was deployed differently. In many places, decisions that prioritised health and decisions that were actually political conflated to the point where the difference between them became indiscernible for people preoccupied with day to day survival. In many cases, measures that aligned with the ideological priorities of particular regimes were adopted and, in many countries, political agendas were opportunistically moved forward in the midst of the pandemic. What is true is that the flow on-effect in those countries that did not adequately respond early meant an unnecessary loss of life, greater inequality, disadvantage and discrimination, and ultimately impacting the world by providing environments conducive to the development of variants.

Different priorities, local conditions, geopolitical and socioeconomic conditions, and leadership influenced different approaches to managing the health emergency. The vast differences in socioeconomic circumstances and living conditions between and within regions and the different types of government highlighted the complexity of responding to global health crises without commitment to a unified global strategy. Among the most vulnerable were the poor, elderly and discriminated against, and those people living in countries with corrupt or weak governments. In countries like the UK and Australia, structural inequalities created by successive conservative governments committed to neoliberal economic policy and individual freedoms worsened. In the US, dramatically failed federal leadership under Trump ensured the country deteriorated into what could only be described as civil conflict and insurrection. In the US, the UK and Australia, the devolution of responsibility to state government levels served to mask inadequate planning and early response bypassing federal responsibilities and allowing internal and external, political blame-shifting.

How the first outbreaks in countries were managed was an important aspect of containing the disease and informed how second and third waves emerged, progressed, and were managed. For example, South Korea had good early results but resisted lockdown, instead relying on efficient tracing leading to significant future waves. Importantly, our analysis provides insights invaluable in preparing for future pandemics. Governments and their leaders needed the capacity and will to take decisive actions, communicate clearly, have scientific literacy and be trustworthy, as trust is needed for communities to follow and be cohesive in the face of a health emergency. Importantly, the survival needs of people in lockdown needed to be addressed. One study published in Nature found that non-pharmaceutical measures (lockdown, physical distancing, closing schools etc) are estimated to have prevented or delayed 530 million cases of COVID-19 across just six countries – China, South Korea, Italy, Iran, France and the US (Hsiang et al., 2020). Another study estimated 3.1 million lives were saved in eleven European countries from March to 4th May in the first wave (Flaxman et al., 2020).

By the end of May, countries were either planning how they would ease restrictions or had already done so, including those countries where numbers of cases were still rising, as saving economies and pressure from business sectors came to the fore. However, by doing so, second and third waves of the pandemic began to emerge as early as June 2020, especially in those countries who did not elect for early suppression measures and eased restrictions, particularly opening international borders, too early. Many countries including the US, India, Brazil and many in Europe, Africa and Oceania were still to feel the full impact of the first wave of the pandemic by the end of May. The history of the world's plagues tells us that second and third waves tend to be far worse than the first and, indeed, that is just what later happened during COVID-19. Many decisions were made in the absence of herd immunity, effective treatments, and uncertainty about whether effective vaccines would eventuate. By the end of the first six months, a multitude of studies were being conducted on vaccines and treatments.

Politicians, royalty and celebrities showed that class and privilege did not protect from COVID-19 although they certainly had access to the best available health care and other resources. New vulnerabilities for people who did not expect to be affected had emerged. At an economic level, a dire future was predicted for the newly unemployed, especially the young (Fronek & Briggs, 2020). In terms of health, we knew that adults and children could be left with chronic illness from COVID-19 and it had yet to be determined how long antibodies would protect people who already succumbed to the disease and recovered.

As countries eased restrictions and citizens travelled home, many governments struggled with how to protect people while dealing with the economic fallout. In the aftermath, one can only be reminded of Beveridge's Evil Giants – want (income support), disease (health), ignorance (education), squalor (housing) and idleness (employment) – the basis of the welfare state established to aid recovery after the devastation of World War 2 – perhaps something world governments should revisit (Beveridge, 1942). A clear pattern was that where provisions were not made for people to eat and sustain housing, it was impossible for them to comply with measures such as lockdown indicating a rethink is needed on universal income provision such as the experiment conducted in Finland. One might ask what would have happened if all governments, in a coordinated and united approach, had imposed a six-week complete lockdown in December 2019, closed borders, imposed mandated health measures and ensured food and income security for all people during that period, a question we pose to Professor Doherty in Chapter 20. Instead by early June, countries that had eased restrictions were dealing with new spikes and, for some, reinstating states of emergency and lockdown restrictions became necessary creating a yoyo effect which further strained economies, and health and psychosocial outcomes while the pandemic spread exponentially.

New Zealand had prioritised lives and acted quickly and decisively. By doing so, the country was close to official elimination status by mid-May which was ultimately reached and forecasted good management of future outbreaks. At the other extreme, Trump and Brazil's Bolsonaro stood out as leaders unconcerned for the well-being of the population, and in the case of Trump, was alleged to have purposefully incited insurrection before and after being legitimately voted out of office. Militarisation of the US, violence, protests over Black American murders by police and overt racism brought the country's political crisis into sharp relief. Other countries such as India essentially had failed lockdowns due to endemic poverty. Without a means to eat and live people could not stay-at-home. By the end of the May, Sweden was all too aware of their wrongheaded approach to the pandemic and the human and social costs of opting for herd immunity in the absence of a vaccine and sought to justify the position taken.

The approach of China, Vietnam and some other Asian countries were the antithesis of ideologies of individualism and minimal state involvement and sparked divisive, discursive positions between maintaining civil liberties and saving lives and between *draconian* measures and free will, raising serious questions about the possibility that the containment of disease may be impossible in open democracies. The UAE had better outcomes allowing people to quarantine at home using ankle monitors rather than confining people in small hotel rooms not designed for quarantine. New Zealand is one country that destroys an assumption that national elimination strategies may not be possible in democracies. It is true to say that in many western cultures, there are stronger beliefs in individual entitlement and personal freedom or liberty, fuelling the infodemic promoted by some that the pandemic was overblown, a belief influenced by the competence of government, the clarity and quality of health messaging and the personal beliefs of leaders. It is interesting to note that the countries with women leaders have been lauded as managing the health emergency effectively and efficiently (Garikipati & Kambhampati, 2020; Hassan & O'Grady, 2020). They tended to respond more quickly and more decisively with clearer communication than many of their male counterparts. Importantly, they also believed in the science. However, the longer-term fate of these countries also depended on a range of complex factors. As world numbers continued to rise in the latter half of 2020, it became clear that the formula that worked had several key elements – early and strict lockdown, early detection of cases and well-managed quarantine, extensive testing and competent tracing and other measures such as mask-wearing. Missing one of these elements and opening too soon in the absence of vaccination failed to control virus spread.

The experiences of countries at the height of the pandemic lend insights into the immense challenges at a macro level which are indeed felt at the micro level. The pandemic made the link between the micro and macro clear. Cultural norms and social behaviour, trust in governments or their failures led social workers around the globe to consider how the macro environment directly affected people at the micro level and how social work practice was shaped within the unique contexts of the health emergency and specific local environments. Amid the terrible toll of this pandemic, there are also many, many reports of community solidarity, people supporting each other and feeling stronger connections with others even when these connections were online or at a distance. Examples range from small neighbourhood acts of kindness to former child soldiers helping their communities as part of a UNICEF program in the Central African Republic. This is a testament to the human spirit, resilience and adaptability.

Before COVID-19 developed into a pandemic, there was report after report of the inevitable tsunami of mental illness and suicides caused by lockdown in many western countries. Without undermining the very real mental health problems experienced by many people and the suicides that did occur, the focus in many countries was on deficit not resilience. Interestingly, a survey conducted in Germany suggested that suicide rates actually declined during the lockdown period. Social workers should strongly consider the role of macro inequalities such as unemployment, discrimination, and social policies and how these external, structural factors intersect with well-being and affect people's mood, and how people actually cope with factors beyond their control. These are important questions to consider in the aftermath of this health emergency. This leads us to another critical question, should we medicalise human responses to this pandemic or ask the question "is it normal to feel this way given these circumstances?" and how important is it to identify and build on strengths, resilience and coping in these circumstances. As we have learned from decades of research on grief and bereavement, knowing the difference between proportionate human responses and mental illness informs our response.

We take up these questions and more in the ensuing chapters of this book. First, we will explore lessons learned from earlier health emergencies in Chapter 3, and then, in Chapter 4, how human dignity, social work values, and human rights frame social work's understandings of health emergencies and our responses to them.

BOX 2.28

REFLECTIVE QUESTIONS

1. Consider the country or state where you now live.
   - In your view, how well did your government and leaders manage the COVID-19 pandemic? What information did you use to come to your conclusion?
   - If there was an outbreak of a new disease, what geographical, political, historical, economic, health and social factors might influence the government's approach to a new health emergency?
   - Who are the vulnerable people in your country or state? And in what way would they be vulnerable in a health emergency?
   - How might the interplay of these factors affect social work roles and how social workers practice?
2. Thinking further about the country where you live, consider the response to COVID-19 against Dickens' eight dimensions discussed in Chapter 1.

References

4Children Uganda. (2020). *Child protection in the context of COVID-19 in Uganda: Coordinating comprehensive care for children*. Catholic Relief Services.

ABS. (2020, June 24). *3303.0.55.004 – Provisional mortality statistics, Jan-Mar 2020*. Australian Bureau of Statistics. https://www.abs.gov.au/ausstats/abs@.nsf/0/0E25B19FEA63D324CA25859000222EBD?Opendocument

Adepoju, P. (2021). Africa is waging a war on COVID anti-vaxxers. *Nature Medicine*, 27(7), 1122–1125.

AIHW. (2016, September 23). *Australian burden of disease study: Impact and causes of illness and death in Aboriginal and Torres Strait Islander people 2011. Cat. No. BOD 7*. Australian Institute of Health and Welfare. https://www.aihw.gov.au/reports/burden-of-disease/illness-death-indigenous-australians/contents/table-of-contents

AIHW. (2019, September 11). *Understanding indigenous welfare and wellbeing*. Australian Institute of Health and Welfare. https://www.aihw.gov.au/reports/australias-welfare/understanding-indigenous-welfare-and-wellbeing

Algaissi, A. A., Alharbi, N. K., Hassanain, M., & Hashem, A. M. (2020). Preparedness and response to COVID-19 in Saudi Arabia: Building on MERS experience. *Journal of Infection and Public Health*, 13(6), 834–838.

Aljazeera. (2020, April 22). Indonesia's coronavirus response revealed: Too little, too late. *Aljazeera*. https://www.aljazeera.com/news/2020/04/indonesia-coronavirus-response-revealed-late-200422032842045.html

Allegri, E. & Di Rosa, R.T. (2020). Dialoghi digitali. La comunità professionale si confronta sulle esperienze in tempo di COVID. In M. Sanfelici, L. Gui, & S. Mordeglia (Eds.), *Il Servizio Sociale nell'emergenza Covid-19* (pp. 179–194). Franco Angeli.

Altman, D., & Valarezo, J. C. (2020, April 24). Deaths and desperation mount in Ecuador, epicenter of coronavirus pandemic in Latin America. *The Conversation*. https://theconversation.com/deaths-and-desperation-mount-in-ecuador-epicenter-of-coronavirus-pandemic-in-latin-america-137015

Amadasun, S. (2020). From coronavirus to 'hunger virus': Mapping the urgency of social work response amid COVID-19 pandemic in Africa. *International Social Work*. https://doi.org/10.1177/0020872820959366

Amnesty International. (2020, June 12). *Southern Africa: Persons with albinism especially vulnerable in the face of COVID-19. Amnesty International*. https://www.amnesty.org/en/latest/news/2020/06/southern-africa-persons-with-albinism-especially-vulnerable-in-the-face-of-covid19/

Andolfatto, D. & Labbé, D. (2020). Faut-il avoir peur du covid? *Revue Politique et Parlementaire le 4 Septembre 2020*. https://www.researchgate.net/deref/https%3A%2F%2Fwww.revuepolitique.fr%2Ffaut-il-avoir-peur-du-covid%2F

Anthony, K. (2020, April 27). Fijian military leader defends government's right to 'stifle' press during Covid crisis. *The Guardian*. https://www.theguardian.com/world/2020/apr/27/fijian-military-leader-defends-governments-right-to-stifle-press-during-covid-crisis

Aung, T., Singh, A., & Prasad, U. (2009). A study of sea–level changes in the Kiribati area for the last 16 years. *Weather*, 64, 203–206. https://doi.org/10.1002/wea.396

Australian Government. (2020). *COVID-19 Australia: Epidemiology Report 24*. Department of Health. https://www1.health.gov.au/internet/main/publishing.nsf/Content/1D03BCB527F40C8BCA258503000302EB/$File/covid_19_australia_epidemiology_report_24_fortnightly_reporting_period_ending_30_august_2020.pdf

Badran, N. C. (2020). A call for action against COVID-19 – Experience of the Social Workers' Syndicate in Lebanon. *International Social Work*. https://doi.org/10.1177/0020872820949626

BBC News. (2020, April 25). Coronavirus: Belarus orphanage seeks help amid 'critical' outbreak. *BBC News*. https://www.bbc.com/news/world-europe-52426260

Beveridge, W. (1942). *Social insurance and allied health services. Beveridge Report*. http://news.bbc.co.uk/2/shared/bsp/hi/pdfs/19_07_05_beveridge.pdf

Burki, T. (2020). England and Wales see 20000 excess deaths in care homes. *The Lancet*, 395(10237), 1602. https://doi.org/10.1016/S0140-6736(20)31199-5

Byamukama, N. M. (2020). *Covid-19 and domestic violence: Four ways out of a double pandemic*. https://www.icglr-rtf.org/covid-19-and-domestic-violence-four-ways-out-of-a-double-pandemic-by-nathan-mwesigye-byamukama/

Caly, L., Druce, J., Roberts, J., Bond, K., Tran, T., Kostecki, R., … Catton, M. G. (2020). Isolation and rapid sharing of the 2019 novel coronavirus (SARS-CoV-2) from the first patient diagnosed with COVID-19 in Australia. *Medical Journal of Australia*. https://doi.org/10.5694/mja2.50569

Chen, N., Zhou, M., Dong, X., Qu, J., Gong, F., Han, Y., … Zhang, L. (2020). Epidemiological and clinical characteristics of 99 cases of 2019 novel coronavirus pneumonia in Wuhan, China: A descriptive study. *The Lancet*, 395(10223). https://doi.org/10.1016/S0140-6736(20)30211-7

Chidambaram, P. (2020, April 23). State reporting of cases and deaths due to COVID-19 in long-term care facilities. *KFF*. https://www.kff.org/medicaid/issue-brief/state-reporting-of-cases-and-deaths-due-to-covid-19-in-long-term-care-facilities/

CNP. (2020, March 29). Lettre ouverte au Ministre des Solidarités et de la Santé, Olivier Véran [Open letter to the Minister of Solidarity and Health, Olivier Véran]. https://sfgg.org/actualites/lettre-ouverte-au-ministre-des-solidarites-et-de-la-sante-olivier-veran/

CNSCBT. (2020a). *The prevention and control of suspected infections with the new coronavirus within Sanitary Units*. Romanian National Centre for the Surveillance and Control of Communicable Diseases. http://www.cnscbt.ro/index.php/ghiduri-si-protocoale/1331-prevenirea-si-controlul-infectiilor-suspecte-cu-noul-coronavirus-in-unitatile-sanitare/file

CNSCBT. (2020b). *Weekly evolution of confirmed COVID-19 cases*. Romanian National Centre for the Surveillance and Control of Communicable Diseases.

Comas-Herrera, A., Zalakaín, J., Litwin, C., Hsu, A., Lane, N., & Fernández, J.-L. (2020). *Mortality associated with COVID-19 outbreaks in care homes: Early international evidence*. LTCcovid.org, International Long-Term Care Policy Network, CPEC-LSE. https://ltccovid.org/2020/04/12/mortality-associated-with-covid-19-outbreaks-in-care-homes-early-international-evidence/

Commonwealth of Australia. (1997). *Bringing them home. National inquiry into the separation of Aboriginal and Torres Strait Islander children from their families*. https://www.humanrights.gov.au/our-work/aboriginal-and-torres-strait-islander-social-justice/publications/bringing-them-home

Cook, M. (2020, April 18). Extreme social distancing: 'Shoot any coronavirus troublemakers'. *BioEdge*. https://www.bioedge.org/bioethics/extreme-social-distancing-shoot-any-coronavirus-troublemakers/13398

Correia, S., Luck, S., & Verner, E. (2020). Pandemics depress the economy, public health interventions do not: Evidence from the 1918 Flu. Available at SSRN. http://dx.doi.org/10.2139/ssrn.3561560

Cousins, S. (2020). New Zealand eliminates COVID-19. *The Lancet*, 395(10235), 1474. https://doi.org/10.1016/S0140-6736(20)31097-7

Craig, A. T., Heywood, A. E., & Worth, H. (2020). Measles epidemic in Samoa and other Pacific islands. *The Lancet Infectious Diseases*, 20(3), 273–275.

Dehning, J., Zierenberg, J., Spitzner, F. P., Wibral, M., Neto, J. P., Wilczek, M., & Priesemann, V. (2020). Inferring change points in the COVID-19 spreading reveals the effectiveness of interventions. *medRxiv*. https://doi.org/10.1101/2020.04.02.20050922

di Ateneo Studi, C. & sulla Famiglia, R. (2020). *La famiglia sospesa.*Vita e pensiero.

Digi24. (2020, February 26). Primul caz de coronavirus în România [The first coronavirus case in Romania]. *Digi24.* https://www.digi24.ro/stiri/actualitate/primul-caz-de-coronavirus-in-romania-1266806

Dinh, L., Dinh, P., Nguyen, P. D. M., Nguyen, D. H. N., & Hoang, T. (2020). Vietnam's response to COVID-19: Prompt and proactive actions. *Journal of Travel Medicine*, 27(3). https://doi.org/10.1093/jtm/taaa047

Djalante, R., Lassa, J., Setiamarga, D., Sudjatma, A., Indrawan, M., Haryanto, B., … Warsilah, H. (2020). Review and analysis of current responses to COVID-19 in Indonesia: Period of January to March 2020. *Progress in Disaster Science*, 6, 100091. https://doi.org/10.1016/j.pdisas.2020.100091

Duckett, S., & Mackey, W. (2020). *Go for zero: How Australia can get to zero COVID-19 cases.* Grattan Institute. https://grattan.edu.au/report/how-australia-can-get-to-zero-covid-19-cases/

Dyer, O. (2019). Measles: Samoa declares emergency as cases continue to spike worldwide. *British Medical Journal*, 367, l6767. https://doi.org/10.1136/bmj.l981

Eades, S., Eades, F., McCaullay, D., Nelson, L., Phelan, P., & Stanley, F. (2020). Australia's First Nations' response to the COVID-19 pandemic. *The Lancet*, 396(10246), 237–238.

Economic Commission for Africa. (2020). A global debate on Africa's COVID-19 lockdown exit strategies. https://www.uneca.org/covid-19-lockdown-exit-strategies

European Commission. (2019). *State of health in the EU – Romania Country Health Profile 2019.* https://ec.europa.eu/health/sites/health/files/state/docs/2019_chp_romania_english.pdf

Eyewitness News. (2020). *'It just got worse': Domestic violence surges under SA lockdown.* https://ewn.co.za/2020/04/29/it-just-got-worse-domestic-violence-surges-under-sa-lockdown

Fainu, K. (2020, April 11). 'We have nothing': Papua New Guinea's broken health system braces for Covid-19. *The Guardian.* https://www.theguardian.com/world/2020/apr/11/we-have-nothing-papua-new-guineas-broken-health-system-braces-for-covid-19?fbclid=IwAR2YNhadpA-hTTfybXKBNAPAJRCt_ZoG9QkREOP8nM3d6Cn0rSkm-3I3R9g

Flaxman, S., Mishra, S., Gandy, A., Unwin, H. J. T., Mellan, T. A., Coupland, H., … Bhatt, S., Imperial College Covid Response Team. (2020). Estimating the effects of non-pharmaceutical interventions on COVID-19 in Europe. *Nature.* https://doi.org/10.1038/s41586-020-2405-7

Folkhälsomyndigheten. (2020). *Första resultaten från pågående undersökning av antikroppar för covid-19-virus* [First results from ongoing study of antibodies to covid-19 virus]. Folkhälsomyndigheten (The Public Health Agency of Sweden). https://www.folkhalsomyndigheten.se/nyheter-och-press/nyhetsarkiv/2020/maj/forsta-resultaten-fran-pagaende-undersokning-av-antikroppar-for-covid-19-virus/

Fronek, P. (2017). Social work in a brave new world. In A. López Pelaez & E. R. Diez (Eds.), *Social work research and practice: Contributions to a science of social work* (pp. 33–50). Thomas Reuters Aranzadi.

Fronek, P., & Briggs, L. (2020). Demoralization in the wake of the COVID-19 pandemic: Whereto the future for young Australians? *Qualitative Social Work.* https://doi.org/10.1177/1473325020973332

Fronek, P., & Rotabi, K. S. (2020). The impact of the COVID-19 pandemic on intercountry adoption and international commercial surrogacy. *International Social Work*, 63(5), 665–670.

Garikipati, S., & Kambhampati, U. (2020). Leading the fight against the pandemic: Does gender 'really' matter? http://dx.doi.org/10.2139/ssrn.3617953

Global Health Now. (2020, May 15). 250 million COVID-19 cases expected in Africa. *Global Health Now.* Johns Hopkins Bloomberg School of Public Health. https://www.globalhealthnow.org/2020-05/250-million-covid-19-cases-expected-africa

Glynn, J. R., Fielding, K., Shakespeare, T., & Campbell, O. (2020). Covid-19: Excess all cause mortality in domiciliary care. *British Medical Journal, 370*, m2751. http://dx.doi.org/10.1136/bmj.m2751

Government of the Hong Kong Special Administrative Region. (2020a). *Government holds inter-departmental meeting on cluster of pneumonia cases in Wuhan* [Press release]. https://www.info.gov.hk/gia/general/202001/02/P2020010200831.htm?fontSize=1

Government of the Hong Kong Special Administrative Region. (2020b). *Government to gazette inclusion of "Severe Respiratory Disease associated with a Novel Infectious Agent" as statutorily notifiable infectious disease under Prevention and Control of Disease Ordinance* [Press release]. https://www.info.gov.hk/gia/general/202001/07/P2020010700603.htm?fontSize=1

Hale, T., Anania, J., Angrist, N., Boby, T., Cameron-Blake, E., Ellen, L., … Zhang, Y. (2021). "*Variation in Government Responses to COVID-19" Version 11.0.* Blavatnik School of Government Working Paper. 23 March 2021. www.bsg.ox.ac.uk/covidtracker

Hart, A. (2020, September 23). How Aboriginal health experts acted first and led the fight against the coronavirus. *The New Daily.* https://thenewdaily.com.au/news/coronavirus/2020/09/23/aboriginal-health-coronavirus/?utm_source=Adestra&utm_medium=email&utm_campaign=Morning%20News%20-%2020200923

Hassan, J., & O'Grady, S. (2020, April 21). Female world leaders hailed as voices of reason amid the coronavirus chaos. *The Washington Post.* https://www.washingtonpost.com/world/2020/04/20/female-world-leaders-hailed-voices-reason-amid-coronavirus-chaos/

Horii, M. (2014). Why do Japanese wear masks? A short historical review. *Electronic Journal of Contemporary Japanese Studies, 4*(2). http://www.japanesestudies.org.uk/ejcjs/vol14/iss2/horii.html?utm_content=buffer47a6e&utm_medium=social&utm_source=twitter.com&utm_campaign=buffer

Hsiang, S., Allen, D., Annan-Phan, S., Bell, K., Bolliger, I., Chong, T., … Wu., T. (2020). The effect of large-scale anti-contagion policies on the COVID-19 pandemic. *Nature.* https://doi.org/10.1038/s41586-020-2404-8

Huang, C., Wang, Y., Li, X., Ren, l., Zhao, J., Hu, Y., … Cao, B. (2020). Clinical features of patients infected with 2019 novel coronavirus in Wuhan, China. *The Lancet, 305*(10223), 497–506.

Investigation Committee of the State Supervisory Commission. (2020, March 19). 关于群众反映的涉及李文亮医生有关情况调查的通报 [Report on the investigation of the situation involving Dr. Li Wenliang]. *CCTV.* http://m.news.cctv.com/2020/03/19/ARTIrEO6nz5wKzeVnNlyBgTM200319.shtml

Johns Hopkins Corona Virus Resource Centre. Johns Hopkins University. https://coronavirus.jhu.edu/

Kangas, O., Jauhiainen, S., Simanainen, M., & Ylikännö, M. (2020). *Suomen perustulokokeilun arviointi* [Evaluation of the Finnish basic income experiment]. Valto. https://julkaisut.valtioneuvosto.fi/handle/10024/162219

Karáth, K. (2020). Covid-19: Hungary's pandemic response may have been worse than the virus. *British Medical Journal*, 371, m4153. https://doi.org/10.1136/bmj.m4153

Kela. (2020). *Basic income experiment.* Kela. https://www.kela.fi/web/en/basic-income-experiment

Klinger-Vidra, R., Tran, B.-L., & Usikyla, I. (2020, April 20). Testing capacity: State capacity and COVID-19 testing. *Global Policy.* https://www.globalpolicyjournal.com/blog/09/04/2020/testing-capacity-state-capacity-and-covid-19-testing

Kompas, T., Grafton, R. Q., Che, T. N., Chu, L., & Camac, J. (2020). Health and economic costs of early, delayed and no suppression of COVID-19: The case of Australia. *medRxiv*. https://doi.org/10.1101/2020.06.21.20136549

Kwegyir Tsiboe, A. (2020). Describing the experiences of older persons with visual impairments during COVID-19 in rural Ghana. *The Journal of Adult Protection*. https://doi.org/10.1108/JAP-07-2020-0026

Lau, J., Sutcliffe, S., & Hiungito, W. (2020). *Lived experiences of COVID-19: Impacts on an Atoll Island community, Papua New Guinea*. ARC CoE in Coral Reef Studies, James Cook University. https://www.coralcoe.org.au/wp-content/uploads/2020/10/Covid-19-report.pdf

Lingam, L., & Sapkal, R. S. (2020). COVID 19, physical distancing and social inequalities: Are we all really in this together? *The International Journal of Community and Social Development*, 2(2), 173–190.

Lone, S. A., & Ahmad, A. (2020). COVID-19 pandemic – An African perspective. *Emerging Microbes & Infections*, 9(1), 1300–1308.

López Peláez, A. & Gómez Ciriano, E. J. (Eds.). (2019). *Austerity, social work and welfare policies: A global perspective*. Thomson Reuters Aranzadi.

López Peláez, A., Marcuello Servós, Ch., Castillo de Mesa, J., & Almaguer-Calixto, P. (2020). The more you know, the less you fear. Reflexive social work practices in times of COVID-19. *International Social Work*, 63(6), 746–752.

Lust, J. (2021). A class analysis of the expansion of COVID-19 in Peru: The case of metropolitan Lima. *Critical Sociology*. https://doi.org/10.1177/0896920521991612

Lyons, K. (2020, February 18). Australia slashes Pacific aid funding for health as region battles medical crises. *The Guardian*. https://www.theguardian.com/world/2020/feb/18/australia-slashes-pacific-aid-funding-for-health-as-region-battles-medical-crises

Maneesh, P., & El Alaoui, A. (2020). How countries of south mitigate COVID-19: Models of Morocco and Kerala, India. *Electronic Research Journal of Social Sciences and Humanities*, 2(II), 16–28.

Marsh, S. & McIntyre, N. (2020). Six in 10 UK health workers killed by Covid-19 are BAM', *The Guardian*. https://www.theguardian.com/world/2020/may/25/six-in-10-uk-health-workers-killed-by-covid-19-are-bame

Mason, R. (2020). "I think I behaved reasonably": Dominic Cummings defends actions in lockdown row. *The Guardian*. https://www.theguardian.com/politics/2020/may/25/i-think-i-behaved-reasonably-dominic-cummings-defends-actions-in-lockdown-row

Mbow, M., Lell, B., Jochems, S. P., Cisse, B., Mboup, S., Dewals, B. G., … Yazdanbakhsh, M. (2020). COVID-19 in Africa: Dampening the storm? *Science*, 369(6504), 624–626.

McCormick, G. (2020, April 8). *The Mexican government's response to Covid-19 is insufficient*. Centre for Strategic and International Studies (CSIS). https://www.csis.org/analysis/mexican-governments-response-covid-19-insufficient

Moreno Mínguez, A., López Peláez, A., & Segado Sánchez-Cabezudo, S. (2012). *The transition to adulthood in Spain. Economic crisis and late emancipation. Social studies collection no. 34*. La Caixa. http://www.publicacionestecnicas.com/lacaixa/34_en/pdf/print.pdf

Muller, S. (2020, April 20). SA lockdown: Coercing the poor, coddling the rich? *Mail & Guardian*. https://mg.co.za/article/2020-04-20-sa-lockdown-coercing-the-poor-coddling-the-rich/

Nhapi, T. G., & Dhemba, J. (2020). The conundrum of old age and COVID-19 responses in Eswatini and Zimbabwe. *International Social Work*. https://doi.org/10.1177/0020872820944998

Nordling, L. (2020, May 6). Unproven herbal remedy against COVID-19 could fuel drug-resistant malaria, scientists warn. *Science*. https://www.sciencemag.org/news/2020/05/unproven-herbal-remedy-against-covid-19-could-fuel-drug-resistant-malaria-scientists

Oksanen, A., Kaakinen, M., Latikka, R., Savolainen, I., Savela, N., & Koivula, A. (2020). Regulation and trust: 3-month follow-up study on COVID-19 mortality in 25 European countries. *JMIR Public Health and Surveillance*, 6(2),e19218. https://doi.org/10.2196/19218

PBS. (2020, June 16). The virus: What went wrong? In M. Gaviria & M. Smith (Producers), *Frontline*. https://www.pbs.org/video/the-virus-what-went-wrong-mk79yu/

Pech, S. (2020, January 29). More than 3000 Chinese from virus-hit Wuhan are in Kingdom. *Khmer Times*. https://www.khmertimeskh.com/684773/more-than-3000-chinese-from-virus-hit-wuhan-are-in-kingdom/

Pei, S., Kandula, S., & Shaman, J. (2020). Differential effects of intervention timing on COVID-19 spread in the United States. *medRxiv*. https://doi.org/10.1101/2020.05.15.20103655

Pirkis, J., John, A., Shin, S., DelPozo-Banos, M., Arya, V., Analuisa-Aguilar, P., ... Spittal, M. J. (2021). Suicide trends in the early months of the COVID-19 pandemic: An interrupted time-series analysis of preliminary data from 21 countries. *The Lancet Psychiatry*. https://doi.org/10.1016/S2215-0366(21)00091-2

Public Health Agency of Canada. (2020, March 25). *New order makes self-isolation mandatory for individuals entering Canada* [Press release]. https://www.canada.ca/en/public-health/news/2020/03/new-order-makes-self-isolation-mandatory-for-individuals-entering-canada.html

Public Health England. (2020). *Disparities in the risk and outcomes of COVID-19*. PHE. https://assets.publishing.service.gov.uk/government/uploads/system/uploads/attachment_data/file/908434/Disparities_in_the_risk_and_outcomes_of_COVID_August_2020_update.pdf

Ramaphosa, C. (2020). *Statement by President Cyril Ramaphosa on escalation of measures to combat the Covid-19 epidemic, Union Buildings, Tshwane*. The Presidency. http://www.thepresidency.gov.za/speeches/statement-president-cyril-ramaphosa-escalation-measures-combat-covid-19-epidemic%2C-union

Romanian Government. (2020a). *DECRET nr. 195 din 16 martie 2020* [Decree no. 195 of March 16, 2020]. President of Romania. Official Gazette no. 212. http://legislatie.just.ro/Public/DetaliiDocumentAfis/223831

Romanian Government. (2020b). *Military Ordinance 7 of April 4, 2020*. Art. 10, Paragraph 2. https://www.unbr.ro/wp-content/uploads/2020/04/Ordonanta-militara-nr.-7-2020-masuri-prevenire-COVID-19.pdf

Romanian Ministry of Internal Affairs. (2020). *Military Ordinance No. 3 From 24/03/2020 on measures to prevent the spread of COVID-19*. https://www.mai.gov.ro/ordonanta-militara-nr-3-din-24-03-2020-privind-masuri-de-prevenire-a-raspandirii-covid-19/

Romanian Ministry of Public Health. (2020). *Order no. 1706/2007 on the management and organization of emergency reception units and compartments from Romania*. https://scjs.ro/legislatie/pdf/OMS%20nr.1706-2007.pdf

Saban, M., Shachar, T., Miron, O., & Wilf Meron, R. (2020). Effect of socioeconomic and ethnic characteristics on COVID-19 infection: The case of the ultra-orthodox and the Arab communities in Israel. *medRxiv*. https://doi.org/10.1101/2020.05.25.20111575

Salvá, A. (2020, May 11). Thailand: The coronavirus suicides. *The Diplomat*. https://thediplomat.com/2020/05/thailand-the-coronavirus-suicides/

Sanfelici, M., Gui L., & Mordeglia, S. (Eds.). (2020). *Il servizio sociale nell'emergenza Covid-19*. Franco Angeli.

Schitea R. (2020, March 15). *Primii 100 de pacienți cu #COVID19 din România. Ce am învățat până acum și ce trebuie să facem în continuare?* [Analysis of the first 100 COVID-19 patients in România. What have we learned so far and what must we do further?] *Raportul De Gardă*. https://raportuldegarda.ro/articol/analiza-primii-100-pacienti-covid19-romania-ce-am-invatat-pana-acum-ce-trebuie-sa-facem-in-continuare/

Setiati, S., & Azwar, M. (2020). COVID-19 and Indonesia. *Acta Medica Indonesiana, 52*(1), 84–89.

Sharma, S., & Paul, A. (2020). COVID-19 India: An insight into the impact of lockdown and community behavioural response. *International Social Work*. https://doi.org/10.1177/0020872820949624

Singh, J.A. (2020). How South Africa's ministerial advisory committee on COVID-19 can be optimised. *South African Medical Journal,* 110(6), 439–442.

Smithson, M. (2020, November 26). Data from 45 countries show containing COVID vs saving the economy is a false dichotomy. *The Conversation*. https://theconversation.com/data-from-45-countries-show-containing-covid-vs-saving-the-economy-is-a-false-dichotomy-150533

Socio-economic Rights Institute of South Africa. (2020). *Submission on the impact of the COVID-19 crisis on housing rights*. Office of the High Commissioner, United Nations Human Rights website. https://search.ohchr.org/results.aspx?k=Submission%20on%20the%20impact%20of%20the%20COVID-19%20crisis%20on%20housing%20rights

Spagnoletti, B. (2020, April 6). Indonesia's lockdown dilemma: Mudik is a safety net for some, but may worsen the Covid-19 public health disaster. *Indonesia at Melbourne*. https://indonesiaatmelbourne.unimelb.edu.au/indonesias-lockdown-dilemma-mudik-is-a-safety-net-for-some-but-may-worsen-the-covid-19-public-health-disaster/

Statsministeriet. (2020, March 11). Situationen kommer til at stille kæmpe krav til os alle sammen [The situation is going to make huge demands on all of us]. *Regeringen*. https://www.regeringen.dk/nyheder/2020/statsminister-mette-frederiksens-indledning-paa-pressemoede-i-statsministeriet-om-corona-virus-den-11-marts-2020/

Steyn, N., Binny, R. N., Hannah, K., Hendy, S. C., James, A., Kukutai, T., … Sporle, A. (2020). Estimated inequities in COVID-19 infection fatality rates by ethnicity for Aotearoa New Zealand. *The New Zealand Medical Journal,* 133(1520). https://www.nzma.org.nz/journal-articles/estimated-inequities-in-covid-19-infection-fatality-rates-by-ethnicity-for-aotearoa-new-zealand

Tashiro, A., & Shaw, R. (2020). COVID-19 pandemic response in Japan: What Is behind the initial flattening of the curve? *Sustainability (Basel, Switzerland)*, 12(13), 5250.

The New Daily. (2020, May 16). Colombian company creates bed that can double as coffin. *The New Daily*. https://thenewdaily.com.au/news/coronavirus/2020/05/16/colombian-company-creates-bed-that-can-double-as-coffin/?utm_source=Adestra&utm_medium=email&utm_campaign=Sunday%20Best%20-%2020200517

Uganda Bureau of Statistics. (2017). *National Labour Force Survey 2016/17*. Uganda Bureau of Statistics.

UNDP. (2020). *Covid-19 in South Africa: Socio-economic impact assessment*. UNDP Republic of South Africa. https://www.za.undp.org/content/south_africa/en/home/library/socio-economic-impact-of-covid-19-on-south-africa.html

UNDP-Uganda. (2020). *Estimating vulnerability to poverty and the dynamics of resilience to shocks: Laying the foundation to leave no one behind in Uganda*. Background paper for the Poverty Status Report 2019. Kampala.

UNHCR. (2020, May 15). *COVID-19 related lockdowns resulted in increased incidences of sexual and gender-based violence against children*. https://www.unhcr.org/en-us/news/briefing/2020/5/5ebe47394/central-americas-displacement-crisis-aggravated-covid-19.html

Vilar-Compte, M., Pérez, V., Teruel, G., Alonso, A., & Pérez-Escamilla, R. (2020). Costing of actions to safeguard vulnerable Mexican households with young children from the consequences of COVID-19 social distancing measures. *International Journal for Equity in Health,* 19(1), 70. https://doi.org/10.1186/s12939-020-01187-3

Wang, S., Wright, R., & Wakatsuki, Y. (2020, November 30). In Japan, more people died from suicide last month than from Covid in all of 2020. And women have been impacted most. *CNN*. https://edition.cnn.com/2020/11/28/asia/japan-suicide-women-covid-dst-intl-hnk/index.html

Wango, G., Wairire, G., & Kimamo, C. (2020). Patterns of development of COVID-19 in low-and-middle income countries: Suggested psychological intervention strategies. *IOSR Journal of Humanities and Social Science*, 25(6), 52–65.

WHO. (2016). *Suicides in the world: Global health estimates. Licence: CC BY-NC-SA 3.0 IGO*. World Health Organization. https://apps.who.int/iris/bitstream/handle/10665/326948/WHO-MSD-MER-19.3-eng.pdf

WHO. (2020, March 11). *WHO Director-General's opening remarks at the media briefing on COVID-19 – 11 March 2020*. World Health Organization. https://www.who.int/dg/speeches/detail/who-director-general-s-opening-remarks-at-the-media-briefing-on-covid-19--11-march-2020

Wiking, M. (2016). *The little book of Hygge: The Danish way to live well. The Happiness Research Institute*. Penguin.

World Bank. (2020a). *COVID-19 to plunge global economy into worst recession since World War II*. https://www.worldbank.org/en/news/press-release/2020/06/08/covid-19-to-plunge-global-economy-into-worst-recession-since-world-war-ii

World Bank. (2020b). *The World Bank in South Africa: Overview*. https://www.worldbank.org/en/country/southafrica/overview

Yang, R., & Castanier, Y. (2020, March 18). Il faut libérer tous les étrangers sans papiers retenus dans les Cra! (We must free all undocumented foreigners held in the Cra!). *Street Press*. https://www.streetpress.com/sujet/1584466767-liberer-tous-etrangers-sans-papiers-retenus-dans-cra-migrants-coronavirus-epidemie-expulsions

Zeberg, H., & Pääbo, S. (2020). The major genetic risk factor for severe COVID-19 is inherited from Neanderthals. *Nature*. https://doi.org/10.1038/s41586-020-2818-3

3

LESSONS FROM PANDEMIC HISTORY

Matthew C. Ward

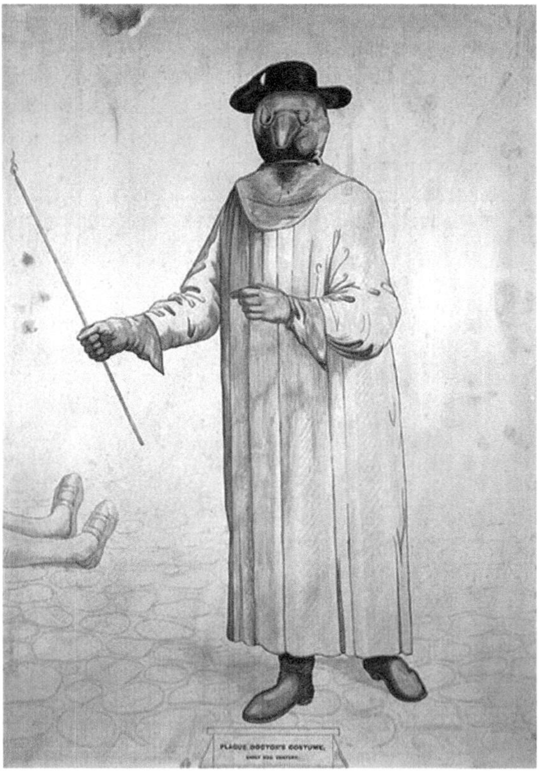

FIGURE 3.0 Bird-beak style mask associated with plague doctors

Source: Wellcome Collection gallery (22 March 2018)

DOI: 10.4324/9781003111214-4

Writing shortly after the Black Death had swept through Europe, the 14th-century Italian scholar Giovanni Boccaccio painted a vivid picture of life in the city of Florence during the pandemic of 1348.

> Each thought to secure immunity for himself… very many, both men and women, abandoned their own city, their own houses and homes, their kinsfolk and possessions, and sought the country seats of others… townsman avoided townsman and that well nigh no neighbour took thought unto other and that kinsfolk seldom or never visited one another and held no converse together save from afar…
>
> *(Boccaccio, 1886, pp. 13–18)*

Although written almost 700 years ago, Boccaccio's description of a city under siege, the rich fleeing to their second homes in the country, the streets deserted, neighbours avoiding each other and conversing only from a distance, sounds eerily like a city under COVID-19 lockdown. As Boccaccio's depiction of the Black Death in Renaissance Florence demonstrates, the experiences of past societies and communities when faced with epidemic and pandemic disease often closely echo the experiences of societies today.

Many, if not most, of the challenges posed by COVID-19 have been faced before, and through the experience of pandemic disease, solutions and policies have been developed. Perhaps the three most fundamental ways in which past epidemics have influenced present practices have been through the development of concepts of quarantine, masking, and vaccination. However, each of these policies posed specific problems which had to be overcome, and they all faced widespread opposition. By examining some of the issues raised by attempts to control epidemic disease in the past, we can contextualise more effectively some of the issues faced by governments and policymakers today.

Quarantine

The idea of a specific process of quarantine had its roots in the 14th-century Italian city-states, in the time of Boccaccio and the Black Death. Because there was no understanding of how infectious diseases spread, and no sense of how long individuals or vessels needed to be isolated to prevent the spread of disease, the standard requirement for quarantine was based on the references to 40 days and 40 nights which repeatedly appear in the Bible. Individuals and vessels arriving from overseas would be forced to isolate completely from the community in which they had arrived for a period of 40 days, *quaranta* in Italian, hence quarantine (Bick et al., 2020).

By the 18th century, the idea of limiting all travel and closely monitoring the movement of peoples across borders had developed much more extensively. The Austro-Hungarian Empire built a permanent line of forts and checkpoints along its extended border with the Ottoman Empire, known as the military border.

The border had official crossing points where travellers could be isolated and examined. In times of plague, which was perceived as being particularly common in the eastern Mediterranean and the lands of the Ottoman Empire, the border could be closed completely, and plague kept out. The border operated with a considerable degree of success for over 150 years between 1710 and 1871 and provides one of the first and most successful examples of international travel restriction (Snowden, 2019).

The concept of quarantine was applied broadly to limit the spread of a range of infections. In North America, *lazarettos*, or quarantine stations, were established to monitor the arrival of all immigrants. Initially, these were relatively small facilities, such as Province Island in the Delaware River outside Philadelphia, but they would eventually develop into large processing stations such as Ellis Island on the East Coast and Angel Island on the West Coast. Over the course of the 19th century, particularly in North America, but also in other parts of the world where there was substantial immigration, immigrants became viewed as dangerous transmitters of infectious disease, and there were extensive attempts to monitor all migrants at the border and to exclude any whom inspectors thought might pose a risk to the community. In these centres, thousands of immigrants could be held and examined in an attempt to prevent the transmission of contagious disease (Kraut, 1994).

As the 19th century progressed and the apparatus of state government became more powerful, the ability to impose an almost all-embracing national quarantine and isolation in times of pandemic developed. In 1918, as *Spanish* influenza swept around the globe, Australia imposed strict quarantine laws. All arriving international travellers were quarantined, and internal quarantine boundaries between the states and territories were also established. While this did not prevent influenza from arriving, the quarantine did delay its arrival by many months, by which time the country was better prepared, and it appears that the virus had also mutated to become slightly less virulent. Many thousands of lives were thereby saved (Cohn, 2018).

The most successful quarantine was implemented by the government of American Samoa in 1918–1919. In order to prevent the arrival of Spanish influenza, the territory implemented a strict all-embracing maritime quarantine, which amounted to the complete exclusion of any arrivals from other islands. Extreme measures were put into effect, which included shore patrols to force back refugees from neighbouring islands struck badly by the pandemic. Neighbouring Western Samoa lost nearly a quarter of its population to Spanish influenza, but American Samoa escaped the pandemic completely. But such policies of complete isolation to exclude disease seem to have worked only effectively in small and relatively isolated locations (Tomkins, 1992).

It was the growing interconnectedness of the world which made the control of infectious disease increasingly difficult in the 20th century. The growth of global trade, from the medieval period onward, transformed the ability of diseases to spread. The Black Death was only able to penetrate throughout Europe because of the expansion of trade networks in the 14th century. In the

19th century, the rapid expansion of trade and the growing speed of transport with the development of steamships greatly facilitated the spread of a wide range of infectious diseases from Yellow Fever to Cholera and Bubonic Plague (Harrison, 2012). Today, the volume and speed of air travel is an unprecedented accelerant of airborne infectious disease.

Cholera was the most feared infectious disease in 19th-century Europe. Between 1830 and 1923, it repeatedly swept throughout Europe. It was feared not only for its very high death rate but also the speed with which it afflicted its victims. A healthy young adult could leave their home in the morning and be struck down within hours, often without being able to return to their home. By evening they would be dead, and because of the speed of the disease death often took place in a more public space. The violent retching and diarrhoea would dehydrate the victim leaving their skin a pale blue (Hays, 2005). All European states sought to exclude the disease, whatever the cost. By the middle of the 19th century, it had proved impossible to exclude cholera by quarantine because the disease was not airborne. Consequently, there was a move away from policies based on quarantine that were designed to prevent sick individuals from entering a population to policies based on isolation that aimed to limit the spread of a disease once it had already entered a community (Barnes, 2014). This distinction is significant because the greatest challenges posed by infectious diseases were when those diseases breached the walls of quarantine and entered the community. Communities might support policies of quarantine because, in general, they involved other people; they kept out strangers. But policies of isolation affected the whole community and frequently promoted intense opposition for many of the reasons seen during the COVID-19 pandemic.

When influenza arrived in the United States in 1918, localities followed a range of different policies. Worried about the impact on civilian morale and desperate to continue the drive for wartime government bonds which saw widespread public gatherings, Philadelphia allowed public meetings, and the city even held a large parade in support of the war bond effort. Before long, over 12,000 Philadelphians had died from the infection (Stetler, 2017). In Wisconsin, health officials initially only warned individuals to avoid theatres and crowded streetcars and ordered school teachers to send home any students who appeared sick. In addition, warning signs were posted on residences where flu cases were suspected. However, as cases of influenza rose quickly, state authorities ordered the closure of all public institutions and the halting of all public activities, from schools to movie theatres to public meetings. However, some local authorities interpreted the state's orders with a degree of discretion and allowed schools and other wartime related public activities to continue (Steven, 2000). St. Louis followed an equally draconian but better enforced policy, demanding that all influenza cases should be reported within two days after the illness was diagnosed and required that infected individuals should isolate in their homes. All public places, from schools to churches and movie theatres, were closed, and public gatherings of any sort were forbidden (Oldstone, 2020).

Masking

The idea of masks, like so much else, had its origins in the Black Death. It was believed that the plague, and other diseases, were spread by *miasmas* in the air and the purpose of plague costumes was to create distance and a barrier between those who had the plague and their carers who feared contamination. Initially, these were just tight masks, often with a sponge soaked in vinegar or a similar substance, designed to filter the air. By the early 17th century, this had developed into the bird-beak style mask associated with plague doctors. But with the exception of plague, and even in cases of plague outside of *pest houses* and *lazarettos*, the use of masks was uncommon until the end of the 19th century (Carmichael, 2006).

With the outbreak of Spanish influenza in the USA in 1918, masks became seen as an important component in the fight against the disease (Peterson, 1989). While not used extensively in previous epidemics, their use had been widespread in wartime hospitals, and modern scientific medicine suggested their utility. In San Francisco, an assemblage of many leading authorities, including the Mayor, Board of Health, and the Red Cross, placed an advertisement in local newspapers urging residents to "*WEAR A MASK* and *Save Your life*" (Crosby, 2003, pp. 103–113). However, there was substantial opposition to such restrictions. Many felt that where restrictions had been imposed, they had failed to stop the emergence of the disease and that, despite the assurances of doctors and health officials, they were ineffective in preventing its spread. Ironically, in believing this, opponents of masking in 1918 may have been, for the most part, correct. Not only were the type of masks worn insufficient, physicians and scientists mistakenly believed that the Spanish Influenza was caused by Pfeiffer's Bacillus (Eyler, 2010). Although it proved impossible to demonstrate a direct connection between the bacillus and the disease, this misapprehension fuelled the conviction that gauze masks could prevent the spread of the bacillus and led to their widespread use, or often misuse. Any protection that the gauze masks provided against a virus, especially when not worn correctly was insufficient. They were often worn loosely around the face and did not cover the nose, and when they were worn it was largely outdoors, not indoors.

The belief that Pfeiffer's Bacillus was the cause of the 1918 Influenza pandemic even led to the development and widespread distribution of vaccines and the inoculation of hundreds of thousands of people. The vaccine offered no protection at all against influenza (Rockafellar, 1986). Indeed, the measures taken to combat influenza in the United States, including the closing of public spaces and the requirement to mask, seem to have had a limited impact because they were not always imposed and enforced effectively. Alfred Crosby has pointed out that the death rates in localities which enforced mask ordinances and strict closing orders and encouraged vaccinations were no lower, and in some cases were higher, than authorities that did not impose such measures. In many instances, he argues, these measures were simply an attempt to be seen to be doing something in the face of an overwhelming pandemic (Crosby, 2003).

Resistance

Disputes about quarantine and mask policies became most intense during the third wave of the pandemic. By this time, individuals and communities had become tired of the extensive restrictions, and their faith in the proposed preventative measures had waned. The public's weariness with the restrictions, and the opposition of shopkeepers and entertainment venues who feared for the loss of revenue such restrictions would cause, meant that even when authorities passed ordinances mandating the wearing of masks, they were often ignored (Luckingham, 1984). The waves of influenza, particularly the belief that the pandemic had been overcome at the end of the second wave, demonstrate how its re-emergence can be even more devastating and make the reestablishment of preventative measures extremely hard. The yoyo effect of ebbs and flows of disease on human behaviour continues to be seen today.

The influenza pandemic of 1918–1919 came in three distinct waves, although they were experienced differently in different parts of the world and even in different regions of the same country. The first wave in the spring and summer of 1918 seems to have been comparatively mild. Its presence went widely unreported, partly because of wartime restrictions, partly because in most countries and jurisdictions influenza was not a reportable disease, and partly because it was not that unusual. The first wave is only visible in retrospect by an examination of death certificates and a thorough investigation of the records of institutions such as the armed forces and prisons. These reveal a much higher than usual incidence of death from influenza and pneumonia in the spring of 1918 (Crosby, 2003).

Sometime in the late summer of 1918, the virus seems to have mutated and became much more virulent. In the United States, the second wave began in ports on the Atlantic Ocean and radiated outwards with devastating impact. The epidemic rampaged across the country in the autumn, but in December, the number of deaths declined dramatically, and most people believed that the pandemic had passed. But then, in January 1919, it returned for a third wave (Morens & Fauci, 2007). Unsurprisingly, the waves of influenza followed a very similar pattern in the United Kingdom although slightly later than in the United States. The second wave was generally the most deadly in both the United States and the United Kingdom, although some regions, such as parts of Scotland, which had seen lower mortality in the second wave, suffered their highest mortality rates in the third wave (Johnson, 2006). Similar waves of influenza appear to have occurred in 2009 when influenza, H1N1, as in 1918–1919, again became a pandemic. In England, the first wave peaked in July 2009 and the second in November. As with the 1918–1919 Influenza, the second wave saw much higher mortality figures (Mytton et al., 2012).

Inequality

Mortality rates can be affected by many different factors. For many infectious diseases, a fundamental factor affecting mortality rates and rates of infection has been poverty (Johnson, 2006). For some epidemic diseases such as cholera, this link has always been very apparent. An outbreak of cholera in London in the 1840s led to substantial efforts to improve sanitation in the poorer parts of the city to reduce the risk of future outbreaks (Thomas, 2010). Such measures were repeated in cities across Europe and North America. For other diseases such as smallpox, the link between poverty and infection has been less apparent, and this may be why smallpox was so widely feared by the wealthy and why such efforts were made to find effective remedies. Rich and poor were equally likely to contract smallpox. However, some evidence shows that the wealthy had a slightly lower mortality rate, possibly due to better and more attentive care (Snowden, 2019).

However, during some epidemics, mortality rates appear to be counter-intuitive. In the Influenza Pandemic of 1918, the African American population in the United States had a lower mortality rate than the population overall. This contradicted patterns for almost every other epidemic disease, where poverty and crowded housing meant that the African American population typically suffered much higher mortality rates (McBride, 1991). One possible explanation for this is that in the spring of 1918, the first and largely unreported wave of influenza had hit the African American community particularly hard. Therefore, much of the African American population had immunity when the second and more deadly wave arrived in the autumn (Crosby, 2003, p. 222).

This should serve as a reminder that possibly the most significant factor affecting mortality rates has been the prior exposure of a community to that disease. When infectious diseases encounter a susceptible population that lacks immunity, the resulting disease spreads unchecked throughout the entire population, in what has been termed a *virgin soil epidemic*. No event illustrates this better than the arrival of European diseases in the Americas in the 16th century. Native Americans had not previously encountered a range of European diseases, from smallpox to bubonic plague, and from measles to influenza (Thornton, 1987). When Native Americans encountered these diseases for the first time, they endured wave after wave of destructive outbreaks. Each successive outbreak weakened the entire community and left it even more exposed to another epidemic of a different disease. During the first century of contact, the Indigenous populations of the Americas may have declined by as much as 95% as a result of repeated epidemics (Dobyns, 1983), a pattern of devastation affecting many colonised peoples.

Vaccination

Perhaps the most deadly disease to strike Indigenous peoples, and perhaps most feared amongst European communities throughout history, has been smallpox. Smallpox was highly contagious and killed around a third of those who contracted it. Those who survived were left with disfiguring pockmarks if they were lucky; if they were less fortunate, complications included blindness. Smallpox was by far the leading cause of blindness in 18th-century Europe (Snowden, 2019). Because of its ubiquity, high mortality, and severe complications, societies attempted to find methods of reducing the impact of the disease.

The initial means of alleviating, rather than preventing, smallpox was *variolation*. This entailed the deliberate infection of a susceptible individual with the disease. Early techniques varied, but many included making a powder from dried smallpox scabs taken from those infected, and breathing them in through the nose, thus infecting the individual with smallpox but generally a mild case. This procedure may have been practised as early as the tenth century in China (Oldstone, 2020). By the 18th century, the practice had evolved. It was more often called *inoculation* but still involved infecting a susceptible individual with the disease by taking pus from a pustule on someone infected. The pus was soaked into a length of thread and then placed in an incision on the patient's arm (Fenn, 2004). The nature of the procedure influenced the naming of the process as inoculation was a horticultural term for a process of grafting, allowing a farmer or gardener to grow different variants on the same rootstock (Oxford English Dictionary, 2021).

In the early 18th century, the wife of the British Ambassador to Turkey, Lady Mary Wortley Montagu, witnessed the procedure in Turkey and had her daughter inoculated by this method. On her return to Britain, many of her friends and acquaintances sought to learn about the procedure. Aided by the increasing interest of the Royal Society in eastern inoculation, Lady Montagu's social position allowed her to convince many of the British elite that inoculation was a preferable alternative to smallpox and to popularise the method (Barnes, 2012). The spread of the practice was made easier when in 1762, English physician Robert Sutton developed a new form of inoculation. Serum was drawn from a smallpox blister and was introduced to those susceptible only by a superficial puncture of the skin (van Zwanenberg, 1978). Sutton's method was viewed as much safer with fewer complications for it had *only* a one per cent fatality rate. The technique became very popular, and Sutton was able to inoculate entire communities, the fear being that one inoculated individual – who after all did have smallpox – could infect the entire community with smallpox (Gordon-Reed, 2008).

The first attempts at broader community inoculation took place in North America not Europe. Smallpox had been relatively uncommon in North America in the 17th century, as low population numbers and the long ocean voyage limited the continent's contact with Europe. When smallpox did arrive, it thus encountered a population which had had little prior exposure to the disease, and severe outbreaks soon developed. To control them, most colonies resorted to strict quarantine and isolation policies (Duffy, 1972). However, when smallpox broke out in Boston in 1721, infecting almost a quarter of the city's population and killing hundreds, the first experiments with inoculation in North America were made. Support for inoculation came from the city's leading Congregational clergy, in particular Cotton Mather, well known for his involvement in the Salem Witchcraft Trials (Peterson, 2019). Mather encouraged Zabdiel Boylston to develop a procedure based on the literature available to him in Boston, and he successfully inoculated several patients. However, as news of his experiment spread, it created outrage. In the ensuing debates, those opposed to inoculation presented fabricated evidence which discredited Boylston's work although he continued with inoculation in secret (Amalie, 2012).

Over the next half-century, opposition to smallpox remained intense, particularly in Boston. However, at the start of the Revolutionary War, the arrival of tens of thousands of British troops directly from Great Britain led to an extensive epidemic that again began in Boston. This would transform attitudes to inoculation. The nascent Continental Army suffered severely, and outbreaks spread throughout the army, threatening to paralyse the American war effort (Becker, 2004). In February 1777, George Washington wrote that,

> Finding the Small pox to be spreading much and fearing that no precaution can prevent it from running through the whole of our Army, I have determined that the troops shall be inoculated. This Expedient may be attended with some inconveniences and some disadvantages, but yet I trust in its consequences will have the most happy effects.
>
> *(Grizzard, 1998, p. 26)*

Over the following months, the Continental Army successfully undertook an unprecedented large-scale inoculation of most of the army. By 1778, the army was essentially free of smallpox. That the army would inoculate all its men during the war created broader confidence in the process. As the war continued, smallpox continued to ravage the civilian population and growing numbers of American civilians also began to seek inoculation. Abigail Adams reported from Massachusetts that "such a Spirit of innoculation [sic] never before took place; the Town and every House in it, are as full as they can hold… I immediately determined to set myself about it, and get ready with my children" (Butterfield, 1963, pp. 45–49). The eagerness with which so many Americans embraced smallpox inoculation in the 1770s successfully overcame the epidemic. However, there was still considerable concern that the death rate from inoculation itself remained around 1%. However, in 1796 English doctor Edward Jenner discovered that inoculation with the mild disease cowpox provided the individual with immunity to smallpox (Rusnock, 2009).

Jenner's discovery was the birth of vaccination, for the word vaccine specifically means derived from cows, from the Latin, *vacca,* meaning cow (Oxford English Dictionary, 2021). The use of a vaccine from cows itself provoked opposition. Opponents of vaccination argued that infecting an individual with material taken from an animal was a moral outrage. They even claimed that some of those who had been vaccinated sprouted horns and began to look like cows (Oldstone, 2020). In the wake of Jenner's discovery, Britain attempted to develop a national vaccine policy that provoked widespread resistance. This opposition became particularly intense in the wake of the Vaccination Act of 1853, which made vaccination compulsory and was enforced by a range of punishments. In 1867, the Anti-Compulsory Vaccination League was founded. It supported the publication of numerous publications. By the 1880s, numerous journals such as the *Anti-Vaccinator*, the *National Anti-Compulsory Vaccination Reporter*, and the *Vaccination Inquirer*, were producing a range of materials and evidence, much of which they fabricated, opposing vaccination, not dissimilar to today's *infodemic*. There were widespread protests across the country, some of which were substantial. In 1885 an anti-vaccination rally in Leicester may have seen 100,000 protestors (Wolfe & Sharp, 2002).

In the 19th century, the experiences of Britain and the United States in promoting smallpox vaccination reveal the importance of public support for government policy. The impact of public confidence in government can be seen most clearly in 1885 when a smallpox epidemic broke out in Montreal. There were nearly 20,000 cases and 6,000 deaths. But these cases were not distributed evenly across the community. Ninety percent of those who died were from the French-Canadian community. The Anglophone population of the region were active supporters of vaccination and had mainly been vaccinated, whereas the more impoverished francophone community, whose trust in the anglophone administration was much more limited, were broadly unvaccinated (Bliss, 1991).

Conflicting interests

Fears and misconceptions about vaccines continued into the 20th and 21st centuries, notably when science and religious, superstitious, political or misinformed beliefs have clashed. In northern Nigeria, attempts to vaccinate against polio met with substantial opposition and mistrust. Datti Ahmed, chairman of the Supreme Council for Shari'a in Nigeria, warned Nigerians against vaccinating their children, claiming that the vaccine had been tainted. He claimed that there was a campaign by western governments against Muslim Nigerians and that they had "deliberately adulterated the oral polio vaccines with anti-fertility drugs and contaminated it with certain viruses which are known to cause HIV and AIDS". Consequently, the vaccination programme in northern Nigeria ground to a halt, and unsurprisingly the disease began to remerge (Yahya, 2007). On occasion, such fears have been linked much more to attempts by the press to sell newspapers. Perhaps most infamously in Britain in the late 1990s, rumours began to circulate in the tabloid press of a link between autism and the MMR vaccine. When the medical journal *The Lancet* published a scientific paper that seemed to support these speculations, anxieties about the vaccine became widespread. Even though *The Lancet's* report was quickly discredited and ultimately withdrawn, popular distrust of the vaccine meant that vaccination rates in Britain plummeted and have not recovered (Horton, 2004).

Disputes and debates about the safety or efficacy of vaccines have clearly hampered attempts to vaccinate the broader community and have increased the incidence of some preventable diseases. However, it was not simply conflicting messages or lack of trust in government policy that could hamper policies attempting to prevent nor limit the spread of disease. Quarantine and isolation policies have also come under repeated attack, particularly since the second half of the 19th century. Some of this opposition has understandably come from within the affected communities, as individuals opposed the restrictive measures imposed upon their lives. In Naples, during the cholera epidemics of the early 20th century, the city's population usually flouted any restrictions attempting to ban public assemblies and limit individual contact with others. But opposition went further. When doctors entered districts looking for patients, angry crowds assembled, fearing isolation and the removal of patients to hospitals. Angry mobs surrounded the doctors who were tending to the sick, and some even had to be rescued by the army (Snowden, 1995). However, in addition to opposition from communities, there has also generally been opposition from business interests, particularly from businesses involved in international trade. In the 19th century, British manufacturers and merchants repeatedly claimed that quarantine and isolation measures were an unwarranted interference by the state in their trade and the free movement of goods and people (Huber, 2006). Such opposition became particularly intense in the wake of cholera in Britain from 1832 onwards. Many British merchants and financiers argued that the strict measures that the government imposed to limit the movement of people and goods in and out of infected locations would destroy the country's economy and were considerably worse than the impact of the disease itself (Bick et al., 2020).

During the Yellow Fever outbreaks, which hit the south-eastern states of the USA in the 19th century, many towns and cities moved to enforce strict quarantines and attempted to limit the arrival of outsiders and monitor train lines. However, they too were opposed by local merchants and railroad corporations who claimed that such quarantines were illegal and created the impression of widespread illegal shutdowns across the South. These restrictions were completely legal, but the impression of widespread shotgun quarantines became commonplace and encouraged people to disregard the restrictions (Huffard, 2013).

Such opposition has, if anything, only intensified over time. During the influenza pandemic of 1918–1919, business interests globally opposed measures limiting movement and preventing public gatherings (Crosby, 2003). Similarly, when moves were taken to restrict travel, following the outbreak of SARS, there was again substantial opposition from a range of business interests. So intense was this opposition that Jacalyn Duffin argued that "when quarantine is invoked on a large, impersonal scale, its economic consequences generate self-righteous ager and unfair exceptions. Powerful elites perceive threats to their wealth and aspirations" (Duffin & Sweetman, 2006, p. 5). Almost every attempt by democratically elected governments to control the spread of disease in the past two centuries has been opposed by business interests.

Even when government policies are clear and policy decisions and made in the light of the best scientific evidence, attempts to limit the spread of disease can still be a dismal failure if local concerns and anxieties are not taken into account. Nowhere is this clearer than in the plague riots that shook Bombay in

1897. Bubonic plague arrived in Bombay in 1896. To combat the plague, the British administration introduced the Epidemic Diseases Act. There were two notable features of the act: firstly, that it sought to protect all those living in India not just Europeans; secondly, that it was one of the most draconian pieces of legislation ever imposed and it completely ignored the cultural practices and even human rights of the civilian population. Convinced of the superiority of western science and medicine, the British began an all-out assault on the plague (Echenberg, 2007).

The government sent out search parties to find anyone who might be sick. These parties had the right to enter any building and subject any individual to an often intimate physical examination. This included the examination of Indian women, often accustomed to seclusion from unrelated men, by white, male doctors. If anyone was suspected of having the plague, they were removed with all their potential contacts to *health camps* where they lived under canvas in cramped quarters with no attention to the mixing of different ethnicities, religions and castes. Even those who died were not spared as post-mortem examinations of suspected plague victims interfered with customary funeral rites and traditions. Outraged mobs soon began to rampage through the city. The city's main hospital was attacked, and the city's Plague Commissioner was assassinated. Wild paranoia began to surface, and rumours circulated that bubonic plague was a poison spread by the British to kill poor Indians and solve the problems of overpopulation and poverty in Bombay. Some even argued that there was a plot by Queen Victoria to sacrifice Indians to the god of plague so that Britain would be spared (Snowden, 2019). With wild rumours such as these circulating, there was fear of any policy that the British administration now attempted. Consequently, attempts to control the plague failed dismally and were counterproductive. The sick were concealed and others fled, helping to spread the disease more widely. Relief of a kind came only when the governor decided to abandon the more draconian measures and launch a more conciliatory campaign, but the damage had been done. Plague continued to rage in India, and over the following 25 years, it killed an estimated 12 million people (Sarkar, 2001).

Similar irrational fears emerged in Africa in response to AIDS. As in India, attempts in Africa to combat the transmission of HIV were hampered because international medical policies often conflicted with the perceptions that many Africans themselves had of the crisis. Initially, many in Africa were unwilling to accept that AIDS was an African illness and argued that it had been imported from abroad by wealthy white tourists and business people. It was perceived as a disease of American and European homosexual men, not heterosexual Africans. Some declared that there was evidence that it been created in western laboratories; others maintained it was a legacy of Apartheid and had been spread by tear gas and was specifically designed to kill the black population (Iliffe, 2017).

When Thabo Mbeki became president of South Africa, he gave credence to many of these ideas. He claimed that poverty, not HIV was the primary cause of

AIDS, and maintained that the antiretroviral drug AZT was toxic and restricted its use. In 2000, he wrote an open letter to Bill Clinton, Tony Blair and Kofi Anan, accusing them of organising a campaign of persecution against those who disagreed with their views of AIDS that was akin to *racist apartheid tyranny*. With the President of South Africa openly avowing such sentiments, popular attitudes in southern Africa to AIDS remained uninformed. Twenty-three percent of South African army recruits said that AIDS was "God's way of punishing sinners". Four percent believed those with AIDS had been bewitched (Johnson, 2010). These failings meant that the HIV and AIDS crisis spread almost uncontrolled in southern Africa to such an extent that Susan Hunter has called AIDS in southern Africa in the 21st century *The Black Death* (Hunter, 2003). A study published in 2008 estimated that over 330,000 South Africans had died as a result of the failure of Mbeki's administration to provide access to drugs and medical care (Ceccarelli, 2011).

AIDS also had another lesson. Mirko Grmek has suggested that the development of international travel and tourism was part of what allowed AIDS to spread across Africa and then internationally spreading rapidly. He concluded that "carriers of bacteria and viruses who in another day may have taken the stagecoach, the long-haul trains, and ships now take to the skies" (Grmek, 1989, p. 21). If the Black Death of the 13th century was spread along the trade routes and caravans that linked the world together, if cholera in the 19th century was spread by steamships plying the oceans, modern pandemics are spread at lightning speed by passengers flying the global skies.

International cooperation

To halt the spread of disease and the emergence of new pandemics, it has become necessary for governments to cooperate evermore effectively. Such attempts at international cooperation are not new and have their roots in the 19th century. The remorseless spread of cholera around the world, spread by global shipping routes, revealed how important it was for countries to cooperate to limit the spread of disease. The development of the International Sanitary Conferences, which met between 1851 and 1894, was designed to help coordinate efforts to limit the spread of cholera epidemics, and in many ways presaged the development of the World Health Organisation (Huber, 2006). The plague outbreak in Bombay was part of a global pandemic, the third major pandemic of bubonic plague, which swept through port cities around the globe from Sydney to Glasgow, from San Francis to Rio de Janeiro, at the turn of the 20th century (Echenberg, 2002).

Nowhere was the global threat of a pandemic shown more clearly than in the coordinated global campaign to control SARS in the early 21st century. The WHO's ability to access a wide range of governmental and non-governmental sources and cooperate in real-time through the internet was crucial in limiting the spread of the pandemic. However, such cooperation can only work if all governments work together (Fidler, 2004). SARS revealed the limits of global cooperation and the fragility of some healthcare systems and almost brought the hospitals in Toronto to their knees. Paul Caulford, the head of Family Medicine and Community Services at Scarborough Hospital in Ontario, wrote of the near collapse of health services in the city. "Despite all our efforts, many hospitals became infected at alarming rates, making non-SARS care too risky. Elective surgery, including that for newly diagnosed cancers, was postponed as operating rooms and outpatient clinics shut down across the city. It would be months before they reopened" (Caulford, 2003).

The most basic lesson that can be taken from a history of disease is that epidemics and pandemics have been a fundamental part of human history. For much of human history, society has been shaped and overshadowed by the spectre of disease (McNeill, 1979). Many of the same problems and issues repeatedly appear in past epidemics, and many of these have reappeared in the COVID-19 pandemic. As the Spanish philosopher George Santayna wrote, "those who cannot remember the past are condemned to repeat it" (Santayana, 1917, p. 284). What is most striking about any survey of past pandemics is how many of the current debates and issues have clear precedents in the past, even the far past. But a study of disease can also demonstrate how effective measures have been developed over the years to overcome the challenges of a range of diseases and the social, economic and political problems that such solutions themselves posed. In particular, the use of vaccination, the awareness of preventative measures such as masking, and policies of quarantine and isolation, have all been used with varying success in the past. However, each had its limitations, and each has provoked different degrees of opposition. Vaccination can be hugely successful and even eliminate a threat, but popular misconceptions can also prevent successful vaccination programmes. Masks can only be effective in certain circumstances and if widely accepted. Quarantine and isolation have been more effective historically in keeping disease out of communities rather than containing it once an outbreak has begun. It is also apparent that governments need to provide clear and consistent information, collaborate with other governments, and most importantly, be open and honest both with their citizens and the governments of other countries.

BOX 3.1

REFLECTIVE QUESTIONS

1. What surprised you most about the history of pandemics?
2. Thinking about COVID-19, are there key lessons we should have learned?
3. What key scientific, social, cultural and political factors have featured in pandemic management throughout history?

References

Amalie, M. K. (2012). Boston's historic smallpox epidemic. *Massachusetts Historical Review*, 14, 1–51.

Barnes, D. (2012). The public life of a woman of wit and quality: Lady Mary Wortley Montagu and the vogue for smallpox inoculation. *Feminist Studies*, 38(2), 330–362.

Barnes, D. S. (2014). Cargo, "infection," and the logic of quarantine in the nineteenth century. *Bulletin of the History of Medicine*, 88(1), 75–101.

Becker, A. M. (2004). Smallpox in Washington's army: Strategic implications of the disease during the American Revolutionary War. *The Journal of Military History*, 68(2), 381–430.

Bick, A., Sluga, G., Ehrhardt, A., Gorman, D., McKenzie, F., Sargent, D., Briffa, H., & King, I. (2020). Nineteenth century. In S. Center & E. Bates (Eds.), *After disruption: Historical perspectives on the future of international order* (pp. 11–23). Center for Strategic and International Studies (CSIS).

Bliss, M. (1991). *Plague: A story of smallpox in Montreal* (1st ed.). HarperCollins.

Boccaccio, G. (1886). *The Decameron of Giovanni Boccacci (Il Boccaccio)* (Holland paper ed.). Villon Society.

Butterfield, L. H. (1963). *Adams family correspondence (Vol. 2)*. Belknap Press of Harvard University Press.

Carmichael, A. (2006). SARS and plagues past. In J. Duffin & A. Sweetman (Eds.), *SARS in context: Memory, history, and policy*. McGill-Queen's University Press.

Caulford, P. (2003). SARS: Aftermath of an outbreak. *The Lancet*, 362, s2–s3.

Ceccarelli, L. (2011). Manufactured scientific controversy: Science, rhetoric, and public debate. *Rhetoric and Public Affairs*, 14(2), 195–228.

Cohn, S. K. (2018). *Epidemics: Hate and compassion from the Plague of Athens to AIDS* (1st ed.). Oxford University Press.

Crosby, A. W. (2003). *America's forgotten pandemic: The influenza of 1918* (2nd ed.). Cambridge University Press.

Dobyns, H. F. (1983). *Their number become thinned: Native American population dynamics in eastern North America*. University of Tennessee Press.

Duffin, J., & Sweetman, A. (2006). *SARS in context: Memory, history, and policy* (Vol. 77). McGill-Queen's University Press.

Duffy, J. (1972). *Epidemics in colonial America*. Kennikat Press.

Echenberg, M. (2002). Pestis Redux: The initial years of the third Bubonic Plague Pandemic, 1894-1901. *Journal of World History*, 13(2), 429–449.

Echenberg, M. (2007). *Plague ports: The global urban impact of Bubonic Plague, 1894-1901*. University Press.

Eyler, J. M. (2010). The state of science, microbiology, and vaccines Circa 1918. *Public Health Reports (1974-)*, 125, 27–36.

Fenn, E. A. (2004). *Pox Americana: The great smallpox epidemic of 1775-82* (2nd ed.). Sutton.

Fidler, D. P. (2004). Germs, governance, and global public health in the wake of SARS. *The Journal of Clinical Investigation*, 113(6), 799–804.

Gordon-Reed, A. (2008). *The Hemingses of Monticello: An American family* (1st ed.). W. W. Norton & Co.

Grizzard, F. E. (Ed.). (1998). *The papers of George Washington, Revolutionary War Series (Vol. 8)*. University Press of Virginia.

Grmek, M. D. (1989). *History of AIDS: Emergence and origin of a modern pandemic* (R. C. Maulitz & J. Duffin, Trans.). Princeton University.

Harrison, M. (2012). *Contagion: How commerce has spread disease*. Yale University Press.

Hays, J. N. (2005). *Epidemics and pandemics: Their impacts on human history*. ABC-CLIO.

Horton, R. C. (2004). *MMR: Science and fiction*. Granta.

Huber, V. (2006). The unification of the globe by disease? The international sanitary conferences on cholera, 1851-1894. *The Historical Journal*, 49(2), 453–476.

Huffard, R. S. (2013). Infected rails: Yellow fever and southern railroads. *The Journal of Southern History*, 79(1), 79–112.

Hunter, S. S. (2003). *Black Death: AIDS in Africa* (1st ed.). Palgrave Macmillan.

Iliffe, J. (2017). *The African AIDS epidemic: A history*. Ohio University Press.

Johnson, N. (2006). *Britain and the 1918-19 influenza pandemic: A dark epilogue*. Routledge.

Johnson, R.W. (2010). *South Africa's brave new world: The beloved country since the end of Apartheid* (Rev. ed.). Penguin.

Kraut, A. M. (1994). *Silent travelers: Germs, genes and the "immigrant menace"*. Basic Books.

Luckingham, B. (1984). To mask or not to mask: A note on the 1918 Spanish influenza epidemic in Tucson. *The Journal of Arizona History*, 25(2), 191–204.

McBride, D. (1991). *From TB to AIDS: Epidemics among urban blacks since 1900*. State University of New York Press.

McNeill, W. H. (1979). *Plagues and peoples*. Penguin.

Morens, D. M., & Fauci, A. S. (2007). The 1918 influenza pandemic: Insights for the 21st century. *The Journal of Infectious Diseases*, 195(7), 1018–1028.

Mytton, O.T., Rutter, P. D., Make, M., Mak, M., Stanton, E.A. I., Sachedina, N., & Donaldson, L. J. (2012). Mortality due to pandemic (H1N1) 2009 influenza in England: a comparison of the first and second waves. *Epidemiology and Infection*, 140(9), 1533–1541.

Oldstone, M. B. A. (2020). *Viruses, plagues, and history* (2nd ed.). Oxford University Press.

Oxford English Dictionary. (2021). Oxford University Press. https://www.oed.com

Peterson, M. (2019). *The city-state of Boston: The rise and fall of an Atlantic power, 1630-1865*. Princeton University Press.

Peterson, R. H. (1989). The Spanish influenza epidemic in San Diego, 1918-1919. *Southern California Quarterly*, 71(1), 89–105.

Rockafellar, N. (1986). "In gauze we trust" public health and Spanish influenza on the home front, Seattle, 1918-1919. *The Pacific Northwest Quarterly*, 77(3), 104–113.

Rusnock, A. (2009). Catching cowpox: The early spread of smallpox vaccination, 1798–1810. *Bulletin of the History of Medicine*, 83(1), 17–36.

Santayana, G. (1917). *The life of reason or the phases of human progress: Introduction and reason in common sense*. Charles Scribner's Sons.

Sarkar, N. (2001). Plague in Bombay: Response of Britain's Indian subjects to colonial intervention. *Proceedings of the Indian History Congress*, 62, 442–449.

Snowden, F. M. (1995). *Naples in the time of cholera, 1884–1911*. Cambridge University Press.

Snowden, F. M. (2019). *Epidemics and society: From the black death to the present*. Yale University Press.

Stetler, C. M. (2017). The 1918 Spanish influenza: Three months of horror in Philadelphia. *Pennsylvania History: A Journal of Mid-Atlantic Studies*, 84(4), 462–487.

Steven, B. (2000). Wisconsin and the great Spanish flu epidemic of 1918. *The Wisconsin Magazine of History*, 84(1), 36–56.

Thomas, A. J. (2010). *The Lambeth cholera outbreak of 1848-1849: The setting, causes, course and aftermath of an epidemic in London*. McFarland & Co.

Thornton, R. (1987). *American Indian holocaust and survival: A population history since 1492* (1st ed.). University of Oklahoma Press.

Tomkins, S. M. (1992). The influenza epidemic of 1918-19 in Western Samoa. *The Journal of Pacific History*, 27(2), 181–197.

van Zwanenberg, D. (1978). The Suttons and the business of inoculation. *Medical History*, 22(1), 71–82.

Wolfe, R. M., & Sharp, L. K. (2002). Anti-vaccinationists past and present. *BMJ: British Medical Journal*, 325(7361), 430–432.

Yahya, M. (2007). Polio vaccines: "No thank you!" barriers to polio eradication in northern Nigeria. *African Affairs*, 106(423), 185–204.

4

HUMAN DIGNITY

Donna McAuliffe with Hilary N. Weaver, Sharon E. Moore and Robert Common

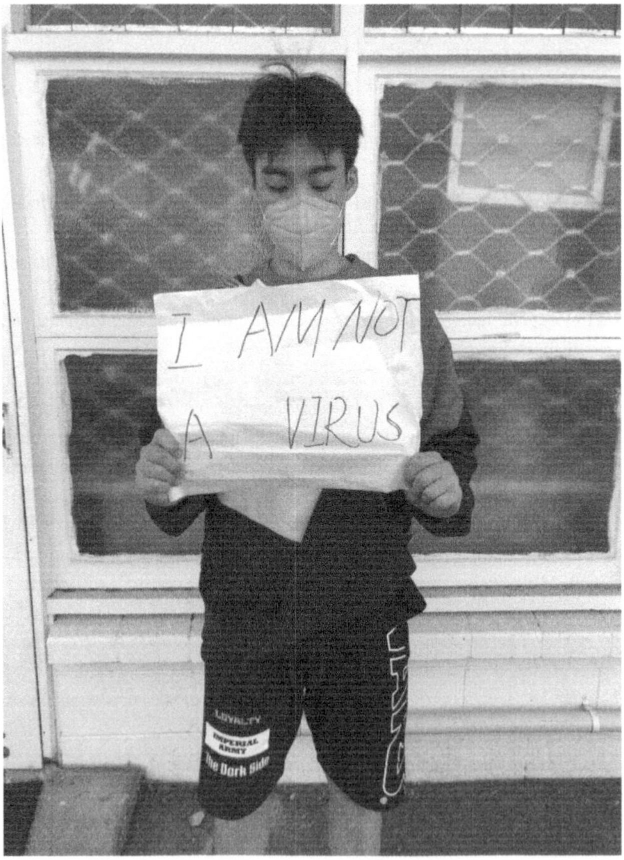

FIGURE 4.0 Protesting against racism

Source: Photograph by Peiching Li

DOI: 10.4324/9781003111214-5

Human dignity, a core social work value, is central to social work practice globally. The definition of dignity is the state or quality of being worthy of honour or respect. Its moral imperative is embedded in the Universal Declaration of Human Rights (UN, 1948, art. 1), the United Nations' Sustainable Development Goals 2015, social work codes of ethics and statements of principles, and is one of the four pillars of the Global Social Work Agenda (Bisman, 2004; Jones & Truell, 2012; UN, 1948; UN, 2015). Nine principles in the revised Global Social Work Statement of Ethical principles (GSWESP) were agreed to by the International Association of Schools of Social Work (IASSW) and the International Federation of Social Workers (IFSW) taskforce in Dublin, Ireland, in 2018 (Sewpaul & Henrickson, 2019). These principles built on the previous Ethics in Social Work, Statement of Principles moving away from its "Euro-north American axis" roots to encompass broader perspectives to reach consensus on the following principles:

- recognition of inherent dignity of humanity
- promoting human rights
- promoting social justice and equity
- promoting the right to self-determination
- promoting the right to participation
- respect for confidentiality and privacy
- treating people as whole persons
- the ethical use of technology and social media
- professional integrity (pp. 1471–1472)

Human dignity, that underpins all other principles, was sorely challenged on many levels during the COVID-19 pandemic and health emergencies such as HIV/AIDS that went before as we found in Chapter 3. Health emergencies bring out the best and the worst of human behaviours as they are times of crises, uncertainty and loss. For example, the mass lockdowns and quarantines implemented by governments in efforts to stem the SARS-CoV-2 virus spread saw the strengths of communities and the desire to care for each other rise to the fore, as well as creating fertile ground for discrimination and violence aimed at people who are labelled as a threat. Marginalised and discriminated people rarely fare well when scapegoats are sought in fractured communities. Blame builds on pre-existing prejudices and the escalating dehumanising of others, for example, the treatment of people with albinism in parts of Africa mentioned in Chapter 2. People of Asian appearance were vilified and subjected to violence by the persistent labelling of the "Chinese virus" by Trump and some other world leaders, as were LGBTQIA+ people by homophobic sentiment voiced by politicians like Putin (Farkas & Romaniuk, 2020; Financial Times, 2020). Refugees, minority religions, people of colour, other groups and entire nations have all been vilified, human rights breached, and human dignity violated. It is also the time when social workers were personally and professionally tested by ethical challenges and tensions between what is happening around them and their professional values, issues that emerged across fields of practice discussed in the ensuing chapters. Upholding human dignity in social work practice from micro to macro interventions is not the least of these challenges.

Human dignity has been described as a "slippery fish" because defining what this important value actually means in practice can be elusive (Borowski, 2007, p. 725). Essentially human dignity involves how we uphold the innate value of all people in practice, ranging from interpersonal engagement to advocacy at structural levels, in ways that ensure respect regardless of status, culture, wealth or other inequalities. Manomano and Mundau (2017) highlight the adjustments needed to contextual and emancipatory thinking, especially when contemporary challenges are overwhelming and people's most basic needs are not being met whether that be access to healthcare, the capacity to feed themselves or to be safe from violence or abuse. Vulnerabilities to loss of human dignity are closely associated with marginalisation, exploitation, racism and discrimination, and their intersections (Chenoweth & McAuliffe, 2020). Although social workers deal with these issues every day, they were intensified during COVID-19 as were the limitations imposed on how social workers could respond. For example, older people denied healthcare based on ageist assumptions addressed in Chapter 10 by Malcom Payne or the denial of basic protections for people on the move discussed in Chapter 11 by Justin Lee and Carmen Monico where practice was constrained by state policies, resources and reduced capacities to deliver the usual services.

As Borowski (2007, p.725) pointed out, social work's commitment to human rights offers a pathway to upholding dignity and stated,

> Human dignity is a norm that legitimizes human rights claims (Dicke, 2002: 118), since human rights follow logically from man's status of worth, of dignity. It is the foundation of the rights and freedoms that are the cornerstones of modern, enlightened societies. Thus, another important way in which social workers foster human dignity is through advancing human rights.

Human rights are embedded in the social work profession's value base (Chenoweth & McAuliffe, 2020; Mapp et al., 2019; Nipperess & Briskman, 2009; Pease et al., 2016). Human rights have also been critiqued for the legalistic language which poses barriers to translating human rights into social work practice and principles which deliver little practical guidance (Schmidt et al., 2020). Schmidt and colleagues (2020) go on to say that a singular focus on dignity to uphold human rights may be insufficient. Their constructivist grounded theory research conducted in the Netherlands developed a theory called the Dignity Circle. They found that people who used services could more easily identify those situations where their dignity was not supported rather than describing situations where their dignity was respected. Four forms of dignity violations were identified – when people felt like an object, for example, treated like a number or labelled; becoming an empty space, that is, their needs are chronically not heard which leads to isolation and an inability to continue to voice concerns; being treated like a child, ignorant and belittled; and finally, viewed as a monster or stigmatised due to looking different, having different norms, being crazy, dirty or a criminal, ultimately affecting self-image.

As a counterpoint, social workers in this study engaged in dignity promotion and "repair" strategies – recognising and treating people as unique redressed the objectification previously experienced; supporting participation in society; treating people as adults helped regain dignity; and finally "professional friendship" defined as long-term non-discriminatory, supportive relationships that still maintained professional boundaries and supported "feeling human". Schmidt et al. (2020) concluded that human dignity is a two-way, circular process, where dignity can be gained or lost in interactive relationships and suggested that social workers also needed to work against oppression at structural levels which is well supported in the literature.

When we consider how social work is always responsive to its context, it is useful to explore how the COVID-19 pandemic brought challenges to social work practice in respect to violations of human dignity and other social work values and ethical principles. It was people with fewer resources, the already oppressed, marginalised and discriminated against who were among the most affected during the pandemic and who are most likely to feel the consequences for many years to come. Loss of employment, income, housing and chronic health conditions for those who were affected by the virus have far reaching impacts. However, strengths were found in those many communities who self-organised, worked together to help and protect each other as well as railing against structural oppression. Joel Izlar further discusses the strengths and challenges in communities working together in Chapter 14. While social workers work with discriminated and oppressed people, many social workers and their colleagues are living the same experience as members of those very same groups. Social workers also needed to engage in self-protective behaviours in their professional role as workers and in their personal lives as citizens.

We explore violations of human dignity through three case studies by co-authors Hilary N. Weaver, Sharon E. Moore and Robert Common which highlight that while pandemic conditions heightened risks, people also took action to reclaim their dignity and rights while at the same time being constrained by the regimes in their countries. Interestingly, contemplating these case studies through a Dignity Circle lens raises questions about how people reclaiming their own dignity might also counter the categories of object, child, empty space and monster at a macro level, while at the same time experiencing antagonists who reassert discursive violations through media and politics. Ioakimidis and Dominelli (2016, p. 435) remind us we must not forget the "structural and political reasons behind the unjustified and colossal contradictions" in the pursuit of dignity. Vulnerability in health emergencies is not exclusively related to disease risks (Farkas & Romaniuk, 2020).

In the first case study, Hilary Weaver explores the experience of Native Americans. In this book we have read examples of how Indigenous Peoples acted quickly to protect their own despite historical and systemic racism, discrimination and oppression. For example, First Australians rallying to protect their vulnerable elders noted in Chapter 2. The Native American experience (see Box 4.1) highlights the strengths of community solidarity and how they took health and safety into their own hands in culturally appropriate ways in the face of government failures.

BOX 4.1

NATIVE AMERICAN EXPERIENCES DURING THE PANDEMIC

Hilary N. Weaver

Native Americans are the Indigenous Peoples of what is now the United States. They are diverse Peoples whose territories and members are bisected by the Canadian and Mexican borders. There are approximately 6.9 million Native Americans belonging to more than 574 Native Nations. While there are 324 reservations or tribally controlled territories, the majority of Native Americans live outside these areas. Native Nations retain elements of sovereignty including the rights to self-governance, determine membership, and develop and run their own health, educational, and judicial systems. Treaties and subsequent legal decisions led to federal responsibility for the health and well-being of tribal members. Despite these legal mandates, the US government has not built an adequate health infrastructure or provided adequate services or funding. Simultaneously, federal laws undermine tribal self-reliance. The pandemic highlighted ongoing tensions between sovereignty and federal paternalism.

Around the world, Indigenous communities often live in an ongoing state of vulnerability to health, economic, and social problems caused by systemic racism, institutional marginalisation, and the power imbalance inherent in colonisation. Long-standing inequities including limited access to food, clean water, and quality healthcare create health disparities and underlying chronic medical conditions that exacerbate vulnerability to COVID-19. The pandemic threatened to overwhelm fragile systems in already socially and economically marginalised communities. In addition to direct health impacts, COVID-19 led to disruptions in education and employment and exacerbated economic and food insecurity.

Native American cultures are grounded in collective cultural values and communal solidarity; factors that make physical distancing and limitations on gatherings and ceremonies particularly painful. During the pandemic many Native Americans found new ways to cultivate well-being and to connect. Having family members at home during lockdowns can facilitate cultural transmission. Some used this opportunity for learning language and participating in cultural practices including dance, music, and gathering medicine.

During the pandemic, Native Americans mobilised various responses including asserting sovereignty to close borders and institute curfews on tribal lands, initiating educational platforms to learn and communicate about COVID-19 in culturally congruent ways, and implementing mechanisms to support well-being under these difficult circumstances. Indigenous communities are exercising practical decision-making power and responsibility, even

(*Continued*)

BOX 4.1 (*Continued*)

NATIVE AMERICAN EXPERIENCES DURING THE PANDEMIC

when federal governments fail. Indeed, some tribal leaders see this crisis as an opportunity to assert cultural, political, and social aspects of nationhood and self-governance in the face of colonial structures and laws. Some envision the possibility of new partnerships, ultimately leading to more just and respectful service delivery systems.

COVID-19 has taken a significant toll on Native Americans, largely due to underlying health disparities and the lack of an adequate infrastructure to support health and well-being, both factors rooted in colonisation and ongoing racism. The pandemic also fuelled a drive for self-determination and building a better future. Native Nations are asserting their power, albeit still within significant colonial constraints, to provide for the well-being of their people and create partnerships grounded in social justice to better serve the health, economic, educational, and social needs of Indigenous Peoples for generations to come.

A salient point is that reclaiming dignity, human rights and justice despite structural and political barriers were underscored by innovation, hope and self-determination in Native American communities during the COVID-19 pandemic.

Racial injustice and state violence are global problems affecting many people (De Genova, 2018; Johnstone & Lee, 2018; Kerr & Cox, 2016). The trauma of Black Americans has its origins not in colonisation but in slavery and ongoing violence, injustice and oppression. The Black Lives Matter movement (see Box 4.2) gained global momentum and highlighted racism around the world during the pandemic. Peaceful protest is a legitimate way of advocating for human dignity and seeking redress for those systemic factors that continue to threaten them, but excessive state violence especially when it results in death is not (Hessel, 2011).

BOX 4.2

BLACK LIVES REALLY DO MATTER

Sharon E. Moore

Trauma, a recurring occurrence in the lived experiences of Black Americans, is defined as "an exposure to an extraordinary experience that presents a physical or psychological threat to oneself or others and generates a reaction of helplessness and fear" (Levenson, 2017, p. 105). For over four centuries, Black residents

(*Continued*)

BOX 4.2 (*Continued*)

BLACK LIVES REALLY DO MATTER

of the US have suffered senseless and deep pain as a result of the negative attributes that have been ascribed to them and the ensuing systematic oppression and inequalities that have affected every area of their lives. Their plight has been compounded by COVID-19. The CDC (2020) indicated that over half a million Americans had died from COVID-19 among whom approximately 15% were Black people. Blacks are 3.5 times more likely to die from COVID-19 than other racial groups and many are frontline workers (Lange et al., 2020). According to the Commonwealth Fund, communities with larger Black populations have disproportionately higher infection and death rates from COVID-19 (Zephyrin et al., 2020). Pre-existing diseases such as diabetes, hypertension, respiratory illnesses, and heart disease contribute to the high rate of COVID-19 deaths among Blacks. Poverty, living in overcrowded households, environmental pollution and inadequate access to health care also contribute to poorer health outcomes among Blacks who become infected with the disease (Burton et al., 2017).

The trauma and grief that Black people are currently experiencing because of the loss of loved ones due to COVID-19 are exacerbated by their historical and contemporary experiences with racism and discrimination. The legacy of the horrific mistreatment that they endured during the era of US slavery, which white America rarely acknowledges, is made even worse as a result of police shootings of unarmed Black men and women. Since 2015, roughly 5,000 Black people have been shot and killed by an on-duty police officer (The Washington Post, 2020). Although Black people make up less than 13% of the US population, they are killed by police at more than twice the rate of White Americans. These shootings are a national occurrence but happen more often in New Mexico, Alaska and Oklahoma which have densely populated areas (The Washington Post, 2020).

In 2020, George Floyd was killed by a white police officer who kept his knee on Mr. Floyd's neck for at least eight minutes and 46 seconds while Mr. Floyd gasped for air and cried out over 20 times that he could not breath. Shortly thereafter he became unconscious and later died (BBC News, 2020). Although there had been scores of police killings of unarmed Black people prior to Mr. Floyd's death and many thereafter, the horrific nature of his death which was video recorded by bystanders caused worldwide outrage and protests. Among those in the forefront of anti-racism, political activism was #Black Lives Matter. This movement was founded in 2013 in response to the murder of Trayvon Martin Shooting Fast Facts (CNN, 2020) and helped to bring international awareness and activism against white supremacy and violence inflicted on Black communities by the state and vigilantes (Black Lives Matter, n.d.). COVID-19 has highlighted the breaches of human rights and lack of human dignity still assigned to Black people in the US.

As Black Americans took to the street, other groups (see Box 4.3) sought to remain hidden for fear of violence, discrimination and being blamed for the spread of disease (Henrickson, 2018). At least 72 countries criminalise the preferences of sexual and gender minorities imposing harsh and unjust sentences which includes whipping, life imprisonment and death sentences in some countries (Bailey, 2012; Healy & Kamya, 2014; Henrickson, 2018). Although the same penalties may not exist elsewhere, discrimination exists in most societies rooted in concepts of normative family structures and in certain fundamentalist religions.

BOX 4.3

THE MARGINALISATION OF LGBTQIA+ PEOPLE DURING PANDEMICS

Robert common

In the 1980s, HIV/AIDS began to tear across the US and the world. In its first decade, over 100,000 lives were lost in a climate characterised by polarisation and stigmatisation rooted in deep political and social division. Discourse surrounding this particular virus labelled HIV a *gay disease* broadening out to an affliction only suffered by *gays and people of colour.* Despite heterosexual people also being affected, warped ideologies persisted with the label leading to violence, discrimination and a profound violation of human dignity and rights. HIV was devastating for all people affected and has gone on to take the lives of many more, as has Hepatitis C and other infectious diseases. Today, people in developed countries with access to good health care live normal lives but many people in the world do not share this privilege. The onset of COVID-19 and the need for urgent action disrupted HIV monitoring and treatment in many countries shining a light on global inequalities (OHCHR, 2020).

The COVID-19 pandemic has layered further inequalities upon LGBTQIA+ people who are already at a structural disadvantage from discriminatory health systems and prejudicial societal views. Taking South Korea as an example, in May 2020 an outbreak in the Seoul district known for being LGBTQIA+ friendly sparked people's real concerns over their privacy triggering pervasive fears of further stigmatisation, in particular, individuals being outed through the country's efficient track and trace programmes (Kim, 2020). Turkey's President Recep Erdogan backed statements made by the Minister of Religious Affairs, Ali Erbas, who inferred that homosexuality *shall bring illness* implying that LGBTQIA+ and same sex partnerships were responsible for the COVID-19 pandemic (AFP, 2020). Within the European Union, the Government of Hungary removed the ability of transgender individuals to alter birth registry language ensuring names match the gender assigned at birth (Gall, 2020). This was achieved on the 19th of May 2020 taking political advantage

(*Continued*)

BOX 4.3 (*Continued*)

THE MARGINALISATION OF LGBTQIA+ PEOPLE DURING PANDEMICS

amid the pandemic as part of a broader homophobic and transphobic political narrative. In Uganda, more than 20 LGBTQIA+ individuals were singled out and violently detained for violating physical distancing requirements not applied to other groups. These are only some examples that have unfolded during COVID-19 (Muhumuza, 2020).

The sense of safety and well-being for many people was eroded by political and social environments as well as the direct health risks and consequences of COVID-19. This pandemic has brought confinement and concomitant mental health issues with it. One such example is research conducted in Portugal that found that young LGTQIA+ felt isolated and demonstrably suffered as a result of lockdown (Macedo, 2020). Many LGTQIA+ individuals draw strength and mutual acceptance from social supports and networks especially youth whose safe spaces were diminished during the pandemic (Paley, 2020). This was also shown to be the case in Canada where isolation from community and closeness was a problem. While the global pandemic has been an undeniable tragedy, it has highlighted the intersectionality of a health crisis with social, emotional and structural violence towards the marginalised. Taking this further, excluding and blaming has been weaponised against some of the most vulnerable in society. The LGBTQIA+ community buried many people in the early days of the HIV epidemic and were blamed by many for its very existence. Lessons learned are seemingly few and far between as the same issues of human rights and dignity arose during COVID-19. Our rights are as indivisible as others, as should be our dignity.

Discrimination based on sexual orientation also poses enormous risks for International workers with diverse orientations when working in certain countries where they would be subjected to unjust and discriminatory laws, immense challenges for social work leaders in certain cultural environments, and for people living in these countries or seeking asylum on this basis (Bennett, 2013). History has shown us that certain groups have been persecuted and denied human dignity based on difference and prejudice when there are economic or health crises.

Conclusion

The three case studies are only some of the many examples where people's dignity has been assaulted across multiple generations on the basis of differences from dominant cultures. Human dignity as a concept has been accepted in social work practice, but there has been little deconstruction to determine how it is incorporated into social work practice and such how such long-standing injustices can be addressed. Upholding human rights is offered as a pathway to human dignity and Ioakimidis and Dominelli (2016) suggest striving for social justice is the key. Just as COVID-19 has amplified many systemic weaknesses, it has done the same for assaults on human dignity.

Many ethical considerations and tensions arose during the COVID-19 pandemic as documented in an IFSW sponsored research project (Banks et al., 2020a, 2020b). Social workers across many countries contributed stories about their struggles in the pandemic environment when services were closed down, home visiting was stopped, use of PPE inhibited clarity of communication, digital means of communication took over face-to-face interactions leading to concerns about quality of assessments, and restrictions on movement leading to isolation and increased mental health concerns. One question in this reporting of the research findings was "how to respect people's rights and dignity when it is difficult to meet them or see their faces" (Banks et al., 2020a, p. 5).

The world media highlighted case after case of decisions being made about who should be afforded the opportunity of treatment such as ventilation and intensive care, over those who were deemed unlikely to survive and therefore not given potentially life-saving treatments. What role do social workers play in the rationing of resources in the midst of a health crisis that has moral decisions at the core? How do we support people who are denied treatment due to limited resources or assumptions made about quality of life? How do social workers provide a safe environment for people too frightened to reveal why they are scared? Do we march on the streets and risk the spread of disease or stay at home in a self-protective bubble? Is it a human right for people to choose not to wear a mask in public versus the protection of self and others and do no harm? How do we support the self-determination of communities in the face of injustice? How do we preserve dignity when there are no resources or when states are in lockdown? How do we uphold human dignity in practice when the odds are against certain groups of people because they are poor and live in housing that is overcrowded and are susceptible to spread of the virus? How do we help preserve dignity for those whose livelihoods and employment crumble in front of them as the economic devastation of the pandemic runs its course through country after country? This chapter has probably raised many more questions than answers about how social workers can uphold human dignity, support the strengths of communities in their day to day work and manage ethical tensions between the personal and professional. We explore some of these issues in the ensuing chapters.

An apt conclusion to this chapter is found in the words of Borowski (2007) who states:

> Social workers are a very privileged lot. What could be more significant than striving through one's day to day work to enhance the human dignity of others?

BOX 4.4

REFLECTIVE QUESTIONS

1. Is it a fair claim that promoting and upholding human rights will ultimately result in promotion of human dignity?
2. How far should individual autonomy and freedom of choice be extended when public health and safety is at risk?
3. How should social workers balance the competing responsibilities of care for self and family, and care for others in the course of their work?
4. Are social workers essential workers in a pandemic?

References

AFP. (2020, April 28). Erdogan defends Turkey religious chief's anti-gay sermon. *The Times of Israel*. https://www.timesofisrael.com/erdogan-defends-turkey-religious-chiefs-anti-gay-sermon/

Bailey, G. (2012). Human rights and sexual orientation. In L. M. Healy & R. J. Link (Eds.), *Handbook on international social work: Human rights, development and the global profession* (pp. 464–471). Oxford University Press.

Banks, S., Cai, T., de Jonge, E., Shears, J., Shum, M., Sobočan, A. M., ... Weinberg, M. (2020a). *Ethical challenges for social workers during COVID-19: A global perspective*. Switzerland. https://www.ifsw.org/ethical-challenges-for-social-workers-during-covid-19-a-global-perspective/

Banks, S., Cai, T., de Jonge, E., Shears, J., Shum, M., Sobočan, A. M., ... Weinberg, M. (2020b). Practising ethically during COVID-19: Social work challenges and responses. *International Social Work*. https://doi.org/10.1177/0020872820949614

BBC News. (2020). George Floyd: What happened in the final moments of his life. BBC. https://www.bbc.com/news/world-us-canada-52861726

Bennett, C. (2013). Claiming asylum on the basis of your sexuality: The views of lesbians in the UK. *The Researcher*, 8(2), 17–19.

Bisman, C. (2004). Social work values: The moral core of the profession. *The British Journal of Social Work*, 34(1), 109–123.

Black Lives Matter. (n.d.). https://blacklivesmatter.com/about/

Borowski, A. (2007). Guest editorial: On human dignity and social work. *International Social Work*, 50(6), 723–726.

Burton, L. M., Mattingly, M. Pedroza, J., & Welsh, W. (2017). *State of the Union 2017: Poverty. Pathways Special Issue*. Stanford Center on Poverty and Inequality. https://inequality.stanford.edu/sites/default/files/Pathways_SOTU_2017_poverty.pdf

CDC COVID Data Tracker (2020). *Center for Disease Control*. https://covid.cdc.gov/covid-data-tracker/#demographics

Chenoweth, L. & McAuliffe, D. (2020). *The road to social work and human service practice* (6th ed.). Cengage.

De Genova, N. (2018). The "migrant crisis" as racial crisis: Do black lives matter in Europe? *Ethnic and Racial Studies*, 41(10), 1765–1782.

Dicke, K. (2002). The foundation function of human dignity in the Universal Declaration of Human Rights. In D. Kretzmer & E. Klein (Eds.), *The concept of human dignity in human rights discourse* (pp. 111–120). Kluwer Law International.

Farkas, K. J., & Romaniuk, J. R. (2020). Social work, ethics and vulnerable groups in the time of coronavirus and COVID-19. *Society Register*, 4(2), 67–82.

Financial Times. (2020). LGBT activists denounce Putin's war on liberal values. https://www.ft.com/content/cc2121f7-a98c-4007-8cf3-ca971ef112ec

Gall, L. (2020, April 3). Hungary seeks to ban legal gender recognition for transgender people. *Human Rights Watch*. https://www.hrw.org/news/2020/04/03/hungary-seeks-ban-legal-gender-recognition-transgender-people

Healy, L., & Kamya, H. (2014). Ethics and international discourse in social work: The case of Uganda's anti-homosexuality legislation. *Ethics and Social Welfare*, 8(2), 151–169.

Henrickson, M. (2018). Promoting the dignity and worth of all people: The privilege of social work. *International Social Work*, 61(6), 758–766.

Hessel, S. (2011). *Time for outrage: Indignez-vous!* (M. Duvert, Trans.). Twelve Hachette Book Group.

Ioakimidis, V., & Dominelli, L. (2016). The challenges of dignity and worth for all: Social work perspectives. *International Social Work*, *59*(4), 435–437.

Johnstone, M., & Lee, E. (2018). State violence and the criminalization of race: Epistemic injustice and epistemic resistance as social work practice implications. *Journal of Ethnic & Cultural Diversity in Social Work*, *27*(3), 234–252.

Jones, D., & Truell, R. (2012). The gglobal agenda for social work and social development: A place to link together and be effective in a global world. *International Social Work*, 55(4),454–72.

Kerr, T., & Cox, S. (2016). Media, machines and might: Reproducing Western Australia's violent state of aboriginal protection. *Somatechnics*, 6(1), 89–105.

Kim, N. (2020, May 11). South Korea struggles to contain new outbreak amid anti-gay backlash. *The Guardian*. https://www.theguardian.com/world/2020/may/11/south-korea-struggles-to-contain-new-outbreak-amid-anti-lgbt-backlash

Lange, S. J., Ritchey, M. D., Goodman, A. B., Dias, T., Twentyman, E., Fuld, J., & Stein, Z. (2020). Potential indirect effects of the COVID-19 pandemic on use of emergency departments for acute life-threatening conditions—United States, January–May 2020. *Morbidity and Mortality Weekly Report*, 69(25), 795–800.

Levenson, J. (2017). Trauma-informed social work practice. *Social Work*, 62(2),105–113.

Macedo, M. (2020, May 18). Covid-19 trouxe solidão e desconforto aos jovens LGBT+. *Noticias. Universidade do Porto*. https://noticias.up.pt/covid-19-trouxe-solidao-e-desconforto-aos-jovens-lgbt/

Manomano, T., & Mundau, M. (2017). Preserving human dignity: Promises and pitfalls – A South African perspective. *International Social Work*, 60(6), 1358–1369.

Mapp, S., McPherson, J., Androff, D., & Gabel, S. G. (2019). Social work is a human rights profession. *Social Work*, 64(3), 259–269.

Muhumuza, R. (2020, April 2). LGBT community raided in Uganda over social distancing. *ABC News*. https://abcnews.go.com/International/wireStory/lgbt-community-raided-uganda-social-distancing-69915445

Nipperess, S., & Briskman, L. (2009). Promoting a human rights perspective on critical social work. In J. Allan, L. Briskman, & B. Pease (Eds.), *Critical social work: Theories and practices for a socially just world* (pp. 58–69). Allen & Unwin.

OHCHR. (2020). *An LGBT-inclusive response to COVID-19*. United Nations Human Rights Office of the High Commissioner. https://www.ohchr.org/EN/Issues/SexualOrientationGender/Pages/COVID19LGBTInclusiveResponse.aspx

Paley, A. (2020, July 31). The coronavirus has shrunk LGBTQ youth's safe spaces. *World Economic Forum*. https://www.weforum.org/agenda/2020/07/the-coronavirus-has-shrunk-lgbtq-youths-safe-spaces/

Pease, B., Goldingay, S., Hosken, N., & Nipperess, S. (Eds.). (2016). *Doing critical social work: Transformative practices for social justice* (1st ed.). Routledge.

Schmidt, J., Niemeijer, A., Leget, C., Trappenburg, M., & Tonkens, E. (2020). The dignity circle: How to promote dignity in social work practice and policy? [De waardigheid-scirkel: Hoe waardigheid te bevorderen in praktijken beleid van sociaal werk?]. *European Journal of Social Work*, 23(6), 945–957.

Sewpaul, V., & Henrickson, M. (2019). The (r)evolution and decolonization of social work ethics: The Global Social Work Statement of Ethical Principles. *International Social Work*, 62(6), 1469–1481.

The Washington Post. (2020). 1000 People have been shot and killed by the police in the past year. *The Washington Post*. https://www.washingtonpost.com/graphics/investigations/police-shootings-database/

Trayvon Martin Shooting Fast Facts. (2020). *CNN*. https://www.cnn.com/2013/06/05/us/trayvon-martin-shooting-fast-facts/index.html

UN. (1948). *Universal declaration of human rights*. United Nations. https://www.un.org/en/universal-declaration-human-rights/

UN. (2015). *Sustainable development goals*. United Nations. https://sustainabledevelopment-un-org.libraryproxy.griffith.edu.au/post2015/transformingourworld

Zephyrin, L., Radley, D. C., Getachew, Y., Baumgartner, J. C., & Schneider, E. C. (2020). *COVID-19 More prevalent, deadlier in US counties with higher Black populations*. To the Point (Blog), Commonwealth Fund. https://www.commonwealthfund.org/blog/2020/covid-19-more-prevalent-deadlier-us-counties-higher-black-populations#:~:text=More%20people%20are%20sick%20with,disproportionally%20burdened%20by%20the%20disease

PART II

Social work practice, issues and responses

5

HOSPITAL SOCIAL WORK DURING THE SECOND WAVE IN CANADA

Barbara Muskat, Shelley Craig, Deepy Sur and Alexa Kirkland

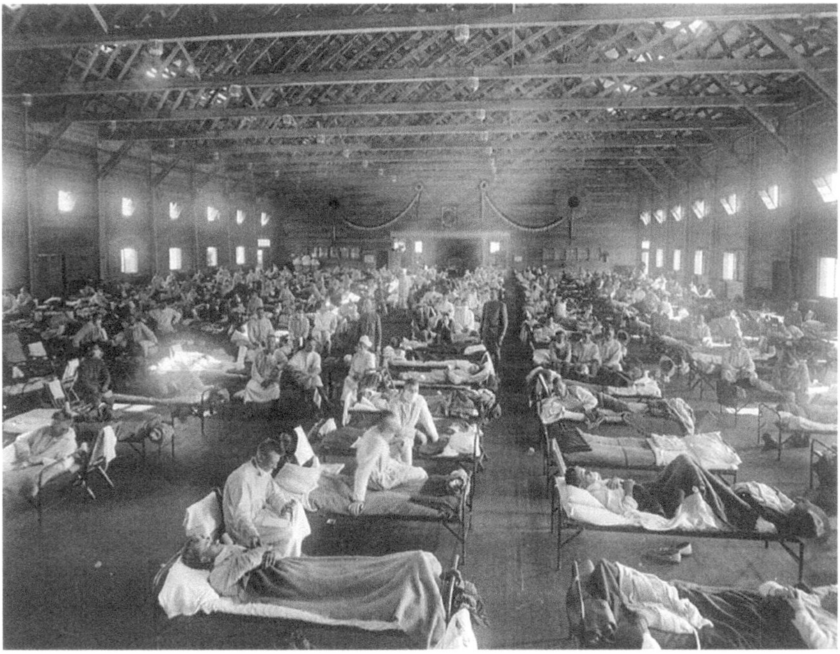

FIGURE 5.0 Emergency hospital during the 1918 influenza pandemic

Source: Photograph National Museum of Health and Medicine

DOI: 10.4324/9781003111214-7

The context of hospital social work

Hospitals are an important setting for social work practice. In North America, social workers have provided services in hospitals for over a century (Craig & Muskat, 2013; Kerson & McCoyd, 2013). In Ontario, 12.6% of social workers are employed in hospital/health care settings, second only to those working in adult mental health/addictions programs (14.9%). Social work positions in hospitals are highly regarded due to valuable employment benefits, competitive salaries, and personal satisfaction (Ontario Association of Social Workers, 2018).

During usual (non-pandemic) times, the roles and duties of social workers in Ontario hospitals focus on direct practice including: conducting psychosocial assessments; delivering counselling/psychotherapy; providing patient and family education; managing discharge planning; linking outpatients with appropriate supports during resource counselling and offering support to interprofessional teams through psychosocial consultation (Craig et al., 2020; Muskat et al., 2017; Ontario Association of Social Workers, 2013). However, emerging research highlights the reprioritising of roles that social workers undertake in response to changes and challenges in health care. Most notably, in recent years, hospital social work services have been called upon to respond to increases in patient medical complexity, high costs of new medical procedures and a focus on shortened hospital stays due to health care funding shortages, both in Ontario, as well as across the globe (Craig & Muskat, 2013; Harslof et al., 2017; Judd & Sheffield, 2010; Nam et al., 2019).

Hospital social work during pandemics

Hospitals are *ground zero* for pandemics. Although hospital social workers modify their work priorities to meet urgent needs there is limited research related to hospital social workers' roles and contributions during pandemics. The SARS crisis generated some exploratory studies and recommendations for social work practice. Gearing et al. (2007) described the need for hospital social workers to be mindful of their own health and emotions, as well as those of their clients, the need for more clarity from multiple levels of governance about guidelines and restrictions (such as visitor policies, personal protective devices and community restrictions), and the role of social workers in offering support to their interprofessional colleagues. Social workers in hospitals in Thailand during SARS (Rowlands, 2007) reported challenges utilising protective face masks, quarantining to prevent spread, helping with contact tracing, supporting the emotional health of the staff and advocating on behalf of discharged patients. The study noted that to address those challenges, social workers drew on their skills in crisis intervention, emergency response, grief counselling and supporting patients and families. Despite a call for the development of theoretical and practice approaches to guide social work during pandemics such as decision-making for potentially limited life-saving therapy, conducting effective psychosocial interventions to patients facing palliative care and probable death, assistance to patients and families with the longer-term effects of the pandemic, and a post-SARS recognition of a need for better preparation (Rosoff, 2008), it appears that standards for hospital social work practice during pandemics have still not been developed. This has resulted in reinvention of roles and responsibilities with each new pandemic (Cheung, 2020).

In 2019–2020, a new disease, not previously seen in humans, coronavirus disease 2019 (COVID-19), arrived in North America (CDC, 2020). COVID-19 is a highly contagious virus, presenting with a wide range and severity of symptoms, including those with the potential to result in hospitalisation, intensive care, ventilator use and death (CDC, 2020). COVID-19 has required a rapid, urgent response by the health care system, placing enormous stress on hospital resources. Research is emerging about the impact of the coronavirus on the social work profession. Levin-Dagan and Strenfeld-Hever (2020) explored the experience of hospital social workers in Israel during the initial stages of the coronavirus pandemic. This work highlights the ways in which social workers have been able to respond to the challenges that accompanied distanced psychosocial support for patients and their families (Levin-Dagan & Strenfeld-Hever, 2020). Social workers noted that an increase in mental health and grief support for patients and families as well as mediating heightened feelings of loss of control were adapted through virtual modalities (Levin-Dagan & Strenfeld-Hever, 2020). Within the Tel-Aviv Sourasky Medical Center, social workers were also established as key members of a new and innovative protocol to allow one person to say goodbye to their dying family member face to face. This practice had not yet been seen in a global context (Levin-Dagan & Strenfeld-Hever, 2020).

COVID-19 in Ontario

The first presumptive case of COVID-19 in Ontario was identified on January 25, 2020 and at the time of this writing the province has confirmed 197,360 total cases, which includes 4,730 deaths (Ontario.ca, 2020). Ontario has experienced a pattern of disease spread similar to other jurisdictions, with an initial wave from February until mid-July 2020, followed by a decrease, largely due to a province-wide lock down on non-essential services and limits on social gatherings. Lockdown rules were eased beginning in August, with a return to the opening of many businesses and resumption of most medical services with continued social distancing and the wearing of masks. A second wave began in September, followed by a large increase in cases by November, resulting in a return to a lockdown in December with business closures and limits in numbers allowed to gather socially. At the time of this chapter, Ontario was fully in the second wave of disease spread with expectations of increasing cases as the province moves into both flu season and winter.

Social work holds a distinctive place in Ontario health care. The Ontario Ministry of Health and Long-Term Care provides, funds and regulates 26 disciplines (beyond physicians and nurses) as regulated health professionals under the *Regulated Health Professions Act, 1991* (RHPA) and *Health Profession Acts* (i.e. *Medicine Act, 1991*; Ontario Ministry of Health, Ontario Ministry of Long-Term Care, 2020a, 2020b). However, social workers are not designated as a regulated health profession in Ontario due to separate regulation and governance by the Social Work and Social Service Work Act (SWSSWA) which is accountable to the Minister of Children, Community and Social Services rather than to the Ministry of Health and Long-Term Care (Ontario College of Social Workers and Social Service Workers, 2015). Despite this differentiated governance structure, many social workers are employed by hospitals, which means they must also abide by those Ministry of Health regulations and in the case of pandemics, encounter similar risks of those in regulated health professions.

In the wake of COVID-19, Public Safety Canada (2020) developed a list of services deemed essential to ensure the health, safety, and economic well-being of the population. It is notable that despite the lack of recognition as a regulated health profession, social workers in hospital settings were designated as an essential service which was not the case in all countries. As essential providers, social workers were advised to continue to do their jobs, as long as they experienced no COVID-19 symptoms, and their employers were obligated to provide appropriate protective equipment and products. However, Public Safety Canada also advised that essential workers who can perform their tasks remotely should do so which applied to some hospital-based social workers. While Public Safety Canada (2020) gave guidance to municipal, provincial, and Indigenous jurisdictions through the definition and list of essential services, they were also clear that this was not a federal order and these jurisdictions still had control over what directives to make to respond to the pandemic. In March, at the start of the first wave of the pandemic, the Ontario College of Social Workers and Social Service Workers issued guidelines for social work practice during the pandemic. Although noting that while some social workers may be permitted to provide in-person services due to low COVID-19 numbers in their locality and/or the nature of the services they provide, the College strongly advised all members, wherever reasonably possible, to provide services by electronic means (OCSWSSW, 2020).

Further adding to the uncertainty, during the height of the first wave of the pandemic in April 2020, the Ontario government announced a temporary pandemic pay benefit for eligible frontline workers (Government of Ontario, 2020). Surprisingly, this benefit was provided to social workers in youth and adult correctional facilities, but not to social workers in hospital settings. Despite advocacy by the Ontario Association of Social Workers (OASW), which included hundreds of letters of support to government ministers, the decision was not reversed. This resulted in disappointment and disillusionment among hospital social workers, who viewed this as devaluing their contributions during these particularly difficult times (Ontario Association of Social Workers, 2020).

Given the scarcity of research regarding pandemic social work practice, the level of uncertainty facing social workers in Ontario during COVID-19 and the lack of evidence-informed practice principles related to hospital social workers during pandemics, the authors developed and conducted an exploratory study of the work of Ontario hospital social workers during the second wave of the COVID-19 pandemic. The survey explored any role changes, the availability of resources available or needed for new job duties, emergent training needs and recommendations for pandemic social work practice in hospitals. The survey received ethics approval by the University of Toronto and was distributed to the membership of the OASW during the second wave of the pandemic, in December 2020. Responses from 150 survey participants are integrated below.

Hospital social work during COVID-19

The first impact of the pandemic was felt in Ontario hospitals in early March 2020. Many elective services were cancelled or postponed or moved to virtual visits or postponements. Inpatient services, such as urgent cardiology procedures, cancer care, complex birthing services, neonatal intensive care, trauma services and emergency medical care continued, albeit simultaneously with increasing COVID-19 treatment. Social workers, as with all hospital staff, were expected to pivot quickly and develop and adopt new approaches to their work. Since no clear directives or templates were provided on how to do this, there was an expected variety of responses to the pivot that involved the setting, focus and approach of hospital social work.

Working in a range of settings

Some social workers were instructed by their institution to continue their work as before, others were informed of changes in their work assignments while others were left to organise this on their own. Social workers generally were expected to or opted to work in-person in inpatient and emergency room settings because of the serious conditions of patients, the urgency and the crisis nature of these medical situations, as well as for support to their physician and nursing colleagues who were working long hours in the face of a new medical crisis with no clear treatment protocols. Those who worked in-person in hospitals described a range of concerns, such as fear of contracting COVID-19 or bringing it home to their families, limits in the availability of personal protective equipment, and exposure to suffering and death in patients and grief and loss in family members. This at times resulted in second guessing their decision about whether or not to work in the hospital (Casey, 2020). Some hospital social workers were redeployed from outpatient to inpatient work and from quieter units to busier units. Other inpatient social workers continued what they were doing pre-pandemic, however, under new conditions. Some social workers described struggles with space to do their work with cramped offices and interviewing spaces becoming more dangerous from a virus exposure perspective, and communication with patients and families becoming more challenging from behind masks.

Working with an evolving focus

A particular area of change and stress for social workers was their involvement in patient-family member contact during strict isolation procedures which had an impact on family visiting and in-person contact with patients. Some social workers described their experiences of being given responsibilities for ensuring families were aware of and adhered to non-visitation policies. A number of social workers described their involvement with developing virtual visiting programs, with new roles including arranging visiting times and managing the equipment required for virtual visitation. This also included being in charge of arranging and holding virtual visits between COVID-19 patients in ICUs who were at the end of life with family members who needed to see their loved one and say their goodbyes. The use of technology for these visits was seen as an asset by some social workers as it allowed family members to be contacted and met with at any time when needed without having to wait for families to travel to the hospital.

In adult hospitals in Ontario, as in hospitals across North America, hospital social workers were also involved in helping to arrange after hospital care with often scarce availability of community-based rehabilitation (with some only providing virtual care) and nursing care beds (Hutchinson, 2020; Shemelia, 2020). This became more complex with refusal of admission to those sites of long stay care until patients test-free of COVID-19 systems, as well as the rapid growth of COVID-19 in the patients and staff in those long-term care settings which resulted in gridlock in hospital beds in acute care settings (Whitten, 2020).

Working virtually

Social workers who worked in outpatient services reported that they were encouraged to work virtually from their homes. This quelled concerns about the risk of exposure to COVID-19 and the potential to pass it on to their family members. But it required them to set up private virtual workspaces and to work around the presence and needs of their family members who were at home due to the concurrent closing of schools and businesses. Social workers described very little institutional support in setting up these new spaces. They often used their home computers and private cell phones and needed to ensure they had home access to medical record systems. While some social workers had already participated in virtual care, in many instances, social workers described very minimal pre-pandemic training and experience in virtual care, with a steep learning curve in setting up and using secure virtual platforms. However, they also described active pursuit of training in virtual clinical work and use of technology. Some social workers described this training as occurring simultaneously as they were learning new, appropriate, and secure technological applications. They were also tasked with educating patients, their families, and groups about how to use these new platforms. Some social workers described stressors that many individuals face in conducting online counselling, such as eye strain, back strain and Zoom fatigue, but they also appreciated that many patients found virtual support to be much more convenient. Concerns were also raised by social workers about the impact of working in isolation from their colleagues and teams, and their limited access to peer support. And together with their inpatient colleagues, respondents described challenges, both practical and ethical, in contacting and working with patients and families who live in situations with limited band width, who do not have access to consistent internet linkages, communication devices or privacy in their homes, as well as those unable to navigate technology due to cognitive challenges.

Working with increased patient mental health concerns

There is a growing awareness of the impact of COVID-19 on the emotional, social and spiritual health of patients and their families (Krasniansky, 2020). A group of social workers in palliative care, together with hospital chaplains described their supportive and spiritual work during COVID-19, particularly in support of fellow staff members. They described how they helped individuals make emotional connections with others, advocated for the rights of those in need, assisted them to reflect on past positive and successful experiences, using the tools of engagement and presence (Alford & Chester, 2020). While generally this work was done through telehealth or other virtual methods, at times social workers needed to conduct visits with hard-to-reach patients. Additional emotional and spiritual approaches were developed for patients on ventilators and unable to verbally communicate (Krasniansky, 2020).

In both inpatient and outpatient settings it was recognised that COVID-19 brought up difficult past experiences and created emotional turmoil for patients and their families. These experiences included past traumas, experiences of abandonment and helplessness and difficult experiences dealing with illnesses, deaths, hospitals and funeral homes. As well there were observations of increased anxiety and fears related to COVID-19 which required increased attention to the potential for emotional and mental health issues in patients and families.

During the first wave, social workers stated that they were often consulted by patients seeking education and information about the coronavirus. Some social workers described the challenges to pivot their role while locating updated, relevant, and accurate information to support their patients during a time of increased anxiety. As the second wave has continued, some respondents stated that there was now a degree of comfortability in locating new information about the coronavirus as well as updated referral processes within their local community agencies.

During this time there was also uptake by social workers in the facilitation of support groups virtually. One example was the adaptation of a perinatal loss group to an online format. This allowed families to attend from home and receive the support they needed around loss during a time surrounded by so much other loss.

Working with vulnerable populations

During the pandemic, hospital social workers increased their support to the most vulnerable populations including the homeless, elderly, and people struggling with mental health issues and addictions. Social workers described helping them secure masks, access to food and to safe spaces, and to family when they lacked access to cell phones or computers. Some social workers employed in rural communities expressed the misconception that all patients have the potential for access to an internet connection. There was also some anxiety among patients when accessing online applications and hospital networks they have never used before. This required creativity and increased coordination between hospital social workers and community resources to serve vulnerable populations with the methods and funding that was available. Many respondents to the survey also expressed that they were supporting patients experiencing increased racism and stigma due to increased positive coronavirus cases in their neighbourhoods. Some social workers expressed the need for more institutional and community support for those experiencing greater health disparities due to racism and issues of equity, diversity, and inclusion, especially because these gaps were increasing, and resources were becoming more limited and restricted due to the pandemic.

At one hospital, social workers gave particular attention to supporting under-housed and homeless patients coming to the hospital's COVID-19 Assessment Centre (Brailsford, 2020). These patients included those with refugee status or those experiencing domestic violence, all situations that made coping with the possibility of having the virus more challenging. These patients could not be sent back to their shelters/drop-in centres or to the streets while awaiting test results. Instead, they were given access to an acute ambulatory care unit where they received case management support from a social worker to coordinate care no matter whether their test results were positive or negative. This included information about food banks and meal programs and direct assistance to find a bed in a shelter. For patients that tested positive, the social workers coordinated with a city-run service that provided a private room and bathroom, as well as monitoring the patient's care. This program's success was built on the social workers' knowledge and connections with services and the development of a well-functioning team approach to care.

Working to support teams and prevent burnout

It is common in hospital social work that there is no backup or relief staff. When a colleague is away from work due to either planned (vacation) or unplanned reasons, coverage is supplied by another social worker. During the course of the first and second waves of the pandemic in Ontario, there was reportedly increased staff absences due to illness in social workers or their family members, as well as due to a paucity of childcare (due to closure of schools and day care facilities). Survey respondents noted that they often experienced exhaustion due to the psychological stress brought on by the pandemic, the acuity of their patients and their need to offer coverage for their colleagues. The social workers who participated in this survey also described a variety of approaches to maintaining their own well-being. These included a variety of methods to maintain connections with and support from their social work and team colleagues. Examples of these self-care initiatives were joining social work support groups on social media; attending daily check-ins and face-to-face or video huddles where it was possible to vent, talk, laugh and be social; and peer support initiatives where they could discuss and receive support related to their clinical work.

Hospital social workers frequently expressed concern about the well-being of their fellow staff, their own well-being as well as worry about their physical health and the health of their own families (Newman-Breman, 2020). The social workers in the study described their involvement in providing emotional support to their team members. This has become even more necessary during the second wave of the pandemic due to the build-up of stress and exhaustion over what has been experienced as an unrelenting crisis. They described this support as being expected from them, yet also within their scope of practice as their knowledge and skills in mental health intervention, mindfulness and trauma-informed care prepared them for this work. This took the form of crisis support to staff and physicians, offering debriefs after difficult losses, and now in the second wave, teaching colleagues how to increase their emotional resilience, offering mindfulness meditations and other stress reducing strategies.

In response to the evolving health crisis and its impact on the mental health of frontline health care workers, the Ontario COVID-19 Mental Health Network (2020) was initiated in March by a community-based psychotherapist, to offer a fast and seamless support network for these individuals. Hospital social workers were among the 900 Ontario licensed mental health professionals who volunteered in this venture. The network was closed in July when the first phase of the pandemic abated. However, social workers described a continuing need for a more robust, easily accessible system of mental health support for hospital frontline staff.

Taken together, the experiences of Ontario's hospital social workers encompassed a range of adaptations to their work to accommodate the increased needs of patients, families and their colleagues during the uncertainty of an evolving pandemic. Their contributions, experiences and insights are helpful in better understanding the roles of social workers during a global crisis, yet further illuminate the importance of cogent and thoughtful preparation. Given the likelihood of future pandemics and the recommendation that medical institutions should be prepared with clear guidelines for all staff (Rosoff, 2008), the uncertainty reported during COVID-19 by Ontario's hospital social workers indicate a need for clear and distinct expectations for social work practice. Despite a call for the development of theoretical and practice approaches to guide social work during pandemics, it appears that these roles have emerged anew in the midst of each crisis, with social workers often struggling to pivot and reprioritise on the fly, leading to reinventing of roles and responsibilities with each new pandemic. There is a need for easily accessible principles for practice for hospital social workers during pandemics similar to principles for practice during other hospital events such as fires, toxic spills, evacuations, or disasters. As stated by one survey participant, "As a profession, it will be important that we debrief on all that we've learned from this pandemic – what worked, what didn't, what was learned, where the gaps were".

Lessons learned and opportunities for greater social work practice effectiveness during future pandemics

Gleaned from the literature and responses from Ontario's hospital social workers, seven principles emerged to support the future state for social work practice during pandemics.

1. *Flexibility and readiness:* Pivot and adapt to use their expertise effectively where needed with the support of clear protocols to ensure seamless transitions during future pandemics (for example, understanding what tasks are considered essential and what tasks can be adjusted to meet new need)
2. *Respond and intervene:* Apply common skills such as crisis intervention, trauma-informed care, end-of-life care, supportive therapies, virtual communication and therapies, and pandemic impacts and mitigation. This requires both individual and hospital commitment to ongoing training and skills development.
3. *Provision of information:* Awareness of community resources that alleviate stressors on well-being, crisis supports and updates to programs and policies related to the pandemic response.
4. *Innovation and Inclusivity:* Innovate to address barriers arising from the medical impact of the pandemic as well as from the needs of vulnerable populations including addressing disproportionality and disparity.
5. *Team support:* Psychosocially support colleagues and staff to continuously maintain strong professional networks, as well as to support the well-being of colleagues and to address staff isolation and burnout.
6. *Enable access:* Create opportunities and advocate for accessibility of services for all clients who may be especially impacted by the pandemic (for example, access to Wi-Fi, advocacy and funding support for electronics, virtual care, etc.).
7. *Designation of social workers:* Officially designate social workers as essential hospital staff with the support of hospital administration to suitably train, compensate and equip social workers with knowledge and materials to pivot seamlessly to emergency conditions.

In summary, increasing the knowledge base around practice principles during pandemics and other crises can translate across workplaces to allow for all social workers to assist patients and their families regardless of the setting. Examining the stories of social work on the front lines and providing platforms for knowledge sharing is a starting point for these emerging principles. These principles may encourage hospital administrators and social workers to be better prepared and have greater certainty about their roles and contributions in future pandemics.

BOX 5.1

REFLECTIVE QUESTIONS

1. How do the issues raised in this chapter relate to health social work in your country?
2. What were some of the challenges encountered by your local hospital social workers during COVID-19?
3. What unique knowledge and skills do social workers need to be prepared for pandemic hospital work?
4. What should health institutions do to better support social workers in pandemic conditions?

References

Alford, G.W. L., & Chester, R. (2020). *Providing soul care in the COVID-19 era.* The Center to Advance Palliative Care. https://www.capc.org/blog/providing-soul-care-covid-19-era/

Brailsford, J. (2020, May 20). *Supporting underhoused and homeless patients during COVID-19.* Women's College Hospital Connect. https://www.womenscollegehospital.ca/news-and-publications/connect/may-20,-2020/social-workers-in-the-aacu

Casey, A. (2020). *Medical social work teams: The impact of the Covid-19 pandemic.* Irish Social Work: Blogging on contemporary social work. https://irishsocialwork.wordpress.com/2020/05/05/medical-social-work-teams-the-impact-of-the-covid-19-pandemic/

CDC. (2020). *Coronavirus and disease 2019 (COVID-19).* Centers for Disease Control. https://www.cdc.gov/coronavirus/2019-ncov/faq.html#Basics

Cheung J. C. (2020). What have hospital social workers been prepared for COVID-19 from SARS, MERS, and H1N1? *Health & Social Work*, 45(3), 211–214.

Craig, S. L., Eaton, A., Belitsky, M., Kates, L., Dimitropolous, G., & Tobin, J. (2020). Empowering the team: A social work model of interprofessional collaboration in hospitals. *Journal of Interprofessional Education and Practice*, 19. https://doi.org/10.1016/j.xjep.2020.100327

Craig, S. L., & Muskat, B. (2013). Bouncers, Brokers, and Glue: The self-described roles of social workers in urban hospitals. *Health and Social Work*, 38(1), 7–16.

Gearing, R.E., Saini, M., & McNeill, T. (2007). Experiences and implications of social workers practicing in a pediatric hospital environment affected by SARS. *Health and Social Work*, 32(1), 17–27.

Government of Ontario (2020, April). *COVID-19, Status of cases.* https://covid-19.ontario.ca/index.html

Harslof, I., Nielsen, U.S., & Feiring, M. (2017). Danish and Norwegian hospital social workers' cross-institutional work amidst inter-sectoral restructuring of health and social welfare. *European Journal of Social Work,* 20(4), 584–595.

Hutchinson, D. (2020, April 20). Social workers playing critical role during coronavirus (COVID-19) crisis. *Click on Detroit.* https://www.clickondetroit.com/health/good-health/2020/04/20/social-workers-playing-critical-role-during-coronavirus-covid-19-crisis/

Judd, R. G., & Sheffield, S. (2010). Hospital social work: Contemporary roles and professional activities. *Social Work in Health Care*, 49(9), 856–871.

Kerson, T. S., & McCoyd, J. L. M. (2013). In response to need: An analysis of social work roles over time. *Social Work*, 58(4), 333–343.

Krasniansky, A. (2020). *Social workers and chaplains at the front lines during COVID-19*. Bill of Health: Harvard Law School. https://blog.petrieflom.law.harvard.edu/2020/04/17/social-workers-chaplains-telehealth-covid19/

Levin-Dagan, N., & Strenfeld-Hever, S. (2020). Reflections on Israeli hospital-based social work with COVID-19 patients and their families. *International Social Work*, 63(6), 766–770.

Muskat, B., Craig, S. L., & Mathai, B. (2017). Complex families, the social determinants of health and psychosocial interventions: Deconstruction of a day in the life of hospital social workers. *Social Work in Health Care*, 56(8), 765–778.

Nam, S.I., Choi, K., & Kim, J. (2019). Role changes of hospital social workers in South Korea. *Social Work in Health Care,* 58(7), 703–717.

Newman-Breman, K. (2020, May 27). *A social worker on how to support our most vulnerable during COVID-19*. Refinery29. https://www.refinery29.com/en-ca/2020/05/9831076/social-worker-coronavirus-pandemic

Ontario Association of Social Workers. (2013). *Social work in hospital-based health care*. Revised 2013. https://www.oasw.org/

Ontario Association of Social Workers. (2018). *A snapshot of social work in Ontario: Key indicators for sustaining a critical profession*. https://www.oasw.org/

Ontario Association of Social Workers. (2020). Final decision made by government on pandemic pay. https://www.oasw.org/Public/Announcements/Final_Decision_Made_by_Government_on_Pandemic_Pay.aspx

Ontario College of Social Workers and Social Service Workers. (2020). Message from the Registrar & CEO regarding COVID-19. https://www.ocswssw.org/2020/03/13/message-from-the-registrar-ceo-regarding-covid-19/

Ontario College of Social Workers and Social Service Workers. (2015). *Response from the Ontario College of Social Workers and Social Service Workers (OCSWSSW) February 2009 in regard to the Health Professions Regulatory Advisory Council (HPRAC) Interim Report to the Minister of Health and Long-Term Care on Mechanisms to Facilitate and Support Interprofessional Collaboration Among Health Colleges and Regulated Health Professionals*. https://www.ocswssw.org/wp-content/uploads/2015/01/HPRAC-Critical-Links-Submission.pdf

Ontario COVID-19 Mental Health Network. (2020). https://covid19therapists.com

Ontario Ministry of Health, Ontario Ministry of Long-Term Care. (2020a). *Health workforce planning branch regulated health professions.* http://www.health.gov.on.ca/en/pro/programs/hhrsd/about/regulated_professions.aspx

Ontario Ministry of Health, Ontario Ministry of Long-Term Care. (2020b). *Understanding health care in Ontario*. http://www.health.gov.on.ca/en/ministry/hc_system/

Public Safety Canada (2020). *Guidance on essential services and functions in Canada during the COVID-19 pandemic*. https://www.publicsafety.gc.ca/cnt/ntnl-scrt/crtcl-nfrstrctr/esf-sfe-en.aspx

Rosoff, P.M. (2008). The ethics of care: Social workers in an influenza pandemic. *Social Work in Health Care*, 47(1), 49–59.

Rowlands, A. (2007). Medical social work practice and SARS in Singapore. *Social Work in Health Care,* 45(3), 57–83.

Shemelia, C. (2020, April). A frontline social worker's perspective on COVID-19. *The New Social Worker*. https://www.socialworker.com/feature-articles/practice/front-line-social-worker-perspective-covid-19/

Whitten, D. (2020). COVID-19 and the social work response-The need for long-term solutions. *Social Work Today*. https://www.socialworktoday.com/news/enews_0520_1.shtml.

6

CHILD PROTECTION AND HEALTH EMERGENCIES IN BOTSWANA

Thabile A. Samboma

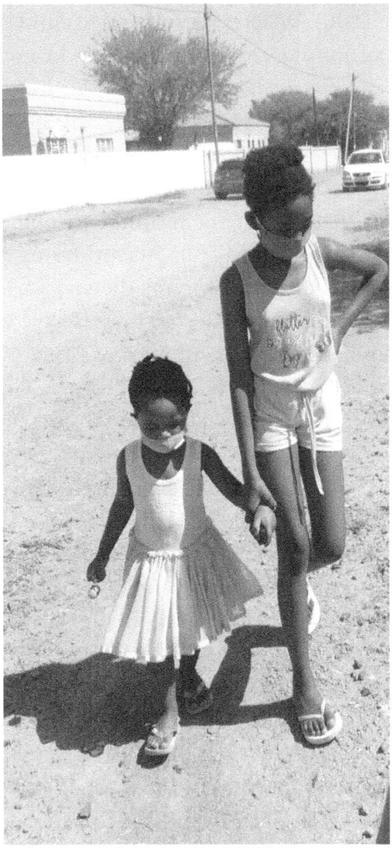

FIGURE 6.0 Children in the village of Tlokweng during lockdown

Source: Photograph by Thabile A. Samboma

DOI: 10.4324/9781003111214-8

Botswana is an upper-middle-income country that has witnessed rapid economic growth for most of its post-independence period since attaining self-governance from Britain in 1966 (Seleka & Lekobane, 2017). Botswana is landlocked in the centre of Southern Africa, bordered by Namibia, Zambia, Zimbabwe and South Africa. Botswana has a relatively young population, of about 2.3 million of which 34.7% of the total population are children less than 15 years of age (CSO, 2017). With such a small population, Botswana is considered to be among the fortunate nations in Africa and has experienced less turbulence in both the political and social aspects of its development.

Since independence, COVID-19 is only the second health emergency to affect the country, the first being HIV/AIDS. Botswana has been dealing with HIV/AIDS for decades with the first case in Botswana diagnosed in 1985. By the early 90s, Botswana had been hard hit by HIV/AIDS leaving many children orphaned and vulnerable, with some children heading households. The Government of Botswana (GoB) defines an orphan as a "child below 18 years who has lost one (single) or both parents (married couples), these parents are either biological or adoptive" (GoB, 2008, 2010). Whereas a vulnerable child is "a child below age of 18 years who; lives in an abusive environment; lives in a poverty-stricken family and cannot access basic services; heads a household; lives with a sick parent(s)/guardian; is infected with HIV and lives outside family care" (GoB, 2008).

Botswana demonstrated a strong commitment in responding to its HIV pandemic by providing universal free antiretroviral treatment to people living with HIV and providing drugs to pregnant mothers through a programme called Prevention of Mother to Child (PMTC). According to Arnab and Serumaga-Zake (2006), the provision of antiretroviral therapy to Botswana citizens and the different HIV/AIDS initiatives and programmes have saved the lives of many parents and children and reduced the number of orphans and vulnerable children. The experience of HIV/AIDS bode well for the GoB's commitment to a COVID-19 response, particularly in relation to the protection of its children.

The GoB reacted quickly and decisively to halt the spread of COVID-19, closing its borders on 24 March 2020. The first confirmed COVID-19 case was reported on the 30th of March. In response, Botswana declared a state of emergency and subsequently imposed an initial 28-day lockdown on the 2nd of April. Later further restrictions on movement were implemented. Lockdown and physical distancing measures adopted by the government severely impacted on the livelihood of Botswana's children. Other direct effects of the COVID-19 pandemic have been minimal in the country, with less than 45 deaths as of December 2020, attributable to fast and decisive action after the first three cases were reported. Although COVID-19 and HIV/AIDS are transmitted differently, their impact affected the lives of children the most.

This chapter discusses child protection in Botswana and explores the impact of COVID-19 on children and those that serve them to prevent and respond to violence, exploitation and abuse against children. For the purpose of this study, child protection in Botswana includes a broad spectrum of activities, projects, programs, policies, within an institutional framework which focuses on the fulfilment of children's rights, implemented by both state and non-state actors.

The child protection framework

To fully appreciate child protection in Botswana, it is important to understand how this sector has evolved over time to its current structures and is still developing to address the needs of children. Agencies in the sector evolved from charity-based institutions that approached children's issues from a charitable mindset to current institutions that employ a range of approaches from needs-based to rights-based programs currently delivered to children and families. In the 1990s when Botswana was hard hit by HIV/AIDS, there was mushrooming of donor funded NGOs that dealt with issues of HIV/AIDS. The economic status of Botswana has since changed and is now rated among middle income countries. This led to the closure of many donor funded NGOs with the remaining struggling financially.

In Botswana, there is an array of government ministries, departments, and committees that work with non-state actors, and faith-based organisations in the interests of children within a legislative framework. The United Nations International Children's Emergency Fund (UNICEF) advises the government, actively participating in the development and review of laws as well as monitoring the well-being of children and promoting that children's rights. Table 6.1 outlines the ministries, departments and committees that protect children.

TABLE 6.1 Child protection institutional framework in Botswana

Ministry of Local Government and Rural Development (MLGRD)	Holds the mandate for child welfare and children's rights. Responsible for social policies, laws and programmes for vulnerable groups – children, women and the poor.
Department of Child Protection (DCP)	Administered by the MLGRD and responsible for children's social protection, identification, assessment and registration of orphans, and to ensure an efficient and effective system of providing material and emotional support services to them.
National Children's Council (NCC)	Established by Section 35 of the Children's Act of 2009 to coordinate, support, monitor and ensure the implementation of sectoral Ministries' activities relating to children with overall responsibility for coordinating policies relating to children, monitoring the implementation of the children's rights and welfare issues.
Children's Consultative Forum (CCF)	Established through Child Act 2009.The forum constitutes ten children's representative from each district.
Department of Social and Community Development (S&CD)	Located in all local authorities and are the largest employer of social workers. Social workers provide generic services, e.g., psychosocial support, counselling and mediation to communities and families, register and maintain the database of orphans, and donate uniforms and food baskets to the needy.
Village Child Committee (VCC)	Educates communities about neglect, ill treatment, exploitation or other abuse of children and to monitor the welfare of children in their respective communities.
Non-State Actors	Civil society Organisations engage with government and other child protection actors to advocate for children and their voice.

(Continued)

TABLE 6.1 Child protection institutional framework in Botswana (*Continued*)

Botswana Police	Have a frontline, central role in protecting children, preventing and investigating crime that violates children's rights.
Magistrate Courts	Under the Child Act 2009, all magistrate courts act as children's courts tasked with overseeing judicial processes related to child abuse and neglect.

In 1995, Botswana ratified the Convention on the Rights of the Child (CRC) and the African Charter on the Rights and Welfare of Children in 2001 (Maundeni, 2009). The Child Act of 2009 incorporates the provisions of the United Nations Charter on the Rights of the Child (UNCRC) which Botswana accented to in 1985. In particular, the new 2009 Child Act has sections on foster care, child trafficking and abduction. The rights enshrined in the CRC run through the Sustainable Development Goals (SDGs) therefore the realisation of these goals must take into account the corresponding rights of children (Wernham, 2018). Several developments to improve child protection have been made in Botswana law including introducing an offence called defilement to protect children under 18, the prioritisation of children's cases that should be quickly dealt with by the courts, raising the marriage age to 21, allowing pregnant girls to attend school, making it illegal to refuse immunisation, and introducing safeguards in border control to curb trafficking.

Critical to children's rights was the development of Botswana's national strategy called Vision 2036 which presents the country's aspiration for its future. One of its four pillars is Human and Social Development which states Botswana will have a safe environment that enables children to grow to reach their potential. This will be achieved by developing strong family support, a safe and secure environment, quality education and health, and the empowerment of children to understand their rights and responsibilities (GoB, 2019). In 2015, Botswana adopted the 2030 Agenda for Sustainable Development which gave Botswana an opportunity to place the protection and interest of children at the heart of policy to ensure all children will be free from fear and violence in all its forms.

The GoB plays an active role in providing social protection by investing in goods and services including education, housing, water and sanitation (Nthomang, 2007). Because the GoB recognises that children are a vulnerable group, several programs to support children have been established. For instance, a feeding program run in all government schools provides children with meals. The Orphan Care Programme (OCP) provides direct benefits for orphans and vulnerable children by ensuring orphans remain in school. Children are provided with appropriate nutritional supplements and are helped to overcome the feeling of loss and trauma following death of parents. There are also special provisions for the children of remote area dwellers provided under the Remote Area Development Programme. Chinyoka and Ulriksen (2020) describe child welfare policy in Botswana as a *familial child welfare regime* where public provision for children reflects a primary commitment to the family. Transfers in the form of coupons are provided for orphans but not for non-orphaned children regardless of how poor they are. Instead, poor families with children are supported through workfare or other (mostly in-kind) payments to adults, and through feeding schemes. The familial benefits are generous per household but not generous per person relative to the national and international poverty lines.

Alternative care in Botswana

In Botswana, there are children living with disabilities, vulnerable children and orphaned children. Based on assessment, some children require alternative care. Alternative care is the "legal temporary transfer of a person below the age of 18 years, who is in need of care, to a place of safety, being an individual, family or residential facility, where provision is made for social, spiritual, psychological, economic, and mental well-being in the best interest of the child" (CSO, 2005).

Kinship care

Kinship care provided by relatives, members of communities and others who have a kinship bond with a child, is the preferred form of care to protect children whose parents are unable to do so (Testa & Rolock, 1999). In Botswana the well-being of children is considered the responsibility of the community where they live, a position reinforced by sayings such as "it takes a whole village to bring up a child". Historically, traditional kinship care by extended family members including aunts, uncles, grandparents, and other relatives, is common throughout sub-Saharan Africa, Botswana included. Extended family members care for children for a variety of reasons including the death of mothers in childbirth and for youth to gain access to education and is a vital coping mechanism in Botswana (Madhavan, 2004). However, due to urbanisation and rapid population growth during the 20th century, the phenomena of child neglect emerged and children living on the streets became a common feature in most urban centres. Additionally, the early 1990s was a nightmare for Botswana as the country was hit hard by HIV/AIDS, severely disrupting traditional family structures and communities. The HIV/AIDS pandemic left many children orphaned.

Institutional care

In Botswana. a child who is a registered orphan will live with their relatives except in extreme cases. The likelihood that a child will be placed in an orphanage is very remote (GoB, 2017). The GoB is of the opinion that children should grow up in families instead of institutions. However, taking into consideration the changes that have taken place in our society, Botswana has since embraced residential care institutions. Maundeni (2009) stated that there are several types of residential care including those for abused, neglected and abandoned children and facilities for children living with disabilities. Botswana has small scale residential facilities that provide a home like setting. These are residential child welfare institutions approved by the GoB, and they include three SOS Children's Villages (Tlokweng, Serowe, Francistown), Childline Botswana, Mpule Kwelagobe Children's Home. The institutions are home to about 625 children across Botswana (GoB, 2017). The private SOS villages aim to provide a home and family for destitute, abandoned and orphaned children housed in family units headed by SOS *mothers*. Childline Botswana, an NGO, was founded in 1990 in response to the escalating number of child abuse cases. Mpule Kwelagobe Centre also provides a home to abused and orphaned children (UNICEF, 2007).

Foster care

Child protection concerns indicate that many children in Botswana are in need of care that can cater for their needs because extended families are no longer coping with the for a variety of reasons. Discussions have alluded to adoption and residential care that do help to a certain extent but face many challenges and are not ideal, whereas statutory foster care provides a system where a child can be cared for and protected. The 2009 Child Act make provisions for foster care arrangements. The government saw it fit to have a pool of foster parents who can provide non-institutional, emergency safe places for children in need of care. The first foster care program was piloted in 2007 by Childline Botswana in collaboration with Ministry of Local Government and Rural development.

Child protection during COVID-19

Like the rest of the world, child protection in Botswana was seriously challenged with COVID-19 in the picture. According to the World Health Organisation, infectious diseases like COVID-19 disrupt the environments in which children grow and develop (WHO, 2020). The virus affected children in three main ways:

1. through infection with the virus itself
2. through the social and economic impacts of control, containment and mitigation measures, intended to reduce or stop transmission of the virus in various contexts and
3. through the potential longer-term effects of the crisis including economic downturn and a delay on progress towards achieving the SDGs (UN, 2020).

Additionally, many of the prevention and control measures adopted by Botswana to contain the coronavirus have resulted in disruptions in the reporting and referral mechanisms of child protection services and challenges in responding, leaving many children and families especially vulnerable.

Child poverty

Even though Botswana's economic status is highly proclaimed, impressive as it is, the story only paints a partial picture of the poverty situation in the country (Lekobane & Roelen, 2020). With respect to children, poverty incidence is higher than it is for adults. Botswana's child poverty is at 20.1% compared to 13.8% for adults (CSO, 2018). Children in Botswana are more vulnerable to poverty than any other population group because they lack both agency and assets. Children are therefore dependent on others to meet their basic needs which are essential for their development (Baaitse, 2020; Trani & Cannings, 2013). The hidden impacts of pandemic response measures, especially the effects of lockdown on family finances and their ability to sustain livelihoods and to make ends meet, further impacted on children's health, nutrition, education, learning, protection, well-being, and increased poverty. For the most marginalised and deprived children, these impacts have the potential to be life-altering and potentially devastating. According to Loperfido et al. (2020), COVID-19 is likely to push children into poverty or increase the depth of poverty for children already living below the poverty line.

According to Lekobane and Roelen (2020), double and single orphaned children experience higher incidences and intensity of poverty compared to children with two living parents. Looking at the Botswana situation, the hardship for children who have lost their parents to HIV/AIDS and now COVID-19 is significant. The government is committed to ensuring that children do not live in poverty and pledged that social protection programs would continue during COVID-19 providing services such as ensuring food baskets were donated.

Child education

Even though Botswana is among the least affected countries by COVID-19, schools across the country closed. During lockdown different schools adopted various alternative measures to teach children such as doing schoolwork online and using various platforms such as WhatsApp, email, skype and so on. Although these are commendable approaches, existing inequalities were exacerbated and children who were already most at risk of being excluded from a quality education were most affected. The digital divide limited many children's access to education, information, staying in touch with friends and family, and enjoying digital entertainment during COVID-19. Furthermore, children of school age are not taught in their mother language which posed obstacles and language barriers to effective communication about staying safe from COVID-19 and other information needed by children. The Government intervened to ensure messages spread by media were broadcasted in various languages.

COVID-19 also showed disparities between public and private schools. Under normal circumstance, institutions of child protection have to work together, but certain things were not done in the best interest of children. For instance, as schools reopened, the government's emphasis was on ensuring that public schools adhered to all COVID-19 protocols whereas private schools were at liberty to open schools provided they felt satisfied. Government inspectors were deployed to schools, however media reports stated that some private schools denied government inspectors access to their premises.

Although Botswana recognises that every child has the right to free basic education, 10%–15% of primary school aged children and 38% of secondary school aged children are not in school (CSO, 2018). Lack of proper education affects many children especially those children in rural areas as in most cases they do not continue their education.

Child health

In Botswana, there is a 90% chance that a child will be born in a health facility with the assistance of trained professionals (GoB, 2017). Although essential services such as health care professionals were not in lockdown, it is still unclear if movement restrictions affected the ability of people to visit clinics and hospitals for their medications. Among the HIV/AIDS patients are children living with the virus who needs routine check-ups. At present, there is no data available on those who have defaulted from taking medication during COVID-19. To curb the virus spread, the GoB set up a mechanism to quarantine COVID-19 patients so that they don't mix with other patients. This move was intended to allow adults and children to continue visiting health facilities and to ensure children could still get their immunisations. It is against the laws of Botswana for a child under five years of age to be denied immunisations and the government emphasised that guardians should continue taking children for their monthly check-ups during COVID-19.

Children with disabilities

Children with disabilities are among the most vulnerable groups of children in Botswana. According to Deen (2014), children with disabilities are segregated in Botswana especially in the educational system which lacks any form of inclusive education. Children have an opportunity to gain formal education only in special schools, most of which are owned by non-governmental organisations. Deen (2014) argues that this is completely contrary to children's rights to inclusive education as guaranteed in international human rights instruments specifically the Convention on the Rights of Persons with Disabilities (CRPD). According to Mitchell and Desai (2003), inclusive education starts with all students with special needs having access to the same educational opportunities as other children.

Although Botswana did not lag in embracing e-learning in schools. Unfortunately, for children living with disabilities, many special education schools, cannot provide e-learning, The infrastructure in schools is not COVID-19 disability friendly and most of the students are from less privileged households with no computers and internet access at home (Mabote, 2020).

COVID-19 was quite a challenging time for children living with disabilities due to restrictions on visiting especially for those children living in residential centres. Visiting restrictions at centres had negative mental health consequences for the children as they lost connections with families. Children with disabilities cannot physically distance as per COVID-19 health protocols as they constantly need support from their caregivers therefore a blanket approach on physical distancing was difficult to uphold and additional safety measures were needed.

Refugee children

Lekobane and Roelen (2020) stated that in terms of citizenship, Botswana is peculiar, non-citizen children have lower poverty incidences than citizens, an unusual situation compared to many other countries worldwide. The majority of non-citizens live in cities or towns where poverty levels are lower and employment opportunities exist. However, loss of employment was a risk during COVID-19 especially for non-citizen children, the majority (60.4%) of whom are from Zimbabwe, 9.9% from South Africa, 14.9% other parts of Africa and 12.6% from elsewhere (Lekobane & Roelen, 2020).

Botswana has not signed the International Convention on the Protection of the Rights of All Migrant Workers and Members of their Families (1990) which affects child refugees. Although non-citizens are reported to experience less incidence of poverty, refugee children face access barriers to services, including schooling and higher education primarily because of their ineligibility for government tertiary student sponsorship (Mmegi Monitor, 2019). As it stands currently, refugee children face significant challenges in engaging in education due to language barriers and cultural aspects taking precedence over policy, especially for refugee children with disabilities, a situation not improved during the pandemic. Refugee children also faced access barriers to health services and essential medicines which made their circumstances in pandemic conditions especially difficult.

Child trafficking

There is an emerging trend of trafficking involving children in Botswana. Children most vulnerable to trafficking are those from unemployed parents, rural poor families, children of agricultural workers and undocumented children from neighbouring countries. Several factors make the children of Botswana vulnerable, among them poverty and lack of education. A report on trafficking in Botswana by the US Department of State (USDS, 2019) pointed to how some parents in poor rural communities send their children to work for wealthier families as domestic servants in cities or in agriculture and cattle farming in remote areas, which increases their vulnerability to child trafficking. Fortunately, with movement restrictions and borders closed there were no new cases of trafficking reported during the COVID-19 period in 2020.

Child labour

In 2016, data published by UNICEF stated that approximately 9% of children in Botswana were engaged in child labour (UNICEF, 2016). The data did not provide information about the sectors, types of activities, and hazards children encounter as child labourers. However, children in Botswana do engage in the worst forms of child labour, including commercial sexual exploitation, cattle herding, and domestic work, each can be a result of human trafficking. According to Bureau of International Labour Affairs (2019), Botswana has made minimal advancement in efforts to eliminate the worst forms of child labour. Upon realising the general lack of awareness on child trafficking issues, the GoB in partnership with other relevant stakeholders embarked on a national campaign on Child Trafficking (UNICEF, 2010)

Key gaps remain in the country's legal framework, including the lack of a minimum age for compulsory education and insufficient prohibitions for hazardous work. In addition, social programs do not always reach intended child labour victims, especially those engaged in cattle herding and domestic work (Bureau of International Labour Affairs, 2019). The government is not able to conduct labour inspections in private farms where child labour is widely believed to exist (USDS, 2018). The lack of accessibility to government social programs which are run monthly by social workers makes children more vulnerable to child labour. Cases of child labour were predicted to increase when COVID-19 restrictions were lifted because of the negative economic impact of lockdown on the families.

Child sexual abuse

COVID-19 quickly changed the context in which children live. Some prevention and control measures, such as home containment, school closures and restrictions on movement, have disrupted children's routines and social support. This meant children remained home with parents, relatives and caregivers. According to Samboma (2020), one would have thought staying home would be ideal for families to bond but unfortunately, the worst happened for some children. Lockdown resulted in increased risks of abuse for children living in unsafe conditions as it was impossible for children to escape abusive parents and guardians due to movement restrictions or closures of safe spaces (Samboma, 2020).

Over the years, there has been a rise in the number of child sexual abuse cases reported in Botswana. Although there is no comprehensive data on child sexual abuse available, reported cases paint an ugly picture of child sexual abuse. For instance, between January and September 2020, police in Kweneng district recorded 107 cases of defilement. Another disheartening statistic is from the Ngamiland district which recorded a total of 528 child pregnancies between January 2020 and November 2020. The number included girls who were still at primary school (Morokotso, 2020). After the first lockdown, the Minister of Basic Education expressed concern that 58 girls returned to school pregnant. It is of paramount importance to note that these are just the few cases that have been reported to relevant authorities, with many cases going unreported.

A study by Rudolph et al. (2017) identified drug and alcohol abuse, parental absence and poverty as factors that increase the risk of a child experiencing sexual abuse. The Kweneng and Ngamiland districts have a high rate of poverty, an element that makes children vulnerable. A study done by International Labour Organization in 2012 at Francistown, situated in the northern part of Botswana, indicated that older men (although there were a few cases of women) use money to obtain consensual sex from young girls (USDS, 2012). Most of these children are from poor families and resort to commercial sex for a living (Kayawe, 2016). Furthermore, it is common in Botswana for parents or guardians to conceal child sexual abuse for various reason but mostly because of commercial gain, stigma and culture.

As well as the broader community, the GoB also wants all children to be educated and informed on child protection concerns within schools and Codes of Conduct for teachers be strengthened to include forbidding sexual abuse and physical and humiliating punishments. Recently during the State of Nation Address, the government committed to ensuring that children and women were protected by prioritizing their issues. The Botswana justice system has been failing children as cases take a long time to go to trial even though the courts claim that children's cases are prioritised but this has not been the case since the inception of Child Act 2009.

Child marriage

Child marriage in Botswana is a hidden problem. The UN Population Fund (UNFPA) partnered with Botswana's Ministry of Health and Wellness in a bid to end child marriages and gender-based violence. As the UNFPA's program specialist, Boago Makatane reported, 1,644 children were in marriage relationships and 3,748 were living in cohabitation in Botswana (Ghanaian Times, 2019). He went on to say that children aged between 12 and 15 years made up 60% of the 1,644 cases while the rest were 16–17 years old, all are below the legal age of consent. There is a very high possibility that COVID-19 may have made children more vulnerable to child marriage even though there is no consolidated data of child marriages taken during lockdown but the rate of child sexual abuse cases is a good indicator of child marriage as child sexual abuse and child marriage are intertwined in many cases.

Challenges during COVID-19

Systemic challenges

Botswana's child protection system is still developing, and a number of barriers exist. For example, the National Children's Council cannot fully execute its mandate due to a lack of finances and the Council felt left out by sectoral ministries during COVID-19 recovery plan engagements. The Children's Consultative Forum, although the voice of children in Tswana culture, currently does not hold much political weight but is a positive step towards realising children's rights in Botswana.

Even though civil societies play a critical role in communities, their benefits are skewed towards urban areas as most NGOs are concentrated in towns and cities with very few in rural areas and, in some places, non-existent. Civil society actors decried a lack of funding during lockdowns, the worst periods during COVID-19. Many civil societies in Botswana depend on European countries for funding. Limited available funds during COVID-19 posed serious setbacks as child protection mandates were hampered. As with many countries that rely on many NGOs to deliver many services, poor coordination of child protection institutions in Botswana is a big problem. Institutions of child protection tend to work in silos producing fragmented service delivery.

Village Child Committees (VCC) do not receive government funding although they are on the front line of child protection. Committees are made up of a village chief, social worker and other members of the community. Committees are elected in an open area, a traditional place of gathering (*kgotla*). Committee members ask about referrals and report cases to the relevant authority. Critical as their function is, they lack capacity and in some parts of the country are not functional.

The police, also frontline workers, experienced a surge in violence against women and children during the pandemic but are ill-equipped lacking the technical capacity to manage the range of child protection issues they face. There are still no proper structures for children's courts eleven years after the implementation of Child Act of 2009, and magistrate courts are still fulfilling this function. There is no doubt that magistrates in Botswana are trained people, however they are not experts in child protection matters. The health emergency heightened these structural weaknesses.

The impact of COVID-19 on social work in child protection services

In Botswana social workers are employed by governmental, non-governmental, and commercial agencies where they provide various services to individuals, families, and communities. Social workers, engaged by the GoB in various departments, are professionals with formal training. The majority of social workers in Botswana are degree holders. Some have Diplomas and Master degrees. Social work education in Botswana is offered by the Department of Social Work in the Faculty of Social Sciences at the University of Botswana (UB) and there are private institutions that offer the same degree. The majority of social workers offer generic services. Their major functions are to implement the Destitution Programme, provide clinical social work, rehabilitation programmes, capacity building for community development, and to intervene with families, work with foster care, adoption and child protection, probation and after care services, and project management.

During lockdowns, social workers were working around the clock distributing food baskets. In response to workload demands, the government engaged 934 temporary social workers to assist in the assessment of those who qualified for food baskets. The majority of the engaged workers were professional social workers while others worked closely with social workers on daily basis. More social workers were deployed to quarantine centres and hospitals to counsel people during this time (BOPA, 2020a). Because the focus of social workers was on distributing food donations to people affected by lockdowns, the provision of psychosocial support and children's safety were overshadowed (Samboma, 2020). To some extent, as government moved swiftly to contain the virus and social workers became food administrators, services that were essential and commendable, the rights and well-being of children were neglected in this period. Child protection agencies experienced strained resources with fewer workers available. Stay-at-home orders made conducting home visits and carrying out other duties difficult. Because children were not going to school, child protection actors such as teachers and counsellors were unable to bear witness or report signs of abuse to the relevant authorities. As well as child protection concerns, there was a general lack of education among communities on how COVID-19 affects children's physical and psychosocial well-being. Under normal circumstances, culturally, it is uncommon to take children for professional counselling which further complicates the care of children.

Social workers in Botswana do not work shifts. During COVID-19 they worked long hours resulting in fatigue. This had a negative impact on their professional obligations as they needed to debrief with their own social support networks and hence were vulnerable to breaking the ethical requirement of confidentiality. Ethical dilemmas and practice challenges were a significant feature of professionals' everyday work during the crisis. Furthermore, the lack of rotational shifts put children in danger when incidents of abuse occurred after hours and some families had to wait for an intervention the next day.

There were health risks to social workers undertaking their duties during the pandemic and there is no risk allowance for social workers. However, social workers employed by government are covered by government compensation if they are hurt while on duty. When a social worker assessing a family for a COVID-19 basket was attacked by the father using a slasher, the nation was left in shock (BOPA, 2020b). As well as indicating the danger for social workers going from house to house in emergency situations, the incident could also be an indication of the severe stress and impact on the mental health of people during the crisis as well as boundary issues for social workers working in the communities where they live.

Conclusion

The main observation in the context of Botswana, is that child protection suffered serious deficits in institutional capacity applicable to all child protection organisations in the Child Protection Institutional Framework. Child friendly infrastructures such as children's courts, disabilities services and other specialised child protection structures need to be established alongside better cooperation and coordination between them, needed for the future. Children's services across health, education and social services sectors have been characterised by a preoccupation with risk and an increasingly bureaucratic and *technical* approach to assessing need. Rather than focusing only on *risky* individuals, all governments must recognise the importance of orienting services to alleviate the precarious and fragile living conditions for some families that create risks to children.

Several challenges to child protection during COVID-19 have been identified in this chapter that require further development. Thus far, there is no consolidated data on how COVID-19 has affected different aspects of children's lives in Botswana. Despite positive responses and new ways of working that could be promoted in the future, the COVID-19 crisis has spotlighted and exacerbated existing problems in the system. For example, to ensure all the rights of children including the right to safety, the technological divide needs to be addressed to ensure access for all children in Botswana. Digital communication with children can provide important access to information and provide safeguards. Capacity building is needed to assist teachers and social workers to overcome their trepidation about technology. While doing so, it is also important to undertake measures to prevent the online abuse of children.

The GoB has made efforts to establish a National Social Protection Recovery Plan to address child vulnerability and provide protection and support for children and young people in the wake of COVID-19. However, caution is indicated when designing social programmes as they are implemented in a variety of distinct political, social, economic and cultural contexts, each of which involves different child protection issues. A one-size-fits-all program, especially as the longer-term impact of COVID-19 has not yet unfolded, will not properly address need. Furthermore, more government investment is needed in child protection especially for training child protection actors and public education about all forms of abuse such as child trafficking and child sexual abuse. When child protection actors lack specialised knowledge and skills in child protection, efforts to protect the rights of children are severely hindered, especially in health emergencies.

BOX 6.1

REFLECTIVE QUESTIONS

1. Think about child protection in your country or state. Who are the actors involved and how are services for children coordinated and delivered?
2. Developing communities help protect children where resources are scarce. Consider how developing community capacity could be part of your social work practice?
3. Thinking about the experiences of children at risk during COVID-19 lockdowns, what lessons need to be brought forward in the next health emergency?

References

Arnab, R., & Serumaga-Zake, P. A. E. (2006). Orphans and vulnerable children in Botswana: The impact of HIV/AIDS. *Vulnerable Children and Youth Studies*, 1(3), 221–229.

Baaitse, D. (2020, February 17). Botswana children are vulnerable to ultra-poverty. *Weekend Post, Insightful*. http://www.weekendpost.co.bw/24855/news/botswana-children-are-vulnerable-to-ultra-poverty/

BOPA. (2020a, May 10). Botswana: COVID-19 social protection to continue. *All Africa*. https://allafrica.com/stories/202005110480.html

BOPA. (2020b, April 30). Daily news: Social worker attacked while assessing family for COVID-19 food basket. *Daily News*. http://www.dailynews.gov.bw/news-details.php?nid=55923

Bureau of International Labour Affairs. (2019). *Child labour and forced labour reports*. https://www.dol.gov/agencies/ilab

Chinyoka, I., & Ulriksen, M. (2020). The limits of the influence of international donors: Social protection in Botswana. In C. Schmitt (Ed.), *From colonialism to international aid: External actors and social protection in the global south* (pp. 245–271). Cham: Springer International Publishing.

CSO. (2005). *Botswana AIDS impact survey II (BAIS II)*. Gaborone, Botswana: Central Statistics Office.

CSO. (2017). *Botswana demographic survey report 2017*. Gaborone Botswana: Central Statistics Office.

CSO. (2018). *Botswana multi-topic household survey report 2015/16*. Gaborone: Central Statistics Office.

Deen, T. (2014, August 18). The myth of inclusive education in Botswana. *AfricLaw: Advancing the Rule and Role of Law in Africa*. https://africlaw.com/?s=The+myth+of+inclusive+education+in+Botswana

Ghanaian Times. (2019, July 1). UN agency partners Botswana to end child marriages: Official. *Ghanaian Times*. http://www.ghanaiantimes.com.gh/un-agency-partners-botswana-to-end-child-marriages-official/

GoB. (2008). *National situation analysis on orphans and vulnerable children in Botswana*. Gaborone: Ministry of Local Government & Rural Development, Government of Botswana.

GoB. (2010). *National guidelines on the care of orphans and vulnerable children*. Gaborone: Ministry of Local Government & Rural Development, Government of Botswana.

GoB. (2017). *Report submitted by the Republic of Botswana to the Committee on the Rights of Child on the Implementation of the UNCRC*. Gaborone: Ministry of Local Government & Rural Development. (MLG&RD), Government of Botswana.

GoB. (2019). *Vision 2036: Prosperity for all*. Botswana: Government of Botswana. Government Printers. https://vision2036.org.bw/

Kayawe, B. (2016). The secret hell of child sex abuse. *Mmegi Online*. https://www.mmegi.bw/index.php/index.php?aid=59927&dir=2016/may/13

Lekobane, K. R., & Roelen, K. (2020). Leaving no one behind: Multidimensional child poverty in Botswana. *Child Indicators Research*, 13. https://doi.org/10.1007/s12187-020-09744-6

Loperfido, L., Burgess, M., Dulieu, N., Orlassino, C., Sulaiman, M., & Arlini, A. M. (2020). *The hidden impact of COVID-19 on child poverty*. London: Save the Children International. https://resourcecentre.savethechildren.net/node/18174/pdf/the_hidden_impact_of_covid-19_on_child_poverty.pdf

Mabote, T. (2020, July 7). COVID-19: Anxiety disorders profound in children living with disabilities. *Global Post*. http://www.gpweekly.com/columns/covid-19-anxiety-disorders-profound-in-children-living-with-disabilities

Madhavan S. (2004). Fosterage patterns in the age of AIDS: Continuity and change. *Social Science & Medicine,* 58(7), 1443–1454.

Maundeni, T. (2009). Care for children in Botswana: The social work role. *Social work and Society*, 7(1). https://ejournals.bib.uni-wuppertal.de/index.php/sws/article/view/41

Mitchell D. & Desai I. (2003). Inclusive education for students with special needs. In J. P. Keeves & R. Watanabe. (Eds.), *International handbook of educational research in the Asia-Pacific region* (pp. 203–216). Dordrecht: Springer.

Morokotso, B. (2020, October 22). Over 500 girls impregnated this year in Ngami. *Sunday Standard.* https://www.sundaystandard.info/over-500-girls-impregnated-this-year-in-ngami/

Mmegi Monitor. (2019, February 25). Failing dreams of Dukwi refugee BGSCE top performers. *Mmegi Monitor.* https://www.mmegi.bw/index.php?aid=79781&dir=2019/february/25

Nthomang, K. (2007, November 17). *Provision of services and poverty reduction: The case of Botswana.* Geneva: UNRISD. https://www.unrisd.org/unrisd/website/document.nsf/(httpPublications)/B8AFAF7E9C8AEB33C1257AF600305225?OpenDocument

Rudolph, J., Zimmer-Gembeck, M.J., Shanley, D.C., & Hawkins, R. (2017). Child sexual abuse prevention opportunities: Parenting, programs, and the reduction of risk. *Child Maltreatment*, 23(1), 96–106.

Samboma, T.A. (2020). Vulnerability of children in Botswana during COVID-19. *International Social Work*, 63(6), 807–810.

Seleka, T. B., & Lekobane, K. R. (2017). Public transfers and participation decisions in Botswana's subsistence economy. *Review of Development Economics*, 21(4), 1380–1400.

Testa, M.F., & Rolock, N. (1999). Professional foster care: A future worth pursuing. *Journal of Child Welfare*, 78(1), 108–124.

Trani, J-F., & Cannings, T. I. (2013). Child poverty in an emergency and conflict context: A multidimensional profile and an identification of the poorest children in Western Darfur. *World Development,* 48, 48–70. https://doi.org/10.1016/j.worlddev.2013.03.005

UN. (2020). Achieving the SDGs through the COVID-19 response and recovery. https://www.un.org/development/desa/dpad/wp-content/uploads/sites/45/publication/PB_78.pdf

UNICEF. (2007). *A world fit for children: Mid- decade review-Botswana progress report.* Gaborone: UNICEF.

UNICEF. (2010). *Thari ya bana. Reflections on children in Botswana.* https://www.unicef.org/infobycountry/files/Thari_ya_bana_2010complete.pdf

UNICEF. (2016). *Findings of the worst form of child labour.* https://data.unicef.org/country/bwa/

USDS. (2012, June 19). *Trafficking in persons report – Botswana.* US Department of State. https://www.refworld.org/docid/4fe30cdf32.html

USDS. (2018). *Trafficking in persons report – Botswana.* US Department of State. https://www.state.gov/reports/2018-trafficking-in-persons-report-2/botswana/

USDS. (2019). *Trafficking in persons report – Botswana.* US Department of State. https://www.state.gov/reports/2019-trafficking-in-persons-report-2/botswana/

Wernham, M. (2018). *Mapping the global goals for sustainable development and convention on the rights of the child.* UNICEF. https://www.unicef.org/documents/mapping-global-goals-sustainable-development-and-convention-rights-child

WHO. (2020). *Q&A on coronaviruses (COVID-19): Can children or adolescents catch COVID-19?* https://www.who.int/emergencies/diseases/novel-coronavirus-2019/question-and-answers-hub/q-a-detail/q-a-coronaviruses

7

FAMILY VIOLENCE DURING THE COVID-19 PANDEMIC

Louise Harms, Eliza Crossley, Elyssa Hudson, Connie Kellett and Lauren Kosta

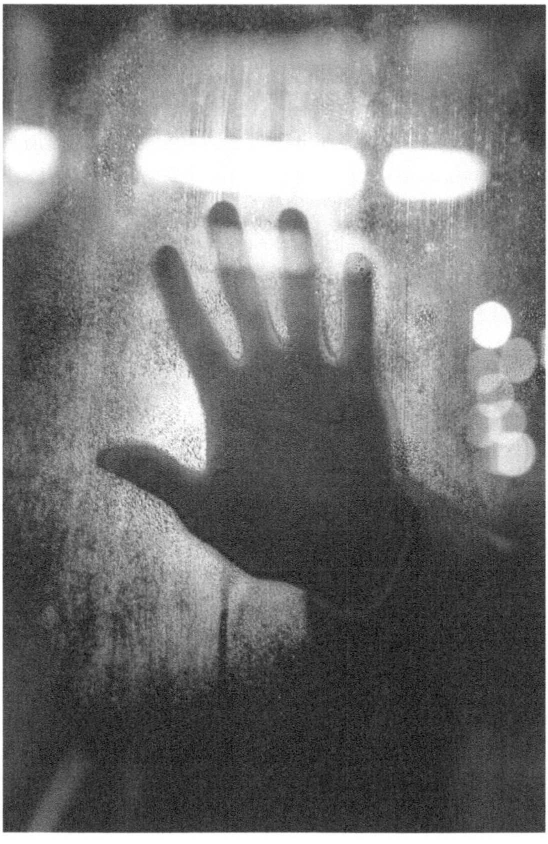

FIGURE 7.0 Family violence is a human rights issue

Source: Photographer Josh Hild

DOI: 10.4324/9781003111214-9

Like all disasters, health emergencies are complex, multidimensional events that can impact upon individual, family, community and global well-being (Drolet, 2019). They require the careful management of physical and mental health concerns in broader social, structural and cultural contexts. In managing particular aspects of one disaster, inadvertently another can be precipitated or exacerbated. This is seemingly the case in managing the coronavirus pandemic and its impact on family violence. The pandemic gives rise to the threats and realities of disease, hospitalisation and treatment, and, for some, death. Alongside this physical threat to life, and the associated trauma, stress and anxiety, specific and necessary public health prevention and intervention strategies have been implemented by many countries to contain virus transmission such strict lockdowns into household environments for extended periods of time. These lockdowns are often coupled with the loss of direct, in-person contact with family, friends, schools, workplaces and support services.

These important emergency management strategies, however, increase the risk factors for family violence – increased time with perpetrators; restricted access to family and friends, to workplaces and support services; financial stress and employment uncertainty; mental health responses such as anxiety, stress and trauma, and increases in alcohol consumption; and reinforced gender roles and expectations. The reported increase in family violence during the pandemic has been termed the *shadow pandemic* (Pfitzner, Fitz-Gibbon & True, 2020), consistent with other emergency contexts where it's referred to as the *hidden disaster* (Parkinson & Zara, 2013). Sophisticated social work responses are required that draw upon existing knowledge of family violence in non-disaster times and knowledge of the unique impacts that health emergencies can have on families and households.

For the purposes of this chapter, we use a widely accepted definition of family violence: "the use of threatening or violent behaviours within families which may be of a physical, sexual, psychological, or economic nature, and includes child abuse and intimate partner violence" (Peterman et al., 2020; van Gelder et al., 2020). Anecdotal evidence from social workers and other practitioners, as well as a small number of empirical studies, strongly suggest that throughout the pandemic there has been an increase in the frequency of family violence. Crucially, this is both in relationships where there is a history of interpersonal violence, as well as in relationships where there has not been violence previously. For social workers, this suggests complex causal pathways and risk factors need to be understood. Therefore, we consider now some of the evidence as to the prevalence and incidence of family violence during this pandemic.

Who is most at risk of family violence during COVID-19?

It is always challenging to have an accurate understanding of the extent of family violence in any community (Meyer & Frost, 2019) and all the more so during a disaster (Molyneaux et al., 2020). The complex nature of victim survivors' reporting of family violence and the difficulties in defining, reporting and data collection are well-noted reasons for the likely under-reporting of its accurate prevalence (Meyer & Frost, 2019).

While a deeper understanding of the complexities of family violence during COVID-19 is yet to emerge, throughout 2020, data from many countries (for example, Mexico, China, France, Lebanon, the United Kingdom and the Asia Pacific region) throughout 2020 indicate increases in family violence, primarily for women and children (Allen-Ebrahimian, 2020; Asia-Pacific Gender in Humanitarian Action Working Group, 2020; Henriques, 2020; Huerta, 2020; Morgan & Boxall, 2020). Moreover, the well-recognised gendered nature of family violence continues to be seen during COVID-19.

In the Australian context, this increase is primarily reflected more through service provider and anecdotal evidence (Pfitzner, Fitz-Gibbon & True, 2020), with police record data showing relatively little change (Morgan & Boxall, 2020). This finding is not surprising, given that women may have felt more reluctant than usual to report violence to the police or lacked the safe opportunity to report, given fears of escalating tensions in locked down households should a perpetrator consequently not be removed from that household. Increases in violence in home environments seems to have been more evident in urban areas rather than rural and remote areas (Morgan & Boxall, 2020), potentially due to the strictest lockdowns occurring in urban settings. Importantly, both data analyses and service providers have demonstrated an increase in the first-time reporting of family violence (Pearson et al., 2020).

Service providers have also voiced concerns that female Aboriginal elders, women and children are at heightened risk of family violence during COVID-19, particularly women who have previously experienced family violence (Johnstone et al., 2020), as are people in LGBTQI+ relationships (Equality Australia, 2020). Some of the particular risk factors include the lack of service and cultural support, access to safe technology, ongoing accommodation, and an inability to connect with their mob. Concerns have also been held for those in disability and aged care residential services, where during lockdown there was no visitor contact. Anecdotally, there were also delays in admissions to aged care, leaving vulnerable people in homes with perpetrators, while some families chose to withdraw residents in favour of home care given the heightened risks of COVID-19 transmission in care facilities.

Understanding the risk factors for family violence in lockdown

As social workers, we have a growing understanding of the risk factors for family violence that can arise during a pandemic. Anecdotal and empirical evidence highlight unique impacts of the various lockdown measures that have been introduced.

For social workers addressing family violence in disaster contexts, it is about understanding a very complex dynamic between gender roles and power on the one hand, and on the other, stress and coping. While family violence in all its forms is never acceptable, understanding the pathways towards it is critical. It is about finding ways to address the reduction of stressors and understanding anger and violence as part of a stress and mental health (PTSD, depression and anxiety) response, while at the same time maintaining the unacceptability of any form of violence.

Case study: the Australian context

In global terms, to date, the COVID-19 disease experiences in Australia have been minimal compared to the infection, hospitalisation and death rates seen in many other countries. Arguably, this is due to the public health management strategies that have been employed, considered to be amongst the tightest measures utilised globally.

Restrictions in the city of Melbourne and state of Victoria were enacted under the state of emergency powers of the Victorian Legislation, the Public Health and Wellbeing Act 2008. Particularly in metropolitan Melbourne, measures have been in place since March 2020. For example, from 9 July 2020, Melbourne residents were in home lockdown for 110 days. There was a five-kilometre restriction on movement and night curfews were imposed. There were only four reasons that people were permitted to be out of their homes: to go to work as an essential worker, to provide care or seek health care, to shop for essentials and to exercise (initially a maximum of 1 hour per day). At all other times, unless people were working in essential services, adults and children were required to be at home, working or home schooling. As we highlight later in this chapter, anyone experiencing family violence was encouraged to leave and reassured of a supportive response. While these lockdown conditions lifted later in 2020, restrictions continued and, already in February 2021, a snap five-day home lockdown was again enacted right across the state of Victoria to contain outbreaks.

We now look at some of the unique risk factors for family violence that have been identified in this context.

Home lockdown

Home lockdowns and movement restrictions meant that for many women and children, the home became a place of further isolation and violence, requiring increased time to be spent with perpetrators of family violence and a simultaneous loss of other private face-to-face contact with networks of family and social support (Morgan & Boxall 2020).

For many households, shared spaces were highly stressful to cope with on a daily basis. Aside from those working in essential services, many adults were forced to work from home or were home unemployed. Parents have had to simultaneously manage working from home with home schooling of their children, with no outside assistance from family members or friends. Stability and routines are known to be so important for well-being during and after disasters (Gibbs et al., 2015). Yet for many adults and children there were major disruptions to daily routines, leading to more stressful and less predictable environments (The Alliance for Child Protection in Humanitarian Action 2019).

Being locked down enabled perpetrators to abuse and control those in their household more easily, monitoring all movement and communication with others. Such forms of coercive control by perpetrators have included efforts to use the COVID-19 restrictions and threat of infection to restrict women's movement, gain access to women's residences and coerce women into residing with them (Morgan & Boxall, 2020; Pfitzner, Fitz-Gibbon & True, 2020). Some perpetrators have also been known to spread rumours that a victim has COVID-19 in order to further isolate them from family and friends (Johnstone et al., 2020). Moreover, where perpetrators have not been living in the same household but share custody of children, some have threatened to infect family members with COVID-19 to increase access to their children (Pfitzner, Fitz-Gibbon & True, 2020).

Such close proximity has also given perpetrators the opportunity to monitor phone and technology use in unprecedented ways, given that privacy and safety of the home environment to talk with others can be so limited, depriving connection with victim survivors' family and social networks (Domestic Violence Resource Centre Victoria [DVRCV], 2020). Practitioners have noted that some women have been restricted in their ability to use their phones, the internet or email to access support service contact (DVRCV, 2020).

Physical distancing requirements – invisibility and loss of connection

Lockdown meant there was less access and visibility to others and often reduced opportunity for the victim to report the violence (Pfitzner, Fitz-Gibbon & True, 2020; Morgan & Boxall, 2020). Many community and social activities (sports, disability support, etc.) for children and caregivers were also ceased during lockdowns. For children experiencing abuse and neglect, their lack of direct classroom contact with teachers or visibility in community activities meant that this may have gone undetected (The Alliance for Child Protection in Humanitarian Action 2019). For some victim survivors, it has meant that other family, friends or neighbours have taken up responsibility for contacting services on their behalf (Morgan & Boxall 2020; Pfitzner, Fitz-Gibbon & True, 2020), acting upon their awareness of the predicaments of women and children.

The financial and employment impacts

The lockdowns also brought about significant changes in many people's employment and financial circumstances, which in turn contribute to increases in family violence (Pfitzner, Fitz-Gibbon & True, 2020; van Gelder et al., 2020). The temporary closure of many businesses and industries meant not only immediate unemployment for many, particularly those on casual employment contracts, it also generated ongoing uncertainty as to the timing and resumption of employment in industries such as hospitality. Meanwhile, other employees have faced increased stress through heightened workplace demand (particularly in health industries) or the competing demands of working from home (Morgan & Boxall, 2020). For some children, the loss of parental income and employment has inevitably meant less resources and food availability. It has also been suggested that there has been an increase in financial abuse due to the stress and uncertainty of household finances (Stewart, 2020). Any of these employment and subsequent financial concerns can exacerbate perpetrators' stress levels, which in turn can generate more anger, conflict and violence (Humphreys, 2020; Lowe, Rhodes & Scoglio, 2012; Sety, 2012).

The stark impact of this financial stress was reflected in a study of Australian women in cohabiting couples ($n = 7446$), who had and had not previously experienced family violence. The report indicated it was not the amount of time isolated with their partner that predicted violence but rather, the "level of financial stress leading into the pandemic was a strong predictor of violence". Importantly, "the probability of first-time violence was 1.8 times higher amongst women who experienced an increase in financial stress" (Morgan & Boxall, 2020, p. 1).

For older people, increases in family violence have been largely attributed to the expectations of support held by adult children who have moved back home due to financial difficulties (Stewart 2020).

Mental health

COVID-19 has also impacted on many people psychologically given its potentially life-threatening nature, as well as the disruption to daily routines, the loss of family and social face-to-face connections, and the ongoing uncertainties of its impact. In this sense, the mental health of all in the community is potentially impacted upon negatively, with fear, depression and anxiety levels known to be heightened (Pereda & Diaz-Faes, 2020). In turn, these mental health factors are associated with increases in family violence, as coping mechanisms of perpetrators are weakened. This has been compounded by longer waiting times to gain access to psychologist appointments and other mental health clinicians, along with the inability to attend face-to-face appointments (Pereda & Diaz-Faes, 2020).

Some perpetrators have preyed on this fear further. As noted earlier, the life-threatening nature of COVID-19 has also been used by some perpetrators to threaten or falsify infection, and thus coerce women into living with them (particularly where children are involved) and threatening that contact could be compromised should the victim survivor become ill.

Reports of increased alcohol consumption

Many have argued that there has been an increase in community alcohol consumption as a coping mechanism for the stress associated with the pandemic and the lockdown, for both victim survivors and perpetrators of family violence (Boxall, Morgan & Rick, 2020; Campbell, 2020; Pereda & Diaz-Faes,

2020; Substance Abuse and Mental Health Services Administration, 2020). In one study, 51% of family violence workers reported an increase in the involvement of alcohol in family violence situations since the COVID-19 restrictions were introduced (Movendi International, 2020). However, some caution must be exercised about the overall high rates of consumption of alcohol, as these rates based upon the increase in alcohol sales in take-away stores (Australian Institute of Health and Welfare, 2020). They must be compared to the reduced consumption of alcohol within licensed premises, which were closed during the lockdown. Recent reports of increased sales need to take into account that bars and restaurants were all closed and highest rates of sales were seen when lockdown restrictions were easing and social gatherings were permitted again. Some early modelling is showing that in Victoria, there has not been the excessive alcohol consumption that was initially reported. However, with perpetrators drinking within the home in more intense and solitary ways, the likelihood of becoming abusive towards family members increases. There is also the lack of social buffers and the requirement to be sober enough to drive home. Alcohol is associated with reduced inhibition, and in complex ways, is a risk factor for increased aggression, impulsivity and violence (Humphreys et al., 2005).

Reinforced gender roles

As with other disasters, gender roles can be reinforced and reverted to during times of great uncertainty (Parkinson & Zara, 2013). In practical terms, many women have had to manage more situational stressors with lockdowns – undertaking home-schooling support roles, on top of often employment and increased home maintenance roles (Boxall et al., 2020; Humphreys, 2020). In behavioural terms, these reinforced gender roles were also noted following extensive bushfires in Victoria in 2009. For example, one study found that the fires challenged men's ability to live up to the perceived social demands of their masculinity, and that these rural men were coping by increased alcohol misuse and aggression. This study identified a form of toxic hypermasculinity, which resulted from post-disaster stress and loss. It led to an increase in and an acceptance of male violence (Parkinson & Zara, 2013) as it was perceived to be as a result of stress and "acting out of character". While this pandemic is different in many ways, anger is a well-recognised dimension of post-traumatic stress responses (Forbes et al., 2015; Kellett, 2019). How it is anticipated and responded to remains less clear, given the harm it can cause both the person with PTSD and family members who are targeted.

Policy and practice responses: preventing and protecting against family violence

Throughout this pandemic, preventing and intervening in family violence have been the responsibility of federal and state governments at the macro level, along with organisational and practitioner level responses at micro levels.

Arguably one of the key interventions has been the financial assistance scheme of the Australian government. An estimated $130 billion (AUD) in funding was mobilised to provide vital safety nets for people experiencing COVID-related hardship through the introduction of, and vitally, the increase in funding for, unemployment (Job Seeker) and employment maintenance (Job Keeper) schemes for a time limited period. These financial buffers played a crucial role in reducing the financial hardship of many people and the loss of many jobs. Maintaining employment not only maintains the financial security of household situations, but it enables the ability to leave an abusive home, travel publicly and access public resources and establish positive relationships outside of it for extended periods of time. It is a protective factor for family violence (Family Safety Victoria, 2018). Women have also been able to access the Crisis Payment for Extreme Circumstances Family and Domestic Violence. This provides up to four small immediate payments within 12 months (each the equivalent of a week's pay of the maximum income support payment) for those needing to separate from family and stay in or leave their home following violence.

At a national level also, the Australian Government promised a funding increase of $1.1 billion for mental health, Medicare and domestic violence support. There was a high level of social and mainstream media communication of family violence awareness and help-seeking options, for both perpetrators and victims (Pfitzner, Fitz-Gibbon & True, 2020). On March 29th, the Australian Government announced a $150 million (AUD) funding increase to predominantly family violence phone counselling services such as 1800 Respect and Mensline Australia. The Federal Government also doubled the number of funded Better Access to Mental Health Care counselling sessions from ten to twenty for 2020.

In the Victorian practice context, all family violence, sexual assault and emergency housing services continued to operate. Victoria Police were required to maintain high levels of response to and prevention of family violence, including maintaining checks on perpetrators and victims, and Magistrates' Courts remained open through online or telephone access (Victorian State Government, 2020) to respond to family violence matters. Changes were made within government to enable ongoing and safe delivery of services. To support the shift to online delivery of service, many staff were provided with additional information and training, and internal high-risk panels were developed within services to review serious perpetrators.

In the non-government sector, a simultaneous shift to COVID-19 measures enabled services to continue to support victim survivors and keep families safe. The ability to escape violent home circumstances was clearly messaged as a priority, seen in addition to the four essential reasons for leaving home. As the Victorian State Government (2020) reiterated,

> Be assured that you have the right to feel safe, access medical support and maintain contact with friends and family. You also have the right to leave the house and won't be fined if you do so.

This ability to escape is closely linked to the availability of secure housing options including the maintenance of independent rental ones. Therefore, a number of important housing interventions were also implemented, with a moratorium on evictions and rental increases, rental assistance, increased funding to short-term accommodation and opportunities to temporarily relocate from high-density, high-rise accommodation where severe lockdowns had occurred. Access to stable housing was a protective factor in decreasing family violence during COVID-19 (Fitz-Gibbon et al., 2020), given the funding of secure hotel accommodation for homeless people in Melbourne throughout the lockdown (Heerde et al., 2020).

In this context of social isolation and physical distancing, technology has played a crucial role as a protective factor, in mediating the social isolation brought about by the physical distancing requirements and providing victim survivors with access to appointments, such as mental health appointments through virtual means has enabled reporting to occur (Pereda & Diaz-Faes, 2020). Smart watches have enabled reporting of family violence, using apps, and being able to access telehealth services which may enable the witnessing by others of family violence, and enabled access to telehealth during walking or shopping outings. (Dick, 2020; Pfitzner, Fitz-Gibbon & True, 2020). General practitioners have also been a critical point of contact to safely disclose family violence during lockdown, particularly for those from higher family violence risk groups such as pregnant women (Central and Eastern Sydney Primary Health Networks, 2020). Some children have had increased opportunity to report family violence occurring within the home, and through their use of online learning technologies throughout the day, which could pick up family violence within the home (Dick, 2020).

Direct practice responses

The Family Violence Multi-Agency Risk Assessment and Management (MARAM) Framework (Family Safety Victoria, 2018) has guided practice across Melbourne and Victoria. Four pillars underpin the MARAM Framework, including a "shared understanding of family violence", "consistent and collaborative practice", "responsibilities for family violence risk assessment and management", and "systems, outcomes and continuous improvement" (Family Safety Victoria, 2018). These pillars shape organisational and direct practice.

Consistent with this is the framework for responding to family violence specifically during disasters, which outlines important practice strategies for social workers, through six key objectives. These are: "increasing awareness and capacity to respond, promoting safety planning, ensuring basic needs are met, providing comfort and support, connecting to long-term services, and promoting psychosocial recovery" (First, First, & Houston, 2017). In many ways, the macro interventions outlined above provide the critical infrastructure and capacity to enact these dimensions for social workers and other family violence practitioners in different practice contexts.

In line with these two frameworks, some of the innovations that have been adopted in practice have been particularly reliant on new ways of communicating. This has been particularly through technology. Clearly, this is dependent on access, acknowledging that many women and children face restrictions with access due to financial barriers or disability, or, lack of public access, as was the case with the closing of public libraries and other public spaces during lockdown, or perpetrators removing access to technology. Preventively, where technology is available, practitioners have sometimes able to conduct video *house tours* with women in high-risk situations, which have enabled more detailed risk assessment and safety planning processes between practitioners and victim survivors. The virtual platforms such as Zoom, Microsoft Teams and WhatsApp have been used for service delivery instead of face-to-face meetings. Practitioners have been able to plan with women when and how to contact them should they feel unsafe using code words and alert systems in text and mobile communications. These practices have helped overcome difficulties both with initiating contact and when privacy cannot be assumed during conversations, for example, where the perpetrator may be in the room. A major phoneline service, 1800 Respect, promoted the use of an app called Daisy, which allows victims to include names of three people they trust. The app allows people to look at information and there is a *quick exit* tab allowing rapid closure of the app without it being recorded in the web browser history. Other mobile services have been developed that do not require users to download an app, making them undetectable on devices. Given perpetrators often use technology to monitor and control women, there has also been a focus on arranging alternative ways to connect through third parties (Family Safety Victoria, 2018).

Changes to the service system itself have occurred to enable greater access and communication. For example, family violence support has been increasingly integrated into other service contexts, such as community medical/general practice clinics and Centrelink (Australia's national social security provider of payments and services), and using these venues have sometimes been used for first-time face-to-face family violence appointments. This highlights the need to ensure that social workers in all practice contexts, not just specialist family violence services, are aware of key assessment, referral and access options. In other countries such as France, staff in pharmacies and other shops are encouraging people to use code words to alert staff when they need help (Usher et al., 2020). Alongside these sources of information, referral and intervention, there has also been an important practice response of countering misinformation during restrictions, such as the false message that police would not respond during the pandemic (Family Safety Victoria, 2018).

For homes where family violence was present in relationships prior to the health emergency, family violence practitioners were required to update safety planning by conducting a new family violence MARAM risk assessment. Family violence risk assessment is dynamic and it is critical to review risk whenever circumstances change. For example, teenagers who are perpetrators of family violence may have temporarily left the family home to stay with a friend as a de-escalation strategy. During the COVID-19 lockdown, they may need to be advised if this is not an option (due to restrictions) and supported to find other strategies.

Practitioners working with adult perpetrators need to also be aware of the signs of change or escalation in violence or any exploitation of the COVID-19 pandemic lockdown measures. Men's behaviour change programs (MBCPs) ceased during lockdown and services have had to adapt under these measures. The online context has been challenging in terms of lacking the central group-work element of MBCPs and there have been concerns about how key principles of such programs such as prosocial peer support (including establishing trust), risk assessment and management, and modelling respectful gendered relationships through the relationship between male and female facilitators could continue to occur under lockdowns (Victorian State Government, 2020). Increased individual contact via case management was utilised as an alternative during periods of lockdown.

Practitioner self-care

Given the nature of family violence work, self-care is always a crucial aspect of social work practice in this field. Prior to the pandemic, the 2017 family violence workforce census showed that nearly one-third of the workforce was considering leaving their job due to burnout (Family Safety Victoria, 2017). It is also a workforce that has been increasingly recognised as one with higher rates of lived experience of family violence (McLindon, Humphreys & Hegarty, 2018), so personal experiences may have also intensified for practitioners. Despite this recognition, for many, self-care has been an even been a harder aspect of practice to maintain. More so than in other disaster contexts, social workers have been insiders to the health and mental health threat of COVID-19 and the lockdown experiences in Melbourne. While social workers in some contexts (hospitals, for example) remained onsite, under the lockdown measures, many others were working from home. This meant a critical boundary between work and home was no longer in place, at a time when services were also experiencing an increase in demand. Using technology to work from home also meant the visibility and privacy of the work in social worker's home environments was encroached upon. Dependent upon the physical make-up of domestic environments for some, it was impossible to separate out space to work from space to live. It sometimes meant that others in the household, including children, were exposed to family violence stories. These could be family violence victim survivors or perpetrators. For most practitioners, ensuring that perpetrators of family violence were quarantined from their personal world was of ultimate importance.

Part of the obligation of workplaces is to support staff to navigate these changes to their working environments and provide a safe working environment irrespective of location. Workplaces have been required to look to the risk of their staff experiencing family violence during their work hours and provide information and supports where this occurs. The Victorian Government has done that for their employees, including making offers to staff to work from alternative locations such as back at their work site, other work locations or the homes of families or friends. The risks from performing family violence work at home have also been addressed. Some of the strategies utilised have included: the introduction of new technologies, tools and training to aid staff protection. For example, headsets that prevent families from hearing the voices of clients, provision of communication platforms that allow home backgrounds to be concealed, additional team and supervisor contact through rituals such as morning stand-up meetings or addition supervision, debriefing and one-on-one contact. In a constructive way, technology has also enabled supervision and debriefing, using platforms like Zoom for team sessions to promote connectedness.

Conclusion

Pandemics are profoundly stressful and uncertain experiences at individual, family, community, national and international levels. Understanding the acute and chronic stressors that are inherent in a health emergency, but also the necessary public health measures, is vital in anticipating family violence prevention and intervention in future health emergencies. Family violence is unacceptable and must be prevented. Ensuring the safety particularly of women and children in these contexts requires social workers to be acutely aware of the complex stress and power dynamics that can come into play. In this chapter, we have highlighted some of the specific experiences and responses in the context of Melbourne, Australia, and we hope that many of these insights may be transferable to other contexts. While the coronavirus pandemic continues to unfold in unpredictable ways, the careful prevention and mitigation of the shadow disaster of family violence that has been left in its wake are important ongoing social work priorities.

BOX 7.1

REFLECTIVE QUESTIONS

1. What has been the impact of the coronavirus pandemic on family violence in your practice context?
2. What measures do you think could be successfully implemented in your community to prevent or minimise the incidence of family violence during and after health emergencies?
3. What strategies could you use to reduce the stress levels of your clients, to enhance family relationships during a health emergency?
4. What self-care strategies are particularly important for social workers who are working in family violence services?

References

Allen-Ebrahimian, B. (2020). China's domestic violence epidemic. *Axios*. https://www.axios.com/china-domestic-violence-coronavirus-quarantine-7b00c3ba-35bc-4d16-afdd-b76ecfb28882.html

Asia-Pacific Gender in Humanitarian Action Working Group. (2020). *The COVID-19 outbreak and gender: Key advocacy points from Asia and the Pacific*. UN Women. https://asiapacific.unwomen.org/-/media/field office eseasia/docs/publications/2020/03/ap-giha-wg-advocacy.pdf?la=en&vs=2145

Australian Institute of Health and Welfare. (2020). *Alcohol, tobacco & other drugs in Australia*. https://www.aihw.gov.au/reports/alcohol/alcohol-tobacco-other-drugs-australia

Boxall, H., Morgan, A., & Brown, R. (2020). The prevalence of domestic violence among women during the COVID-19 pandemic. *Statistical Bulletin no. 28*. Canberra: Australian Institute of Criminology. https://www.aic.gov.au/publications/sb/sb28

Campbell, A. (2020). An increasing risk of family violence during the COVID-19 pandemic: Strengthening community collaborations to save lives. *Forensic Science International: Reports, 2*, 1–3. https://doi.org/10.1016/j.fsir.2020.100089

Central and Eastern Sydney Primary health networks (2020). *Domestic violence and COVID-19: Pregnancy is a risk factor*. https://www.cesphn.org.au/news/latest-updates/3964-domestic-violence-and-covid-19-pregnancy-is-a-risk-factor

Dick, S. (2020). How smartwatches are saving the lives of women and children. *The New Daily*. https://thenewdaily.com.au/news/national/2020/11/19/domestic-violence-smartwatch/?utm_source=Adestra&utm_medium=email&utm_campaign=Morning%20News%20-%2020201120

Domestic Violence Resource Centre Victoria. (2020). *COVID-19 and domestic violence. The Link*. Melbourne: DVRCV. https://thelookout.org.au/family-violence-workers/covid-19-and-family-violence/covid-19-and-family-violence-faqs

Drolet, J. (Ed.) (2019). *Rebuilding lives post-disaster*. New York: Oxford University Press.

Equality Australia. (2020). *LGBTIQ+ Communities and COVID-19: A report on the impacts of COVID-19 on Australian LGBTIQ+ communities and building a strong response*. Melbourne. https://equalityaustralia.org.au/wp-content/uploads/2020/04/Report-re-COVID19-and-LGBTIQ-Communities.pdf

Family Safety Victoria. (2017). *Census of workforces that intersect with family violence*. Melbourne: Victorian Government.

Family Safety Victoria. (2018). *The family violence multi-agency risk assessment and management framework*. Melbourne: Victorian Government. https://www.vic.gov.au/maram-practice-guides-and-resources

First, J. M., First, N. L., & Houston, J. B. (2017). Intimate Partner Violence and Disasters: A Framework for Empowering Women Experiencing Violence in Disaster Settings. *Affilia, 32*(3), 390–403.

Fitz-Gibbon, K., Pfitzner, N., Walklate, S., Segrave, M., Meyer, S., & True, J. (2020). *Victorian Governments response to the COVID-19 pandemic: Submission to the Public Accounts and Estimates Committee, July 2020*. Monash University: Monash Gender and Family Violence Prevention Centre. https://www.parliament.vic.gov.au/images/stories/committees/paec/COVID-19_Inquiry/Submissions/45a._Monash_Gender_and_Family_Violence_Prevention_Centre.pdf

Forbes, D., Alkemade, N., Waters, E., Gibbs, L., Gallagher, C., Pattison, P., Lusher, D., MacDougall, C., Harms, L., Block, K., Snowdon, E., Kellett, C., Sinnott, V., Ireton, G., Richardson, J., & Bryant, R. A. (2015). The role of anger and ongoing stressors in mental health following a natural disaster. *Australian and New Zealand Journal of Psychiatry, 49*(8), 706–713.

Gibbs, L., Block, K., Harms, L., MacDougall, C., Baker, E., Ireton, G., Forbes, D., Richardson, J., & Waters, E. (2015). Children and young people's wellbeing post-disaster: Safety and stability are critical. *International Journal of Disaster Risk Reduction, 14*(Part 2), 195–201.

Heerde, J., Patton, G., Young, J., Borschmann, R., & Kinner, S. (2020). Adolescent and young adult homelessness during the COVID-19 pandemic: Reflections and opportunities for multi-sectoral responses. *Parity, 33*(10), 1–5.

Henriques, M. (2020). Why Covid-19 is different for men and women. *BBC Future.* https://www.bbc.com/future/article/20200409-why-covid-19-is-different-for-men-and-women

Huerta, C. (2020, July). COVID-19 and Mexico's domestic violence crisis. *Pursuit.* https://pursuit.unimelb.edu.au/articles/covid-19-and-mexico-s-domestic-violence-crisis

Humphreys, C. (2020, August). Poverty is trapping women in abusive relationships. *Pursuit.* https://pursuit.unimelb.edu.au/articles/poverty-is-trapping-women-in-abusive-relationships

Humphreys, C., Regan, L., River, D., & Thiara Ravi, K. (2005). Domestic Violence and Substance Use: Tackling Complexity. *The British Journal of Social Work, 35*(8), 1303–1320.

Johnstone, A., Foster, H., Smith, K., & Friedlaner, L. (2020). *Experiences of Indigenous Women impacted by violence during COVID-19.* Haymarket: Women's Safety NSW. https://apo.org.au/sites/default/files/resource-files/2020-06/apo-nid306542.pdf

Kellett, C. S. (2019). *Experiences of anger following the 2009 Black Saturday bushfires: Implications for post-disaster service provision* (Unpublished doctoral thesis). The University of Melbourne, Australia.

Kumar, A. (2020). COVID-19 and domestic violence: A possible public health crisis. *Journal of Health Management, 22*(2), 192–196.

Lowe, S., Rhodes, J., & Scoglio, A. (2012). Changes in marital and partner relationships in the aftermath of Hurricane Katrina: An analysis with low-income women. *Psychology of Women Quarterly, 36,* 286–300.

McLindon, E., Humphreys, C., & Hegarty, K. (2018). "It happens to clinicians too": An Australian prevalence study of intimate partner and family violence against health professionals. *BMC Women's Health, 18*(1), 1–7.

Meyer, S. & Frost, A. (2019). *Domestic and family violence: A critical introduction to knowledge and practice.* New York: Routledge.

Molyneaux, R., Gibbs, L., Bryant, R., Humphreys, C., Hegarty, K., Kellett, C., Gallagher, H. C., Block, K., Harms, L., Richardson, J., Alkemade, N., & Forbes, D. (2020). Interpersonal violence and mental health outcomes following disaster. *BJPsych Open, 6*(1), E1. https://doi.org/doi:10.1192/bjo.2019.82

Morgan, A., & Boxall, H. (2020). *Social isolation, time spent at home, financial stress and domestic violence during the COVID-19 pandemic.* https://www.aic.gov.au/sites/default/files/2020-10/ti609_social_isolation_DV_during_covid-19_pandemic.pdf

Movendi International. (2020). *COVID-19 Australia: Alcohol's role in family violence revealed.* https://movendi.ngo/news/2020/06/03/covid-19-australia-alcohols-role-in-family-violence-revealed/

Parkinson, D. & Zara, C. (2013). The hidden disaster: Domestic violence in the aftermath of natural disaster. *Australian Journal of Emergency Management, 28*(2), 28–35.

Pearson, E., Cowie, T., & Butt, C. (2020, September 24). Record family violence offences and COVID fines drive crime rate surge. *The Age.* https://www.theage.com.au/national/victoria/record-family-violence-offences-and-covid-fines-drive-crime-rate-surge-20200924-p55yqz.html

Pereda, N., & Diaz-Faes, D. (2020). Family violence against children in the wake of COVID-19 pandemic: A review of current perspectives and risk factors. *Child and Adolescent Psychiatry and Mental Health, 14*(40).

Peterman, A., Potts, A., & O'Donnell, M., et al. (2020). *Pandemics and Violence Against Women and Children*. Center for Global Development (Working Paper 528). Washington, DC: Centre for Global Development. https://www.cgdev.org/publication/pandemics-and-violence-against-women-and-children

Pfitzner, N., Fitz-Gibbon, K., & True, J. (2020). *Responding to the "shadow pandemic": practitioner views on the nature of and responses to violence against women in Victoria, Australia during the COVID-19 restrictions*. https://bridges.monash.edu/articles/Responding_to_the_shadow_pandemic_practitioner_views_on_the_nature_of_and_responses_to_violence_against_women_in_Victoria_Australia_during_the_COVID-19_restrictions/12433517

Sety, M. (2012). *Domestic violence and natural disasters*. http://www.adfvc.unsw.edu.au

Stewart, E. (2020). *Coronavirus has made financial abuse more common; experts say. Here's what to do about it*. https://www.abc.net.au/news/2020-08-15/coronavirus-financial-abuse-domestic-violence-money/12554234

Substance Abuse and Mental Health Services Administration (2020). *Intimate partner violence and considerations during COVID-19*. https://www.samhsa.gov/sites/default/files/social-distancing-domestic-violence.pdf

The Alliance for Child Protection in Humanitarian Action. (2019). *End violence against children, UNICEF, WHO, COVID-19: Protecting children from violence, abuse and neglect in the home*. https://www.unicef.org/sites/default/files/2020-05/COVID-19-Protecting-children-from-violence-abuse-and-neglect-in-home-2020.pdf

Usher, K., Bhullar, N., Durkin, J., Gyamfi, N., & Jackson, D. (2020). Family violence and COVID-19: Increased vulnerability and reduced options for support. *International Journal of Mental Health Nursing*, *29*, 549–552.

van Gelder, N., Peterman, A., Potts, A., O'Donnell, M., Thompson, K., Shah, N., & Oertelt-Prigione, S. (2020, April). COVID-19: Reducing the risk of infection might increase the risk of intimate partner violence. *The Lancet*, *21*. https://doi.org/10.1016/j.eclinm.2020.100348

Victorian State Government. (2020). *Interventions for people who use violence*. Melbourne: Department of Health and Human Services. https://www.vic.gov.au/interventions-people-who-use-violence

8

FAMILIES AND THE COVID-19 PANDEMIC

Perspectives from the UK

Gabriela Misca, Janet Walker and Gemma Thornton

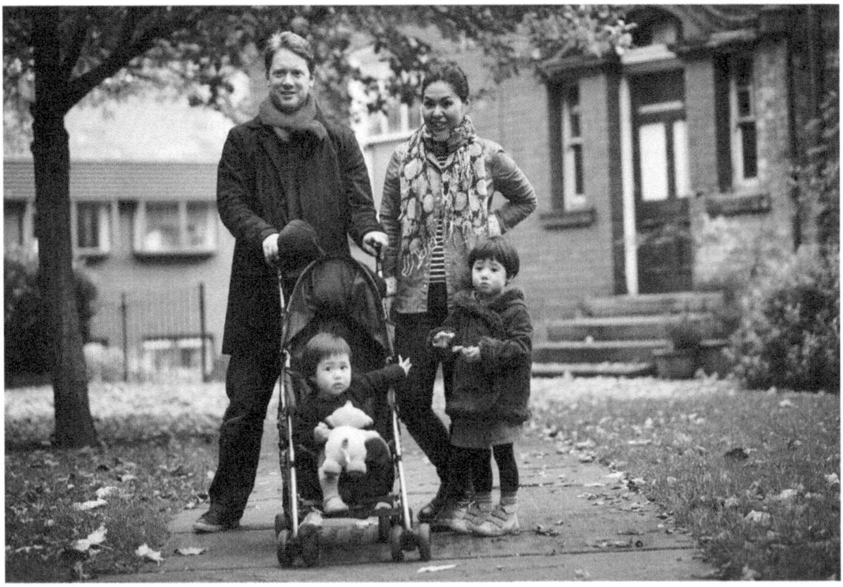

FIGURE 8.0 Families experienced varying levels of stress and adaptation in lockdown conditions

Source: Photograph courtesy of Relate UK

DOI: 10.4324/9781003111214-10

COVID-19 and the UK context

By May 2021, more than 4.4 million cases of COVID-19 had been recorded in the UK, and over 127,000 people had died within 28 days of testing positive (BBC, 2021). The emergence of new variants extended lockdowns, reinforcing the need for governments to impose continued restrictions. While lockdowns had the desired impact of reducing the spread of COVID-19 in the UK, there were wide-ranging consequences for families whose freedoms were severely curtailed, necessitating adaptation to a *new normal*.

As the virus took hold a vaccine was regarded as the only way to beat the pandemic and open up the world economy. Two vaccines were approved by December 2020, Astra Zeneca and Pfizer, allowing the roll-out of a widespread vaccination programme. Between December 2020 and April 2021, the UK had given the largest number of vaccine doses per 100 people in the world, just ahead of the USA (BBC, 2021). The Westminster Government aimed to vaccinate the entire adult population by the end of July 2021 to reduce the spread of the virus and death rate and release UK citizens from months of heavy restrictions on their daily lives. There were, nevertheless, continued warnings from health and scientific experts that the pandemic would continue. Hopefully, citizens could live with it, by probably receiving booster vaccinations every year and maintaining some physical distancing measures.

The impacts on UK families

While every individual has their own story about life during and after the ravages of the pandemic, emerging evidence on a number of key impacts were prevalent across society, irrespective of an individual's or family's personal circumstances, and we refer to these in turn.

Inequalities and ethnicity

While the coronavirus was no respecter of geographical boundaries or ethnicity, evidence of social inequalities in relation to COVID-19 emerged in Spain, the USA and the UK (AQuAS, 2020; Bambra et al., 2020; Chen & Krieger, 2020). Data from England and Wales found that people from Black, Asian and Minority Ethnic (BAME) groups accounted for 34.5% of 4,873 critically ill COVID-19 patients in the period ending April 16, 2020, yet only 14% of the population of England and Wales are from these backgrounds (ICNARC, 2020).

The interaction between racial and socioeconomic inequalities and the increased risk of mortality amongst COVID-19 patients from BAME groups became obvious as the pandemic continued, due to inequalities found in the social determinants of health, the conditions in which people live and work (Bambra et al., 2020). For example, lower-skilled occupations and occupational inequalities were associated with an increased risk of contracting COVID-19 and increased mortality. BAME groups are disproportionally represented in lower-paid jobs, such as in the service sector including cleaning, retail, delivery services, and public transport. While the majority of workers were asked to work from home during the pandemic, those in lower-paid jobs were designated as key/essential workers and required to go to work. Not only were the BAME groups at higher risk of contracting COVID-19, they had higher exposure to it than those who could work from home. Health inequalities were further aggravated by poor housing and overcrowding, and repeated and lengthy periods of lockdown meant that these problematic conditions were worse for families living in deprived urban communities.

Death in isolation and unresolved grief

The most evident impact has been the high death rate. For the families and friends of those who died, life changed irreversibly. One of the most upsetting consequences of the pandemic was isolation from family. Relatives were prohibited from visiting family members admitted to hospital and the elderly people in care homes for fear of the disease spreading. By prohibiting visitors to hospitals and care homes, thousands of people died without loved ones being with them or allowed to say goodbye.

Furthermore, because funerals could only be attended by very few people, many family members and friends were prohibited from paying their respects and sharing in the normal end-of-life rituals. Death took people away with little opportunity for families to grieve together. One funeral company described the "emergence of a pandemic of unresolved grief and loss, the effects of which will take years to heal" (Co-Op Funeralcare, 2020). This way of death in modern society has been described as cruel and inhuman, and the psychological cost will be felt for many years to come.

Managing underlying health conditions and shielding

People with underlying health conditions were at particular risk; deemed vulnerable and required to shield, they and often those caring for them were not allowed to go out for essential food shopping or minimal exercise for months on end. A study by Westcott et al. (2021) of cystic fibrosis sufferers found that anxiety levels rose during the period of lockdown, although most participants coped well. Shielding was shown to have had a disruptive effect on people's independence, confidence, social relationships, education and employment. Participants who were relatively young may have developed resilience as a result of managing their medical problems in everyday life and be able to adapt more readily to restrictions, and to stay connected with friends via social media (Westcott et al., 2021). Despite having well-developed coping strategies, the researchers recommended that well-being and mental health assessments of people with underlying health conditions should form part of standard clinical care.

In June 2020, the British Association of Counselling and Psychotherapy reported that 35% of those shielding said their mental health worsened during the pandemic, and that this percentage was higher amongst those aged over 60 (Kinmond, 2020). Increased feelings of uncertainty and lack of control emphasised the importance of offering therapeutic support.

In March 2021, a charity involved with supporting people with disabilities warned that the impact of shielding would continue long after restrictions are lifted (SCOPE, 2021). Those shielding and living alone had to manage reductions in support provided by carers and the risk that carers might be carriers of the coronavirus. Moreover, those shielding have had very limited possibilities to engage in physical exercise, with negative impacts on physical health with knock-on negative impacts on mental health. SCOPE indicated that people who had been shielding may take a while to feel safe going outside and will need support in improving both their physical and mental health.

Isolation and loneliness

Pandemic mitigation measures increased the loneliness and isolation of people living alone, many of whom were isolated from family and friends during lengthy periods of lockdown (Mental Health Foundation, 2021). Although no substitute for human contact and the warmth of human touch, technology which supports contact via Zoom calls and FaceTime enabled many people to stay in contact with family and friends.

The Office for National Statistics (ONS) in the UK has been researching people's well-being and social inequalities for nearly a decade. During the first month of lockdown in April 2020, the equivalent of 7.4 million people said their well-being was affected by feeling lonely (ONS, 2020). Working-age adults living alone were more likely than the average to report loneliness both *often* or *always* over the past seven days, as was the case for those in *bad* or *very bad* health in rented accommodation, or those who were either single or divorced/separated. Using measures which distinguished between chronic loneliness and lockdown-loneliness, the data revealed that people in Great Britain who were married, cohabiting or in a civil partnership were less likely than the average to report either chronic or lockdown loneliness, while those who were either single or divorced/separated were more likely to say they had been lonely. The findings suggest that younger people and those living alone were at the greatest risk of lockdown loneliness. This is not surprising and indicates that household composition and relationship status are associated with loneliness. As early as the first month of lockdown, when people in the ONS survey were asked about their biggest concern, those described as chronically lonely and those who were lockdown-lonely cited the impact of the pandemic on their well-being as the single biggest concern. As the pandemic and the restrictions on daily living continued into 2021, long-term loneliness was associated with an increased risk of mental health problems, including depression, anxiety and severe stress.

Mental health concerns

The social isolation and physical distancing rules had a differential impact on individuals and households, with some managing to flourish despite restrictions on personal freedoms while others became increasingly distressed. The emerging evidence suggests that mental health issues escalated, and domestic abuse increased. In April 2020, the World Health Organization warned that new restrictive measures, such as self-isolation, lockdown, and quarantine may lead to an increase in loneliness, anxiety, depression, insomnia, harmful alcohol and drug use, self-harm, or suicidal behaviour (WHO, 2020). A study undertaken in Italy, Spain and the UK using a number of standardized measures of mental health estimated that around 42.8% of the populations in these countries were at high risk of stress, anxiety, and depression as a result of economic inactivity and their exposure to negative economic shock, and suggesting that the consequences on mental health would be worse in developing countries (Codagnone et al., 2020).

A narrative review by Fegert et al. (2020) looked specifically at the mental health consequences for children and young people. They found that numerous mental health threats for children and young people are associated with the pandemic and subsequent restrictions. They urged child and adolescent psychiatrists to ensure continuity of care during all phases of the pandemic. In their view, the mental health risks would disproportionately affect children and adolescents who were already disadvantaged and marginalized. They suggested that more research was required to assess the longer-term implications of the restrictions on the mental health of children and young people.

Nine months into the pandemic, data published by the Mental Health Foundation (2020) indicated that almost half of the UK population had felt anxious or worried in the previous two weeks, rising to 64% in people with pre-existing mental health conditions. A quarter of people reported feeling lonely, and feelings of loneliness were higher in younger people and the unemployed, full-time students and single parents. The study also reported that almost half of the people were feeling unable to cope with the uncertainty of the pandemic, a quarter were worried about coping with self-isolation, and nearly half were worried about the mental health of their children. The indications were that the longer the pandemic continued, the greater the worries people had about the impact on their well-being.

Family violence

Lockdowns around the world led to an increase in cases of domestic violence where women and children had no escape from their abusers during quarantine (Chandra, 2020; Graham-Harrison et al., 2020; Kumar, 2020). Kumar and Nayar (2020) argued that providing psychosocial support for individuals and families would be increasingly important. For some, the financial hardships of redundancy and unemployment were themselves triggers for mental ill-health, extreme worries about the future and increased domestic abuse.

In November 2020, police in England and Wales recorded crime data showing an increase in offences of domestic abuse during the pandemic (ONS, 2020). While it cannot be determined whether this increase was directly attributed to the pandemic, the Metropolitan Police in London recorded an increased number of calls relating to domestic abuse during lockdown likely due to families spending more time together at home. There was also an increase in the demand for domestic abuse victim support services, especially via helplines. The ONS data showed that between April and June 2020, the number of offences flagged as domestic abuse by police increased each month, coinciding with the first lockdown period, and then with the easing of lockdown from May onwards when it may have been safer to contact the police.

The Centre for Women's Justice (CWJ, 2020) reported that increases in domestic abuse were evident around the world, including in China, the USA, Brazil, France, Australia and the UK. The CWJ pointed out that confining people under one roof for long periods of time was a key factor in the rise of domestic abuse. In addition, the ability of victims to seek social and practical support was severely limited by the stay-at-home restriction. Even in families with no history of domestic abuse, the pressures of coronavirus and lockdown restrictions led to tensions which resulted in abuse (Sharma & Borah, 2020). The United Nations referred to the rise in domestic abuse during COVID-19 as a *shadow pandemic*, reported further in Chapter 7 (BBC, 2021).

Parents with children at home

Families with dependent children, especially those living in smaller spaces, had other challenges to overcome. While they were less likely to experience intense isolation and loneliness during lockdowns, they had to manage every aspect of life within the confines of their home, including home-working and home-schooling. Juggling work, parenting and educating children were a particular challenge for parents, especially for lone-parents and those with limited or no access to computers. Only children of key/essential workers and children with special needs were able to attend school during the pandemic. The majority had to stay at home, often with limited space in which to study and to play. Families with access to outside spaces had a significant advantage over those living in apartment buildings with no easy access to the outside world. Bedrooms and kitchens became offices and school rooms, with little of the normal routines that separate home life from work and school. This was extremely difficult for children with special educational needs unable to comprehend the restrictions, and for parents who themselves were disabled or suffering physical or mental ill-health. Parents had to find new ways to maintain healthy boundaries for their children and relate to them appropriately, particularly in lockdown.

Advice for parents became available online with tips for healthy parenting routines. Many schools helped parents with home-learning, and the Westminster government provided laptops to assist with children's education. It will be some time before the impacts of lockdown on family life and children's education will be fully understood.

Impact on frontline and keyworkers

The UK has not had to resort to mass graves for coronavirus victims as was necessary elsewhere but death with dignity was severely lacking. The restrictions on how the end-of-life was managed have had long-lasting consequences for frontline workers, especially health and social care professionals who nursed and cared for very sick people day in and day out, watching large numbers of people die. Personal testimonies illustrated the profound feeling of helplessness amongst care workers, nurses and doctors. Health and social care professionals had to balance COVID-safety and protecting their own well-being with the need to provide continuing support and intensive care to sick and vulnerable people.

Concerns about the well-being of frontline workers have been expressed in many countries. The families of first responders in China, for example, were found to have increased concerns about the safety of the person working on the frontline (Li et al., 2020). Sleep problems and anxiety symptoms were common (55% and 49%, respectively) and higher levels of depression and Post Traumatic Stress Disorder (PTSD) were indicated compared with the rest of the population. Two US physicians, Kusin and Choo (2021), highlighted the challenges faced by parents on the front-line, describing the ways in which work and home lives became intertwined and disrupted. Parents lost their regular childcare and worried constantly about the risks of the disease penetrating their homes. They described how their daily routines changed with less focus on personal hygiene, disrupted sleep cycles and a sense that they were *just surviving*.

Emerging findings from the *Families Un-Locked* study

There is no doubt that the pandemic has had socially, psychologically and economically devastating impacts across the globe, and that the UK has suffered a greater incidence of disease and more deaths per head of the population than many other countries. The world picture in 2021 remains serious, with new waves in Europe and rising death rates in countries such as Brazil and India. COVID-19 is expected to continue to threaten lives and livelihoods for a long time to come, certainly until the world population has been vaccinated. There is widespread belief that daily life will never return to pre-pandemic norms. It is within this context of this serious, highly infectious and deadly disease, capable of endless mutations, that we consider the evidence relating to how families and individuals adapted to serious stress, drawing on data from an ongoing UK research study (Misca, 2020, 2021; Misca & Thornton, 2021).

The *Families Un-Locked* study led by Dr Gabriela Misca at the University of Worcester in partnership with Relate (www.relate.org.uk) was launched in

August 2020 to collect longitudinal data through repeated surveys on the medium and long-term effects of pandemic-related stressors on families and relationships. It is employing a mixed method design, eliciting participants' reflections and recollections of their behaviours and feelings during the first and strictest lockdown from March to June 2020. Data were collected post this lockdown, through a purposefully designed survey. Given the exploratory nature of the study and the unprecedented circumstance of the lockdown, this included questions about respondents' relationships in general, during the lockdown and the following period, and assessing key variables related to family and relationships, coping, health and well-being (Misca & Thornton, 2021, for description of study methodology). Since November 2020, the study is being concurrently replicated in Australia with colleagues from Griffith University and Relationships Australia to enable international comparisons.

Research data reported in this chapter were collected during the first phase of the study (August-November 2020), see Misca and Thornton (2021), and comprised 772 participants' retrospective self-reports about their use of positive and negative coping (behaviours, feelings) during the first lockdown as compared to before the pandemic.

Focus on keyworkers

Here, we focus on data from a subsample of keyworkers. Out of the total sample ($N = 772$), 30% ($n = 206$) of respondents reported that during the first lockdown, they were employed as *keyworkers* who continued to work in health and emergency services, social care, including care for the elderly, police and fire rescue, education and childcare as well as transport, food processing and essential provision. Just over a quarter of the keyworkers (26%) worked in frontline care. The vast majority of keyworkers were in a couple relationships (85%), and just under half (44%) had a partner working as keyworker, in *dual-keyworker* couples.

In order to compare keyworkers' couple relationships and parenting with those who were not in keyworker roles during lockdown, we split the couples in the overall sample ($n = 631$) by keyworker status: 14% of respondents were in dual-keyworker couples; 32% of total couples were in partnerships with one keyworker, and in 54% of all couples neither partner was a keyworker. Almost two-thirds (64%) of dual-keyworker couples and almost half (45%) of couples with one partner employed as a keyworker had children under 18 living in the same household. By contrast, just under a third (31%) of non-keyworker couples had dependent children. By using the (reduced) school provision for keyworkers' children during lockdowns, keyworker families experienced a higher risk of exposure to COVID-19 – via increased physical contacts through both their work and their children's school attendance, thus adding to the sources of stress experienced by keyworker families.

Around a third of respondents who were in keyworker couples (44% of dual- and 33% of one-keyworker couples) reported a pre-existing diagnosis of a mental health condition compared with 35% of non-keyworker couples. When comparing these couples, the strain on keyworker couple relationships was evident, with significantly more dual-keyworker couples (45%) and one-keyworker couples (39%) arguing more ($X^2 = 14.759$, df = 6, $p < .022$). Also, more dual-keyworker couples reported that they had been growing apart (43%) and had felt tension/strain (68%); and almost half (45%) felt less positive about their relationship and less close than the one-keyworker and non-keyworker couples, although these differences did not reach statistical significance in our sample, they are important findings. Moreover, a third of dual-keyworker couples agreed that "things were bad already and the lockdown has made it worse" and almost half (47%) agreed that "lockdown put a real strain on our relationship".

The impact of the pandemic on keyworkers' families

An analysis of the qualitative data revealed the extent to which keyworkers highlighted the impact of lockdown on their mental health, due to a double effect of heavy, stressful workloads and the absence of the (usual) support mechanisms due to lockdown. Comments such as the following were common: "Vastly increased workload. Extreme tiredness. Re-occurrence of stress and anxiety. Unable to do the things that help me manage my mental health" (education keyworker).

People referred to the impact of frontline work stress spilling into their couple relationships, particularly salient in the testimonies of dual-keyworker couples: "My husband's job being very stressful and us not getting on and not supporting each other" (NHS dual-keyworker couple), and; "Not feeling like we're a team in our marriage. Feeling criticised" (social care keyworker), and, "My partner and I both struggled and were not able to support each other" (NHS dual-keyworker couple).

Some keyworkers lived apart from family members to keep them safe, but this added to the stress of the family left at home: "Missing my husband who was [isolating] in a hotel for 8 weeks" (partner of NHS keyworker).

Although comparisons between keyworker and non-keyworker parents did not reach significance, more non-keyworker parents reported feeling overwhelmed by their childcare responsibilities (78%) and felt anxious about their children's education (85%). The children of many keyworkers were able to attend school during lockdown unlike most other children. Keyworker parents spoke vividly about the difficult choices that they had to make: "Feeling like I'm not a good parent, not giving enough attention – not doing as well as I can in my job – ignoring my child so I can do my job" (social care keyworker). Some parents described the inadequacies of the support they received for their children, and while home-schooling was often referred to as a struggle by parents generally, keyworker parents saw it as a luxury they did not have:

> Being a keyworker and my children going to 'daycare' at school where they were not taught but 'supervised' in their learning. Not being able to

> home-school because of work. I strongly believe that keyworkers' children were disadvantaged during lockdown as we did not have the luxury of home-schooling.

Keyworker parents also spoke about the support they gave their children to cope with the unusual situation of going to school by themselves:

> Holding down a stressful job and being a mum to two children who coped so well attending school despite none of their friends being there. Instilling confidence in my children so that they could attend school during lockdown and cope with this change.
>
> *(Social care keyworker)*

At times they felt compelled to *hide* their own stress and to be there for their children:

> Keeping up appearances for my children – hiding anxiety/stress. Talking things through with older child [3yrs]. Making good use of the spare time – activities with children, tidying, decluttering house.
>
> *(NHS keyworker)*

An NHS keyworker in a dual-keyworker couple spoke about the compound effect of the strains they felt due to demands of their work while protecting themselves and their families, children and friends:

> Not feeling supported/understood by my partner when having to isolate for two weeks with the children. Not feeing able to carry out my job … Not seeing family members or support friends in person. Trying to filter what the children are exposed to re the virus while continuing to send them to nursery. Allowing others (friends/family/colleagues) to express their anxieties to me without being consumed by them or disregarding them. Seeing other people lose loved ones.
>
> *(NHS keyworker)*

And,

> Volunteering to work on COVID ward in NHS. Difficult with thirteen patients with dementia and COVID and making sure they were all happy and comfortable with minimal staffing levels. Partner furloughed and drinking alcohol whilst I am working from home.
>
> *(NHS keyworker)*

Like other families, keyworkers worried about their extended families: "My elderly father was critically ill in another country (India) and I couldn't visit him due to fear of COVID and entry restrictions." (NHS keyworker); "Unable to visit parent in care home. Unable to visit parent in hospital. Unable to visit sibling at home. Supporting son through a level cancellation. Supporting husband through changes in job situation/furlough period. Added workload in job" (social care keyworker).

They also worried about passing the virus to their families: "Caring for my mum who was shielding, concerned I would carry virus into her home" (NHS keyworker). "I am an ITU [Intensive therapy Unit] nurse. Wearing personal protective equipment (PPE) – feeling claustrophobic/panicky. Worried about passing COVID to the people I love." (NHS keyworker). It was also difficult to see their families worrying for them: "Seeing [my] elderly parent worry for my health" (social care keyworker).

Nevertheless, keyworkers spoke about their jobs as a source of strength and *doing one's duty*: "As a keyworker in school I have just kept going, even though holidays. I've been tired but just kept on going. I felt like I was making a difference and doing my bit for the national cause" (education keyworker).

However, some felt let down by their employer and by the government: "I feel less cared for by my employer" (social care keyworker); "Frustration at Government in Westminster" (Police keyworker). Keyworkers also spoke about burn-out: "Tired during days off due to 15-hour days when working" (NHS keyworker); "After six months of lockdown I am feeling burned out" (NHS keyworker). While some shared what can be interpreted as signs of *moral injury*:

> [I felt] guilty for colleagues who were on the front line during the lockdown (NHS). I saw very poor leadership.... Flip flopping advise, e.g. mask, no mask mandatory, holiday travel quarantine vs no quarantine, counting COVID deaths & understanding of COVID virus infection management.
>
> *(NHS keyworker)*

The impact of the COVID-19 pandemic through a *family resilience* lens

While the negative impacts of the pandemic have been considerable, adapting to and coping with severe restrictions on daily life over many months was a challenge for everyone, irrespective of their living arrangements. The ability of families to cope with stress is a core factor indicating whether a family is functional. Resilient functioning requires the maintenance of healthy relational boundaries which are neither enmeshed nor entirely rigid. Patterns and levels of family functioning before the pandemic will have influenced how family members coped and adapted to the challenges. Some families coped better than others, and individuals within the same family unit varied in their level of coping behaviour. The ability of the family unit to provide emotional guidance and support is key for successful functioning and the extent to which the family is able to navigate unprecedented circumstances (Walsh, 2016, 2020).

In order to explore the impact of the pandemic on family life, it is helpful to perceive family units as interconnected individuals who are reliant upon one another, thus framing the impact as primarily affecting individuals and then feeding into their family systems. This flow from context to individual into the shared system is multidirectional; the family system affects members, who then operate as individuals in the wider societal context. Family functioning affects its members and is, in turn, affected by them connecting various interpersonal relationships with wider contextual factors such as poverty, psychological and physical health, employment, caring responsibilities, inequalities, and the practicalities of everyday life.

It is important for social workers to understand how far families are able to provide hope and how many foster despair and stress. We can expect the feelings and reactions of each family member to influence the feelings and reactions of others in the same household, even when individuals create a distinct and separate life. We have long understood that family members are influenced by circular and continual interchanges of emotion (Ackerman, 1972).

Family vulnerabilities

Families are normally regarded as a place of safety, of nurturing and support where the effects and experience of a crisis, such as the pandemic, intersect with individual, situational and circumstantial factors. Not all homes offer a safe haven as the evidence about domestic abuse has revealed. The Archbishop of Canterbury drew attention to this before the pandemic: "In almost all circumstances of human life, the greatest source of hope and the main location of despair, is found in the family" (Welby, 2018, p. 63).

Individuals and families in the UK were differentially equipped to face the threat of coronavirus, and we would expect those with the most social, economic, and psychological assets to be more likely to fare well (Walsh, 2020). Families who had built up resilience through weathering previous crises had a greater ability to find positives which strengthen bonds and clarify priorities (Walsh, 2016). Conversely, the Children's Commissioner for England report (2020) pointed out that pre-existing vulnerabilities were exacerbated during the pandemic with poverty, unemployment, mental health issues and domestic abuse all increasing to varying extents due to the pressures which arose during the crisis. The report discussed the toxic trio of domestic abuse, addiction and severe parental mental health issues as affecting 2.2 million children in England prior to the pandemic and demonstrated how this situation increased. The report recommended the prioritization of contact with social workers and children's centres but professional contact with families was thwarted by the *stay at home* rule which prevented home visits. Cessation of contact by social work professionals is likely to have increased the risk of harm.

By examining the stresses and the ways in which families coped with them, we can develop a picture of relative resilience and consider how professionals can best help people adapt to new circumstances. A survey conducted in June 2020, as the UK population was emerging from the first lockdown, found that disadvantaged groups reported more suicide ideation (Kousoulis et al., 2020). The researchers drew mixed conclusions. The majority of people had coped with a difficult experience and demonstrated a measure of resilience in meeting challenges. Disadvantaged groups were more likely to have experienced increasing pressure and deterioration in their circumstances. The Mental Health Foundation report (Kousoulis et al., 2020), concluded that in addition to the provision of mental health services, the social determinants of well-being need to be recognised and societal inequalities reduced.

The UK Household Longitudinal Study (Daly et al., 2020), a large cohort study, found vulnerability and resilience to be influenced by factors such as gender, employment and pre-existing challenges including financial insecurity and lone parenthood. Xue and McMunn (2020) reported that women were completing more housework and childcare during the pandemic, on average 15 additional hours per week, and most couples did not reduce their employment hours even though the majority were working from home. Women reported higher distress than men related to the number of additional hours spent on household responsibilities. In families in which men contributed more to household activities, both partners reported lower distress. A picture emerges of households in which partners support one another through a more equitable approach to household responsibilities, reporting better functioning, suggesting that resilience is increased through connectedness and mutual support (Walsh, 2016).

Parenting during the pandemic

Becoming responsible for education through home-schooling presented many parents with novel challenges. The majority chose to exercise, spend time outdoors and access green spaces as a way of coping. These positive coping choices reflect a resilient organisational process of flexibility to adapt, with families doing what they could under restrictive circumstances. Daly et al. (2020) reported that 96% of parents experienced improved or consistent relationships with their children and 97% reported close or very close relationships with their children. Protective factors included financial security and the appropriate space to work at home effectively, while lone parents tended to report increased financial vulnerability, although 25% of those who were in deprived circumstances still reported improved relationships with their children. Cheng et al. (2021) found that working parents indicated higher financial distress and poorer well-being than adults without children, highlighting the additional responsibilities experienced by parents.

Parents' reactions to change are likely to determine children's experience and reactions. Crescentini et al. (2020) examined the link between parental coping and its impact on children in Italian families and found that parents who felt depressed and anxious reported that their children displayed similar symptoms. Significantly, nearly a quarter of parents reported moderate to severe post-traumatic stress symptoms. Parents with children with more complex additional needs reported increased stress for themselves and more psychosocial problems for children. These findings were replicated in families with pre-existing mental health diagnoses (Misca & Thornton, 2021), single parent families and low-income families, reflecting similar findings from a study in the UK (Cheng et al., 2021). Unsurprisingly, the research suggested that families with more coping resources reported better well-being than those with fewer resources.

Spanish parents who reported distress and feeling depressed or anxious, were found to adopt more avoidant parenting practices, with less structure and focus for children in their everyday life (Romero et al., 2020). When parents identified as being vulnerable, specifically showing anxiety and depression, their children's behavioural changes were characterised as displaying conduct problems, emotional problems and hyperactivity. Conversely, parents who reported lower stress and fewer difficulties with their children were likely to have engaged in more daily activities and spend greater time on home-learning (Romero et al, 2020). Children coped well when parents were able to offer structure, attention and care, adapt to the circumstances and manage their own emotions.

Parental coping is clearly a predictor of children's well-being. Evandrou et al. (2021) also examined whether conflict and stress increased when family members had moved due to the pandemic. They found that conflict had increased when households had changed, despite the reasons for doing so being varied, such as students returning home from university, or grandparents moving in to help with childcare. These families reported higher interpersonal conflict and stress than families whose living arrangements were unchanged.

Protective factors: religiosity/spirituality

Spirituality has been identified as an important factor in the development of resilience (Walsh, 2016). Outlining the multitude of losses experienced during the pandemic: deaths, physical contact, livelihoods, hopes, dreams and normalcy, Walsh (2020) underlines how belief systems are key to how the pandemic has been understood, constructing meaning through familial lenses. Core beliefs help family members seek a new sense of adjusted reality. Organised religion provides a belief system present within the family system and in the religious structures and practices outside the family. Attending online church services was far higher than would normally be the case for services in church. The Archbishop of Canterbury's Easter sermon in 2020 had a combined audience of more than 5 million. One study (Centre for the Study of Christianity and Culture, 2021) found that the closure of churches in the UK had a serious negative impact on individual and societal well-being.

Looking to the future

The coronavirus pandemic has had enormous impacts on all individuals and families and the consequences may linger for years to come. Furthermore, the death rates amongst BAME groups have shone a spotlight on racial inequality in the UK. A report published in March 2021 from the Commission on Race and Ethnic Disparities (2021) highlighted acute geographical inequality, with the most concentrated pockets of deprivation being amongst ethnic minority groups, particularly those of Pakistani, Black Caribbean and Black African heritage. The Commission also commented that, contrary to popular belief, ethnic minority groups have high levels of aspiration, resilience and optimism.

COVID-19 has exposed the nation to individual loss and collective trauma, unprecedented since the Second World War. As the pandemic spread, increased concerns were expressed by social care and health professionals about the mental health consequences. The pandemic has drawn attention to the differences which influence coping and resilience. Recognising these is very important for those practitioners working in social care. Individuals and families experiencing mental health issues, living in poor and overcrowded homes and without adequate financial resources found it much harder to be resilient.

The pandemic has increased the level of community support which has been organized and offered to individuals and families unable to manage everyday life. Charities have encouraged local initiatives and volunteers have shown remarkable kindness. Families have also had to care for others in ways which they may not have done previously.

It is important to note, however, that the research emerging during the pandemic was for the most part confined to studies conducted remotely using internet surveys. The potential implications of this are that participants were more likely to share certain characteristics: IT literacy, internet access, less chaotic home lives, time available, and willingness to take part in research. It is probable that some groups are less well represented in the data, limiting the generalisability of conclusions. Further research is essential.

BOX 8.1

REFLECTIVE QUESTIONS

1. What were the impacts of the pandemic on families in your country?
2. As keyworkers, what effective self-care practices should social workers adopt?
3. What are the limitations of emerging research on the impacts of the pandemic on families?

References

Ackerman, N.W. (1972). *The psychodynamics of family life: Diagnosis and treatment of family life.* New York: Basic Books.

AQuAS. (2020). *Coronavirus SARS-Cov-2 interactive map.* Catalan Agency for Health Quality and Assessment. http://aquas.gencat.cat/.content/IntegradorServeis/mapa_ covid/atlas.html

Bambra, C., Riordan, R., Ford, J., & Matthews, F. (2020). The COVID-19 pandemic and health inequalities. *Journal of Epidemiology and Community Health*, 74(11), 964–968.

BBC. (2021, May 17). COVID-19 in the UK. How many coronavirus cases are there in your area? *BBC News*. https://www.bbc.co.uk/news/uk-51768274

CWJ. (2020). *COVID-19 and the surge in domestic abuse in the UK.* Centre for Women's Justice https://www.centreforwomensjustice.org.uk/new-blog-1/2020/11/10/covid-19-and-surge-in-domestic-abuse-in-uk

Chandra, J. (2020, April 2). Covid-19 lockdown: Rise in domestic violence, police apathy: NCW. The Hindu. https://www.thehindu.com/news/national/covid-19-lockdown-spike-in-domestic-violence-saysncw/article31238659.ece

Chen, J. T., & Krieger, N. (2020). *Revealing the unequal burden of COVID-19 by income, race/ethnicity, and household crowding: US county vs ZIP code analyses. Harvard Center for Population and Development Studies Working Paper Series 21 April 2020.* 19(1). https://tinyurl.com/ya44we2r

Cheng, Z., Mendolia, S., Paloyo, A. R., Savage, D. A., & Tani, M. (2021). Working parents, financial insecurity, and childcare: Mental health in the time of COVID-19 in the UK. *Review of Economics of the Household*, 19, 123–144. https://doi.org/10.1007/s11150-020-09538-3

Children's Commissioner. (2020). *Childhood in the time of COVID.* Children's Commissioner for England. https://www.childrenscommissioner.gov.uk/report/childhood-in-the-time-of-covid/

Codagnone, C., Bogliacino, F., Gómez, C., Charris, R., Montealegre, F., Liva, G., Lupiáñez-Villanueva, L., Folkvord, F., & Veltri, G. A. (2020). Assessing concerns for the economic consequence of the COVID-19 response and mental health problems associated with economic vulnerability and negative economic shock in Italy, Spain, and the United Kingdom. *PLoS ONE*. https://doi.org/10.1371/journal.pone.0240876

Commission on Race and Ethnic Disparities. (2021). *Report 2021.* https://assets.publishing.service.gov.uk/government/uploads/system/uploads/attachment_data/file/974507/20210331_-_CRED_Report_-_FINAL_-_Web_Accessible.pdf

Co-Op Funeralcare. (2020, July 4) A nation in mourning report: Is the UK heading towards a grief pandemic? *Co-op Funeralcare Media Report.* https://www.coop.co.uk/funeralcare/nationinmourning

Crescentini, C., Feruglio, S., Matiz, A., Paschetto, A., Vidal, E., Cogo, P., & Fabbro, F. (2020). Stuck outside and inside: An exploratory study on the effects of the COVID-19 outbreak on Italian parents and children's internalizing symptoms. *Frontiers in Psychology*. https://doi.org/10.3389/fpsyg.2020.586074

Daly, M., Sutin, A., & Robinson, E. (2020). Longitudinal changes in mental health and the COVID-19 pandemic: Evidence from the UK Household Longitudinal Study. *Psychological Medicine*. https://doi.org/10.1017/S0033291720004432

Evandrou, M., Falkingham, J., Qin, M., & Vlachantoni, A. (2021). Changing living arrangements and stress during Covid-19 lockdown: Evidence from four birth cohorts in the UK. *SSM – Population Health*, 13, 100761. https://doi.org/10.1016/j.ssmph.2021.100761

Fegert, J.M., Vitiello. B., Plener, P., & Clemens, V. (2020). Challenges and burden of the Coronavirus 2019 (COVID-19) pandemic for child and adolescent mental health: A narrative review to highlight clinical and research needs in the acute phase and the long return to normality. *Child and Adolescent Psychiatry and Mental Health*. https://doi.org/10.1186/s13034-020-00329-3

Graham-Harrison, E., Giuffrida, A., Smith, H., & Ford, L. (2020, March 28). Lockdowns around the world bring rise in domestic violence. The Guardian. https://www.theguardian.com/society/2020/mar/28/lockdowns-world-rise-domestic-violence

ICNARC. (2020, April 17). *Report on COVID-19 in critical care*. London: Intensive Care National Audit and Research Centre. https://www.icnarc.org/

Kinmond, K. (2020, June 19) *Coronavirus: The impact of shielding on mental health and wellbeing*. British Association of Counselling and Psychotherapy. https://www.bacp.co.uk/news/news-from-bacp/2020/19-june-coronavirus-the-impact-of-shielding-on-mental-health-and-wellbeing/

Kousoulis, A., McDaid, S., Crepaz-Keay, D., Solomon, S., Lombardo, C., & Yap, J., et al. (2020, July). *Coronavirus: The divergence of mental health experiences during the pandemic*. Mental Health Foundation. https://www.mentalhealth.org.uk/coronavirus/divergence-mental-healthexperiences-during-pandemic

Kumar, A. (2020). COVID-19 and domestic violence: A possible public health crisis. *Journal of Health Management*, 22(2), 192–196.

Kumar, A., & Nayar R. (2020). COVID 19 and its mental health consequences. *Journal of Mental Health*, 30(1). https://doi.org/10.1080/09638237.2020.1757052

Kusin, S., & Choo, E. (2021). Parenting in the time of COVID-19. *The Lancet*, 397(10269). https://doi.org/10.1016/S0140-6736(20)32755-0

Li, W.-H., Feng, Z., Xu, L., Cheng, P., Zhang, L., & Li, L.-J. (2020). The psychological impact of COVID-19 on the families of first-line rescuers. *Indian Journal of Psychiatry*, 62(9), 438-444.

Mental Health Foundation (2020). *Wave 8: Late November 2020*. https://www.mentalhealth.org.uk/our-work/research/coronavirus-mental-health-pandemic/key-statistics-wave-8

Mental Health Foundation. (2021). *Loneliness during coronavirus*. https://www.mentalhealth.org.uk/coronavirus/loneliness-during-coronavirus

Misca, G. (2020, September 28). *Families un-locked: New study exploring the long-term impacts of the pandemic on families and relationships*. https://www.worcester.ac.uk/about/news/2020-families-un-locked-new-study-exploring-the-long-term-impacts-of-the-pandemic-on-families-and-relationships

Misca, G. (2021). *Study finds lasting impacts on families during COVID-19 pandemic*. https://www.worcester.ac.uk/about/news/academic-blog/study-finds-lasting-impacts-on-families-during-covid-19-pandemic.aspx

Misca, G., & Thornton, G. (2021). Navigating the same storm but not in the same boat: Mental health vulnerability and coping in women university students during the first COVID-19 lockdown in the UK. *Frontiers in Psychology*. https://doi.org/10.3389/fpsyg.2021.648533

Romero, E., López-Romero, L., Domínguez-Álvarez, B., Villar, P., & Gómez-Fraguela, J. A. (2020). Testing the effects of COVID-19 confinement in Spanish children: The role of parents' distress, emotional problems and specific parenting. *International Journal of Environmental Research and Public Health*, 17(19). https://doi.org/10.3390/ijerph17196975

SCOPE. (2021, March 18). *The impact of shielding will continue long after the roadmap finishes* https://www.scope.org.uk/news-and-stories/lasting-impact-of-one-year-shielding/

Sharma, A., & Borah, S. B. (2020) COVID-19 and domestic violence: An indirect path to social and economic crisis. *Journal of Family Violence*. https://doi.org/10.1007/s10896-020-00188-8

The Centre for the Study of Christianity and Culture. (2021). *Churches, Covid-19 and communities; Experiences, needs, and supporting recovery*. University of York https://churchesandcovid.org

The Office for National Statistics (ONS) (2020, June 19). *Coronavirus and the social impacts on Great Britain*. https://www.ons.gov.uk/peoplepopulationandcommunity/healthandsocialcare/healthandwellbeing/bulletins/coronavirusandthesocialimpactsongreatbritain/19june2020

Walsh, F. (2020). Loss and resilience in the time of COVID-19: Meaning making, hope, and transcendence. *Family Process*, 59(3), 898–911.

Walsh, F. (2016). Applying a family resilience framework in training, practice, and research: mastering the art of the possible. *Family Process*, 55, 616–632.

Welby, J. (2018). *Reimagining Britain: Foundations for Hope*. Great Britain: Bloomsbury Continuum.

Westcott, K.A., Wilkins, F., Chancellor, A., Anderson, A., Doe, S., Echevarria, C., & Bourke, S.J. (2021). The impact of COVID-19 shielding on the wellbeing, mental health and treatment adherence of adults with cystic fibrosis. *Future Healthcare Journal*. https://doi.org/10.7861/fhj.2020-0205

WHO. (2020, April 15). *Coronavirus disease 2019 (COVID-19) Situation report, 86*. World Health Organization. https://www.who.int/docs/default-source/coronaviruse/situation-reports/20200415-sitrep-86-covid-19.pdf?sfvrsn=c615ea20_6

Xue, B., & McMunn, A. (2021). Gender differences in unpaid care work and psychological distress in the UK Covid-19 lockdown. *PLoS ONE*, 16(3). https://doi.org/10.1371/journal.pone.0247959

9

DISABILITY AND HEALTH EMERGENCIES

Tarek Zidan

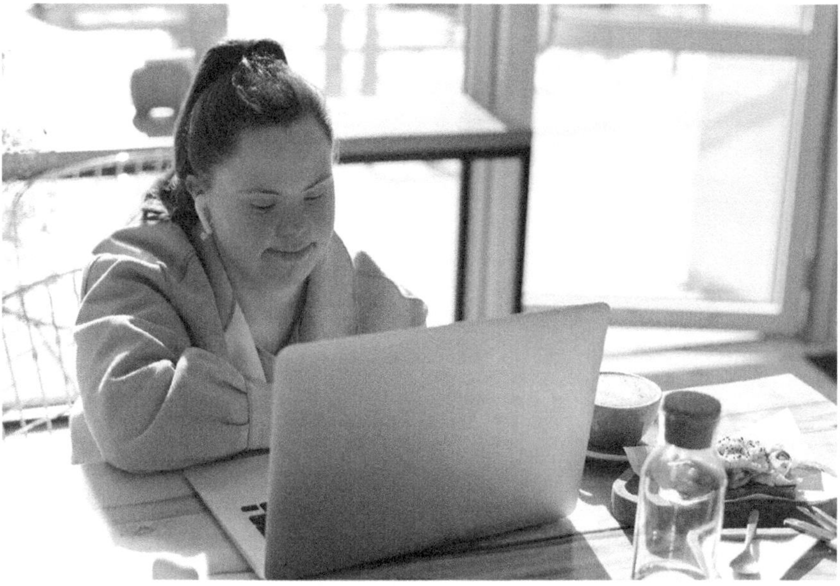

FIGURE 9.0 The capacity of people living with disability to work from home and who have access to resources and technology has helped them to survive and thrive during COVID-19

Source: Photo by Cliff Boot

DOI: 10.4324/9781003111214-11

According to the Johns Hopkins Coronavirus Resource Center, more than two million people worldwide had lost their lives from COVID-19 and over 100 million confirmed cases were reported on the 31st of January 2021, and numbers were continuing to rise (Johns Hopkins Coronavirus Resource Center). Infections were spreading and outbreaks occurring in many parts of the world, and at the time of writing this chapter, one million new cases had been recorded in the previous six days.

Disparities and risks to people with disabilities during COVID-19

The global emergency response to COVID-19 with regards to planning and response, and access to medical care for persons with disabilities has been mixed, highlighting disparities in care, outcomes and the value placed on life and human dignity especially for people with disabilities who are homeless, living in residential and psychiatric facilities or in prisons (OHCHR, 2020). The pandemic introduced unique and unprecedented threats to disability communities around the world in terms of trauma and stress in addition to the fear of infection by COVID-19 and its health consequences. Concerns included discrimination in favour of non-disabled people in care systems, as well as physical, emotional and educational impacts of isolation, and the deaths and illnesses of loved ones and community members (Lund et al., 2020)

Several issues contributed to this disparity. Pre-existing problems such as access to health care, access to equipment, and the provision of sufficient physical personal care and other assistance (depending on the disability) were made more evident during the COVID-19 pandemic as governments and general society implemented actions to address the virus. Countries worldwide have attempted various methods to make coronavirus education, prevention, and safety more accessible and useful for disabled citizens. Nevertheless, systemic issues of ableism and other prejudice and discrimination hindered those efforts especially amongst medical providers and others who are not living with a disability (Goodenough, 2020).

The Office of the United Nations High Commissioner for Human Rights (OHCHR, 2020) described the impact of COVID-19 on persons with disabilities in health, living conditions, income and employment, education, and personal safety. According to the OHCHR (2020), persons with disabilities have faced all types of discrimination. They made strong recommendations and highlighted promising programs worldwide such as those that appropriately allocated resources. Recommendations to address discrimination included:

- Prohibit the denial of treatment on the basis of disability
- Ensure priority testing
- Promote research on the impact of COVID-19 on people with disabilities
- Identify and remove barriers to treatment (including accessible environments)

- Ensure continued supply and access to medicines
- Training and awareness of health workers to prevent discrimination
- Consult and actively involve people with disabilities (OHCHR, 2020, p. 2)

Some recommendations made would be expensive for some countries and no suggestions were made as to how initiatives could be funded. In Nepal, for example, the exact numbers of people with disabilities is not known and there were few resources and inadequate infrastructure prior to the pandemic (Pandey, 2020; Panthee et al., 2020). On 19 July 2020, Nepal had recorded only 57 COVID-19 cases. However, by August 31st, just six weeks later, the number of cases grew to over 38,000, with 221 deaths. With escalating numbers, people with disabilities were reported to feel neglected and helpless. Additionally, Pandey (2020) reported the lack of facilities heightened due to the pandemic's impact. Nevertheless, even in existing facilities, people were at risk, for example, the case of a medical specialist with a disability who became infected with coronavirus. He believed he was infected by a security guard who had mild symptoms and interacted with several others before realising he was infected (Pandey, 2020). Jalali et al. (2020) reported the impact of COVID-19 on persons with disabilities in Iran, amongst the worst affected in the region in the early stages of the pandemic with 44,000 infected people by 31 March 2020. People with disabilities in the already impoverished country had even greater difficulty obtaining food and other supplies especially when caregivers required quarantine, further restricting assistance for individuals with disabilities and their ability to survive.

In contrast, the UK, a well-resourced country, has found itself amongst the top five worst-affected countries in the world. Eskyte et al. (2020) described the difficulties for people with disabilities amongst UK residents in terms of ease of movement especially when accessing public streets during that country's coronavirus response. Repeated lockdowns and other restrictions made obtaining necessities extremely difficult for many people. People with disabilities were not generally identified amongst the most vulnerable at the beginning and were generally absent from planning in a country that has had a failed response to managing the pandemic. Mandated masks were not required to be transparent in the UK and most other countries which made it much more difficult for pedestrians with disabilities to ask for the help of others and deaf or hearing-impaired people to read lips. Over half of the adults with disabilities who responded to a survey in the spring of 2020 reported difficulties obtaining regular medicines, food, and other necessities (Office for National Statistics [ONS], 2020). People who struggled and whose carers could not reach them for many reasons were left alone and isolated from the rest of the population. Although mask exceptions were granted to some people, the public was generally not aware of these exceptions. This lack of knowledge increased unwarranted criticism and hostile behavior from the public towards those people who were unable to wear masks and were exercising an allowed exception, increasing their distress during this period.

Aurora (2020) reporting on statistics from the Office for National Statistics, UK, described the disparity between disabled men and disabled women in COVID-19 mortality rates. Coronavirus infected women with significant disabilities were 3.2 times more likely to die than infected non-disabled women. Infected men with significant disabilities were 2.5 times more likely to die than infected non-disabled men. Aurora (2020) cited a disabled women's group who attributed the men/women disparity to greater psychological stress and feelings of isolation experienced by women. She concluded that the significantly disabled had less access to adequate medical care due to greater poverty and a general lack of support during the pandemic.

All people are vulnerable to impairment at some point in their lives whether from birth, trauma, illness or old age, while disability stems from sociopolitical impacts and how barriers are addressed (Bickenbach et al., 1999). Around the world, many people with disabilities live in residential care facilities, such as nursing homes and specialist institutions. This includes young people inappropriately placed in aged care institutions due to lack of support to live independently and children with disabilities who still live in institutional settings to receive the medical and rehabilitation services they need. Glynn et al. (2020) explained that many older residents in institutions have additional underlying health challenges that make them more vulnerable to COVID-19. Residential care facilities and community care also expose people to care providers who regularly move between multiple clients, constantly rotating shifts and whose job requires close personal contact with people vulnerable to disease. It is was these workers who were provided with less training and less access to personal protective equipment (PPE) than frontline hospital workers, placing themselves and the people they work with at risk.

The Australian Associated Press highlighted the efforts of the Australian Royal Commission into Violence, Abuse, Neglect and Exploitation of People with Disability (Australian Government, 2020; Goodenough, 2020). Public hearings collected the experiences from 40 people with disabilities, witnesses and caregivers who gave evidence of their increased feelings of isolation, frustration about inadequate communications from authorities, and increased difficulties in obtaining PPE and other daily necessities during lockdowns as well as other episodes of neglect and abuse. This leads us to the first case study which describes the experience of disruption in the life of one young man during lockdown, drawn from a telephone interview conducted by an MSW student intern in April 2020.

Case study 1

This case describes the experience of a young man in his late teens with an Intellectual Developmental Disability (IDD) and an Autism Spectrum Disorder (ASD) and the impact of COVID-19 on his life. It should be noted that some people with autism prefer identity-first rather person-first language. At the beginning of 2020, he lived in a group home and was actively involved in an adult day program for individuals with an IDD. His treatment plan included steps and measures for agency staff to appropriately manage his ASD. However, in mid-March, onsite programming was suspended due to the proliferation of COVID-19 across the US. The loss of such a program is significant for individuals and can result in unwanted adverse outcomes like feelings of isolation which hurts their mental health. For individuals with ASD, routine is a mainstay of that person's daily life activities and disruptions to routines pose significant challenges and adjustment.

The young man enjoyed his time in day programming and attendance was very important to him. During the interview, he indicated that he struggled with boredom and had become listless after the closure of the day program. It became much more difficult for him to follow instructions from group home staff and to achieve his previously independent tasks such as daily/weekly chores of sweeping, making his bed, doing his laundry, and keeping his room clean. Caregivers began spending more time with him to compensate for the lack of day programming and other community activities, made worse by the extended nature of pandemic measures. Caregivers compensated with new activities that he liked doing such as drawing and working colors and playing games like Uno. Still, this young man is just one example of the negative impact that COVID-19 continues to have on our IDD and ADD people in the US and elsewhere at both local and national levels.

This case study clearly shows the importance of planning and responses at all levels to meet the needs of people with disabilities in health emergencies and to find creative ways of ensuring needs that are met when health risks require restrictive methods. These barriers also challenged social workers in the field to address inclusion, complex needs and how to best support families and caregivers.

Discrimination, ethics and decision-making

Abrams and Abbott (2020) argued that the words used to describe COVID disease and related complications perpetuate discrimination against those with disabilities. Abrams and Abbott (2020) specifically challenged the phrases *pre-existing conditions* and *underlying health conditions*, arguing that although these seem to be harmless terms, they have provided excuses for healthy people to view the virus with less concern. Abrams recalled a television interview with the UK Prime Minister Boris Johnson in which strategic government inactions was discussed. The strategy, of nonaction or relying on herd immunity, would allow the virus to take its natural course within the population, accepting the related loss of life. Of course, the losses would primarily be of older people, and those people with pre-existing conditions or other health issues. The interview prompted a reaction from disabled commentators who expressed that they felt expendable, given they are amongst the people with such conditions. Abrams and Abbott (2020) defined three uses of the phrase *pre-existing conditions*. The first is a simple acknowledgement of an additional medical problem. The second use distinguishes a person with such conditions from what is deemed *normal*. The third use identified a moral distinction relative to desired actions or treatment which opens the gate tor discrimination.

Abrams and Abbott (2020) wrote of the letters sent to several families and organisations, notifying that resuscitation should not be expected for people seriously ill with COVID-19 and that plans should be made for that reality. The subjective decision-making for rationing care was frightening for people who fell into group that feared they may not receive care when needed. Abrams and Abbott (2020) acknowledged that the coronavirus presented few new issues, as society has a long history of prioritising who is eligible for medical care. However, the rationing of care should not select who should live and die, strictly based on perceived societal value and utility. They further argued against the thought of disability as a deprivation of something good, thus causing harm that is a source of pain and suffering. Indeed, disability can be a source of pain and suffering, but not necessarily so, as often it is lack of resources, societal restrictions and attitudes which create distress. Many able-bodied people including health care providers think of disability as worse than death. Because societal norms are not often questioned and easily absorbed, people with newly acquired disabilities can struggle with adjustment to new and dramatic changes in life and roles which takes time to resolve. When higher nursing home (and community) deaths are attributed to the deceased's pre-existing disabling or medical condition, Abrams and Abbott (2020) argued that such attribution obscured poor living conditions in nursing homes as contributing factors. Perhaps it also signals a failure of governments to properly implement appropriate policy, resources and oversight.

The UK public was temporarily concerned when a young girl died of COVID-19 until she was subsequently confirmed to have had pre-existing conditions, according to Hoskin and Finch (2020a) who encouraged social workers in the UK to join with other stakeholders to raise concerns about legislative protections for the disabled that were being eroded with the pandemic response. Hoskin and Finch (2020a) described a scoring measurement that denied hospital admission to those with chronic medical conditions and disabilities. Family members of those with learning difficulties were receiving *do not resuscitate* letters.

Hoskin and Finch (2020b) also noted nursing home COVID-19 deaths were initially not included in the coronavirus death counts, leaving the impression of a lesser concern for, and interest in, deaths of those residents. Abrams and Abbott (2020) reported that the England and Wales death count from coronavirus infections increased by 41% when care homes began to be included in the overall count, and Hoskin and Finch (2020b) further noted that death counts of people with learning disabilities and autism were also delayed. Hoskin and Finch (2020b) mentioned the early government response that permitted local administrators to temporarily suspend legal requirements for support systems to the disabled, thus reducing needed support. However, most local public workers did not implement these authorised suspensions, instead responding to the expressed concerns of people with disabilities and those who support them. The legislation also suspended educational obligations of local administrators towards disabled and special needs students at local schools. This left families without support for educating these students. Many disabled people and their sponsors were concerned about how easily their legally protected support systems were now vulnerable to the new whims of government.

Examples of negative COVID-19 impacts on persons with disabilities in the US and globally were compelling and overwhelming. In July 2020, one troubling example of discrimination during COVID-19 occurred in Texas (Cook, 2020). A father of five with quadriplegia and brain damage from a prior heart attack was denied treatment and life sustaining measures when he became ill with COVID-19. His family wrote to the federal Office for Civil Rights at the Department of Health and Human Services and said,

> Statements made directly to Mr. Hickson's wife, Melissa, by the treating professional indicate clearly that the determination to withhold life sustaining measures was predicated on the discriminatory notion that Mr Hickson's disabilities made his life unworthy of continued life sustaining measures, including provision of nutrition and hydration.
>
> *(Cook, 2020)*

The problem of health practitioners holding more negative views about quality of life that do not align with a person's reality has long been recognised (Andrews et al., 2020; Dorsett & Fronek, 2007). A person with a disability has likely developed effective coping skills that make perceived disadvantages much less significant and what constitutes quality of life differs from person to person, disabled or not.

One of the main issues in medical resource allocation is the basis on which decisions are made. Andrews et al. (2020) provided examples of three different approaches to rationing medical care in ethics and political philosophy: utilitarianism, egalitarianism, and prioritarianism or the priority view. The utilitarian or practical method assigns subjective quality of life measurements for estimated remaining life and then allocates resources to maximise the quality of remaining life years. This method depends on determining the quality of life, and persons without disabilities usually make that determination. The quality-of-life perceptions of persons with disabilities may be significantly different. The egalitarian approach allocates resources more randomly, for example, through a lottery system. Although a lottery would allow equal opportunity to win resources, resources would not necessarily be allocated to those most in need and likely to benefit from the allocation. The prioritarian example favored medical attention towards younger people because they would be more likely to enjoy a full life, whereas older people have already experienced a full life.

Rationing in health emergencies, especially during a global pandemic where resources are indeed scarce poses many ethical and practical dilemmas in situations where hospitals and health workers are overwhelmed which creates an environment that through urgency and resource scarcity can serve to justify discriminatory actions. There have been many reports about the distress experienced by health workers faced with these dilemmas and the personal costs they experience. Andrews et al. (2020) discussed moral trauma and the personal burden on medical care providers implementing any healthcare rationing method as well as the impact on families. Andrews et al. (2020) recommended transparency in the decision process which fosters greater understanding and more acceptance of decisions and provides a framework for appeal, if appropriate.

In the US, the issues of rationing medical care are not new to the coronavirus pandemic. Many reports and publications, often from conflicting perspectives, were written about the events at Memorial Medical Center and its Life Care facility in New Orleans, Louisiana, after Hurricane Katrina struck in August 2005 (Bailey, 2010; Fink, 2009, 2014; Kahn, 2007; Kahn & Siegel, 2007; Robertson, 2009). Kahn and Siegel (2007) illustrated some of the difficulties faced by medical professionals in times of crisis. The rising floodwaters in the days after the Hurricane passed prompted the medical facility's evacuation, where 57 critical care, palliative and longer-term patients were resident on the seventh floor and not included in evacuation planning. Evacuation proceeded moving patients from other floors to boats or the roof's helipad.

Nevertheless, after days without power, the life support of seven critical care patients dependent on respirators was maintained by the remaining hospital staff conducting manual ventilation. Driven by urgency, fatigue, fear and little chance of evacuation, there was discussion between remaining staff about what to do with patients including those who were not critically ill. If palliative patients were given sufficient morphine to last until the patient died naturally, there was a risk that the morphine drip would be exhausted before the person's death that would leave the person in acute suffering until their ultimate death. According to additional reporting by Fink (2014), the staff decided to provide lethal injections of the pain reliever morphine and midazolam, a quick sedative. One of the people that died as a result was a man with paraplegia who was hospitalised for colostomy surgery. This and other actions raised extreme concern for families about informed consent and other issues. As people died before the staff left, their bodies were moved to a chapel's central location. When the disaster mortuary team arrived, they found 45 bodies. That was more than they found at any other medical facility in New Orleans. Autopsies on the bodies found several with excessive morphine in their system. After nearly a year of investigating, Louisiana Attorney General, Charles Foti, announced the arrest of Dr Anna Pou and two nurses. They were charged with homicide attracting a punishment of death by lethal injection (Fink, 2014).

A grand jury declined to prosecute Dr Pou. Fink (2014) mentioned a juror who noted there were no witnesses to Dr Pou injecting patients. Bailey (2010) reported that Dr Pou had many supporters who argued that she was a hero, not a murderer, because she did not abandon her patients. Instead, she stayed with them as long as she could in the days after the Hurricane. She assisted in evacuation for all considered able to be safely evacuated. The American Medical Association ultimately commended her for her service to New Orleans. However, also noted was a disaster experts' panel for America's Institute of Medicine disavowed euthanasia's appropriateness during disasters. After being cleared by the grand jury, Pou's later advocacy for laws that protected the actions of medical workers in emergency and disaster situations (Fink, 2013; Nossiter, 2007). The State-level protections prevented civil liability for acting in good faith in disaster scenarios. Prosecutors were encouraged to obtain advice from a medical panel to decide whether to seek criminal convictions. Pou has since worked to pass laws on the management of patients in disasters including during pandemics and argued that informed consent was not possible during disasters (Fink, 2009). As Fink (2013) highlights, the Katrina aftermath clarified an ethical duty to prepare for emergency situations. Hoskin and Finch (2020a) acknowledged that medical providers have a long history of making difficult health care rationing decisions towards the best benefit and welcomed public discussion of the issues. The concern of family members of those people who died at Memorial hospital did not align with the actions of Dr Pou. Although it is certainly clear that health professionals are faced with terrible decisions in emergencies, the cases of people with disabilities in the UK, events at Memorial hospital and Mr Hickson's denial of treatment raise serious questions about ethics, decision-making in emergency situations and the precedents these events have set for future disasters that have been legitimised.

Where to from here?

Globally, the needs of people with disabilities have not been sufficiently met during COVID-19 despite efforts of social workers and caregivers. Like other groups, people with disabilities, are likely to remain vulnerable in the pandemic's aftermath. The COVID-19 pandemic and prior disasters raise many issues that must be debated before the next pandemic. Abrams and Abbott (2020) explained the goal related to the COVID-19 response should not aspire to return to *normal* as soon as possible for people with disabilities due to issues they faced long before this current pandemic. Nevertheless, Abrams and Abbott (2020) also noted older legislation in the US, such as the Americans with Disabilities Act that provided accommodations generally useful in pandemic conditions. For example, many public buildings have automatic door openers for the disabled that allows people to enter buildings without touching doorknobs. The authors reported the development of many online systems and software solutions that have enable people with disabilities who have access to technology to work remotely when quarantined and expand employment opportunities. Hoskin and Finch (2020a) also noted some bright spots from the coronavirus response. Persons with disabilities, who were more accustomed to staying at home, appreciated the expanded services now generally available to accommodate so many others also now staying at home. They expressed that it is unfortunate that it took a pandemic to generate empathy towards those persons with disabilities.

This brings us to the second case study, an intensely personal reflection from one social work graduate student on their experience as a person with a disability during the COVID-19 pandemic.

Case study 2

The current COVID-19 pandemic has had a profound effect on society at large, the likes of which we have never seen. As a person with a disability, the impact has been even more significant. For example, many persons with disabilities have compromised immune systems that make functioning in a pandemic that much more complicated as many are afraid even to leave their homes. For me, it has been a challenge both physically and mentally. I am also a professional who helps others with disabilities. My job mostly requires me to provide in-person services. This has made the need to be diligent in protecting self and others but with the added risk of having a disability. It frequently crosses my mind about the impact of respiratory disease on my health given my physical limitations, not getting regular exercise, and its effects on my lungs and respiratory system. Even though, I do not have a compromised immune system, there is still added risk because of these factors.

This, in turn, has had a profound effect on my mental health, adding to the sense of isolation and depression that the pandemic has seemingly brought on everyone. I have found it necessary to increase my mental health treatment due to the stress and anxiety. The pandemic has brought on sessions that often cover issues relating to the struggles of functioning in a society that is not built for persons with disabilities are now intensified and cover a more significant overarching theme of how one fits into that same capitalist system. Nevertheless, we are asked to risk much more to act as another, needing to function regardless of disability in the greater system. A capitalist system that already inherently puts individuals with disabilities at massive disadvantage forces many to now risk sickness and even death to put food on the table.

The pandemic effects will have a long-lasting effect on our mental health as a society. However, I have hoped that some good will come of the situation, specific to those with disabilities. The pandemic has forced many companies to allow employees to work from home. The long-term implications of this may significantly impact opportunities for those with disabilities to hold jobs and who might not otherwise be able to due to mobility issues outside of the home.

A second good that may come of the pandemic is the ability to connect with others virtually. I have been fortunate to maintain close connections with my friends worldwide through virtual happy hours and maintaining everyday communication through text conversations with that same close-knit group of friends.

While the current novel COVID-19 pandemic has had its significant challenges, people with disabilities are healthy, resilient people. We are used to adapting to conditions that are not ideal, yet somehow finding a way. Some of us are lucky enough even to thrive. My hope is when we make it through the other side of this pandemic, society will be more comfortable, understanding, inclusive, and willing to find a way to work with those who have their challenges.

This case study should reinforce that the erroneous assumptions made by some politicians, law and policymakers, and clinicians should have no place in speaking for people with disabilities who have their own voice and deserve to be included and be afforded the same rights and dignity as all other people.

Conclusion

Research gaps remain about the impact of COVID-19 on people with disabilities. Time will allow research into the long-term implications of COVID-19 including vaccine distribution, safety and effectiveness. Disparities for the disabled and intersections with ethnicity, gender and socioeconomic disadvantage in health emergencies requires research attention to inform evidence-based programs in recovery and to promote equal access to quality medical care. The greatest disparities are global, as people with disabilities are reliant on the resources their countries afford to them, although the neglect of people with disabilities was also keenly felt in first world countries.

Research will not solve issues of injustice and the treatment of persons with disabilities in health care systems but actions to implant disability ethics to end prejudice and discrimination that undermines the well-being and lives of individuals with disabilities during pandemics will. According to Singh (2020), to protect the rights of persons with disabilities during pandemics, social justice must be advanced for all people, with and without disabilities, and public health experts and policymakers cannot ignore disability. Understanding disability rights and social justice are crucial in defeating the COVID-19 pandemic and its aftermath. It is imperative to maintain disability ethics in medical settings to understand structural discrimination and to promote equitable practices, respect for disability culture, and ways to safeguard healthcare for persons with disabilities equally during health emergencies as well as in non-health emergency conditions. Equal allocations of resources for persons with disabilities should not be solely focused on the judgements of others about quality of life nor disregard the need for informed consent and other considerations. Quality of life is unquestionably subjective.

Decisions based on battlefield triaging need urgent re-examination for future ethical care. Discourse that describes the pandemic as *a war* may inadvertently support such responses, and stereotypical assumptions must be questioned. Persons with disabilities should be included, not excluded, from risk management planning and response. Disability ethics can be implemented in medical models of care by removing prejudices and safeguarding the adequate protection of all people's interests, including those with disabilities (Singh, 2020). Additionally, health care providers, psychologists, and social work practitioners must remain vigilant of the marginalisation of the disability community during this global ordeal and work to address neglect and disadvantage in all communities in every country to end all types of discrimination, systemic and institutional, along with other forms of injustice and oppression (Lund et al., 2020). It is timely for social workers and other professionals to advocate for the recommendations of the OHCHR (2020) and stand with people with disabilities to raise awareness about injustice and unethical practices. The non-disabled have ethical and professional obligations to reject ableism, treat everyone with equal consideration, accept the complexity of every individual's circumstances and to listen to the voices and concerns of people with disabilities especially in challenging times (Lund & Ayers, 2020).

BOX 9.1

REFLECTIVE QUESTIONS

- What are some of the assumptions made by non-disabled people about people with disabilities that you have heard? And how does this affect inclusion in society?
- How might social workers support individuals and families who are subjected to care rationing and what professional dilemmas are presented in this work?
- How do social work's professional ethics and recommendations concerning the rights of people with disabilities inform social work practice at micro, mezzo and macro levels of intervention?

References

Abrams, T., & Abbott, D. (2020). Disability, deadly discourse, and collectivity amid coronavirus (COVID-19). *Scandinavian Journal of Disability Research*, 22(1), 168–174.

Andrews, E. E., Ayers, K. B., Brown, K. S., Dunn, D. S., & Pilarski, C. R. (2020). No body is expendable: Medical rationing and disability justice during the COVID-19 pandemic. *American Psychologist*. http://dx.doi.org/10.1037/amp0000709

Aurora, M. (2020, August 13). Disability and COVID-19: A deadly virus made worse by discrimination. *Yahoo/News*. https://news.yahoo.com/disability-coronavirus-discrimination-ons-135611408.html

Australian Government. (2020). *Royal Commission into Violence, Abuse, Neglect and Exploitation of People with Disability*. https://disability.royalcommission.gov.au

Bailey, R. (2020). The case of Dr Anna Pou: Physician liability in emergency situations. *AMA Journal of Ethics*. https://journalofethics.ama-assn.org/article/case-dr-anna-pou-physician-liability-emergency-situations/2010-09

Bickenbach, J. E., Chatterji, S., Badley, E. M., & Üstün, T. B. (1999). Models of disablement, universalism and the international classification of impairments, disabilities and handicaps. *Social Science & Medicine*, 48(9), 1173–1187.

Cook, M. (2020, July 26). Coronavirus futility in Texas. *BioEdge*. https://www.bioedge.org/bioethics/coronavirus-futility-in-texas/13484

Dorsett, P., & Fronek, P. (2007). Shifting sands: Changing the way we think about practice. *SCI: Psychosocial Process*, 20(1). https://www.academia.edu/6150027/Shifting_sands_Changing_the_way_we_think_about_practice

Eskyte, I., Lawson, A., Orchard, M., & Andrews, E. (2020). Out on the streets – Crisis, opportunity, and disabled people in the era of Covid-19: Reflections from the UK. *ALTER, European Journal of Disability Research*. https://doi.org/10.1016/j.alter.2020.07.004.

Fink, S. (2009, August 1). The deadly choices at Memorial. *The New York Times*. https://archive.nytimes.com/www.nytimes.com/2009/08/30/magazine/30doctors.html

Fink, S. (2013). *Five days at memorial: Life and death in a storm-ravaged hospital*. New York: Crown Publisher.

Fink, S. (2014, February 8). Hurricane Katrina: After the flood. *The Guardian*. https://www.theguardian.com/world/2014/feb/07/hurricane-katrina-after-the-flood.

Glynn, J. R., Fielding, K., Shakespeare, T., & Campbell, O. (2020). Covid-19: Excess all-cause mortality in domiciliary care. *BMJ*. https://www.bmj.com/content/370/bmj.m2751

Goodenough, C. (2020, August 14). Disability inquiry on COVID-19 impact. *The Islander*. https://www.theislanderonline.com.au/story/6879717/disability-inquiry-on-covid-19-impact/

Hoskin, J., & Finch, J. (2020a, June). Covid-19, disability and the new eugenics: Implications for social work policy and practice. *Social Work 2020 under COVID-19 Magazine*. https://sw2020covid19.group.shef.ac.uk/2020/06/02/covid-19-disability-and-the-new-eugenics-implications-for-social-work-policy-and-practice/.

Hoskin, J., & Finch, J. (2020b, July 28). How disabled people have been completely disregarded during the coronavirus pandemic. *The Conversation*. https://theconversation.com/how-disabled-people-have-been-completely-disregarded-during-the-coronavirus-pandemic-142766

Jalali, M., Shahabi, S., Lankarani, K. B., Kamaili, M., & Majgani, P. (2020). COVID-19 and disabled people: Perspectives from Iran. *Disability & Society*, 35(5), 844–847.

Johns Hopkins Coronavirus Resource Center. https://coronavirus.jhu.edu/map.html

Kahn, C. (2007, February 16). New Orleans hospital staff discussed mercy killings. *NPR*. https://www.npr.org/templates/story/story.php?storyId=5219917

Kahn, C., & Siegel, R. (2007, July 24). Jury sides with doctor in Katrina "mercy killings". *NPR*. https://www.npr.org/templates/story/story.php?storyId=12205440

Lund, E. M., & Ayers, K. B. (2020). Raising awareness of disabled lives and health care rationing during the COVID-19 pandemic. *Psychological Trauma: Theory, Research, Practice, and Policy*, 12(1). https://doi.org/10.1037/tra0000673

Lund, E. M., Forber-Pratt, A. J., Wilson, C., & Mona, L. R. (2020). The COVID-19 pandemic, stress, and trauma in the disability community: A call to action. *Rehabilitation Psychology*, 65(4), 313–322.

Nossiter, A. (2007, July 25). *Grand jury won't indict doctor in hurricane deaths. The New York Times*. https://www.nytimes.com/2007/07/25/us/25doctor.html

OHCHR. (2020, April 29). *COVID-19 and the rights of persons with disabilities guidance*. Office of the United Nations High Commissioner for Human Rights. https://www.ohchr.org/Documents/Issues/Disability/COVID-19_and_The_Rights_of_Persons_with_Disabilities.pdf

Office for National Statistics (ONS). (2020). *Coronavirus and the social impacts on disabled people in Great Britain*. UK: Office for National Statistics. https://www.ons.gov.uk/peoplepopulationandcommunity/healthandsocialcare/disability/articles/coronavirusandthesocialimpactsondisabledpeopleingreatbritain/may2020

Pandey, L. (2020, August 31). *Coronavirus in Nepal a double threat for disabled people. DW News* https://www.dw.com/en/coronavirus-in-nepal-a-double-threat-for-disabled-people/a-54769845?maca=en-NL-Corona-Compact

Panthee, B., Dhungana, S., Panthee, N., Paudel, A., Gyawali, S., & Panthee, S. (2020). COVID-19: The current situation in Nepal. *New Microbes and New Infections*, 37. https://doi.org/10.1016/j.nmni.2020.100737

Robertson, C. (2009, September 11). Review of patient deaths after hurricane. *The New York Times*. https://www.nytimes.com/2009/09/12/us/12hospital.html

Singh, S. (2020). Disability ethics in the coronavirus crisis. *Journal of Family Medicine and Primary Care*, 9(5), 2167. https://doi.org/10.4103/jfmpc.jfmpc_588_20

10

AGEISM, OLDER PEOPLE AND COVID-19

Malcolm Payne

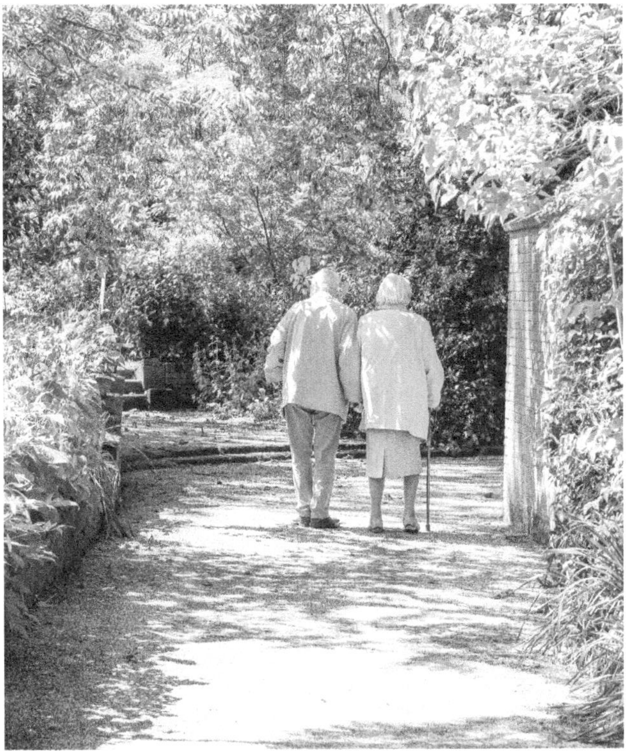

FIGURE 10.0 A walk through the park. Arboretum Trompenburg, Rotterdam, the Netherlands

Source: Photographer: Micheile Henderson on Unsplash

DOI: 10.4324/9781003111214-12

Older people are more susceptible to COVID-19 and more likely to die if they catch it. The older they are, the more likely people are to die from the disease. That susceptibility intersects with other susceptibilities, for example of black and minority ethnic groups and of people with pre-existing health conditions. People in these groups, therefore, are even more likely to contract the disease and die from it as they grow older.

Part of the susceptibility is that some frail older people live in care homes, or, a jargon phrase, *long-term care facilities* (LCTFs), that provide support in the activities of daily living or provide nursing, mainly for older people and also some younger people with disabilities. Transmission of the disease is easier in residential care because people with high susceptibility to COVID-19 are clustered together, often in crowded conditions where controlling virus transmission is difficult.

In this chapter, I examine the significant impact of the COVID-19 pandemic on older people's lives, policy and service responses to it and on healthcare and other services for them. End-of-life care for older people was also affected by the pandemic. The most vulnerable older people are housed and cared for in LTCFs as part of social care provision. There is evidence of serious dislocation and failings in planning, policy-making and service provision. In a concluding comment, I argue that the poor public policy responses and service provision demonstrates ageism.

Older people and COVID-19

Older people's susceptibility to contracting the disease and die from it was known from the early stages of the pandemic. An early report of the source outbreak in China found that no deaths occurred in the group aged nine years and younger, but eight percent of cases aged 70–79 years died, and 14.8% of those aged 80 years and older (Wu & McGoogan, 2020). Later experience confirmed the susceptibility of older people, particularly of men in the 70–79 and 80+ age groups (Chen et al., 2020; Lithander et al., 2020; Mallapaty, 2020). Older people suffer higher mortality than others for all causes and usually have higher levels of co-morbidity (that is, having several adverse health conditions at the same time) than younger people, so this pattern in COVID mortality is not unexpected (Promislow, 2020). Lithander et al.'s (2020) study also found that older people presented to healthcare services atypically or not with the same symptoms as younger people and the pattern of symptoms was often not picked up by the widely used World Health Organization (WHO) *suspected case definition*. Older people, therefore, needed to be assessed differently from the routine for younger people. It is not clear how carefully this distinction was applied in many countries.

All these factors had consequences for older people during the 2020 pandemic in two ways. First, older people, especially if they were also affected by other risk factors, became targets of concern and protection in policy and healthcare and social responses to the pandemic as it developed, although sometimes ineffectively. Second, older people themselves reacted emotionally, psychologically and in their social relations to their understanding of the situation.

COVID-19 and older people's lives

Older people's lives were inevitably affected by the pandemic and official and informal responses to it. These responses developed as the pandemic extended its reach. The main issues for vulnerable populations, including older people especially if there were intersections with other risk factors in their lives, were the need for information targeted to be useful to them, problems accessing services, deprioritisation of routine healthcare and social services, discrimination against particular groups, such as migrants and Roma people and stigma and legal as well as financial barriers to maintaining people's safety (European Centre for Disease Control and Prevention, 2020b). Clear and accurate information about the risks to them and guidance about actions they should take were needed to enable them to use their own coping skills and experience of life to deal with the health consequences and then to adapt their way of life in other respects. Information appropriate to older people's needs was often not available.

A picture of people's reactions, some social consequences of the pandemic and official responses to it were offered by an annual survey of intergenerational relationships in the UK (Gardiner et al., 2020). The survey concluded that the impact of COVID-19 on older people led to a *U-shaped* pattern of change compared with the pre-pandemic situation. The virus itself determined physical health outcomes but the shape of the pre-COVID economy drove economic impacts. Older people were more at risk of health consequences, but their financial position was more stable than younger people in the working population who were more affected by economic disruption. Government responses, however, often pursued maintenance of the economy in ways that did not focus on older people's needs.

Disruptions in healthcare and other services for older people caused by policy responses to the COVID-19 pandemic were considerable. In England, for example, Propper et al. (2020) found that between February and May 2020, 16.8% of people over 50 years of age had hospital treatment cancelled and 10% were unable to visit or speak to their GP. Care-seeking behaviour also changed with three-quarters of people who needed contact with community health services unable to contact them or deciding not to do so. Most people, however, continued to receive medication in the community. People with worse health status and those living in deprived areas were most affected by these disruptions to community services.

The pattern of healthcare problems affecting older people and the economic consequences affecting young people is exemplified in a survey of the pandemic's financial consequences for older people in the UK (Crawford & Karjalainen, 2020). Nearly 20% of people aged 52 years and older had a worse financial position by July than before the outbreak. Twenty-nine percent of people in work before the outbreak and *just getting by* at that time were worst off compared with 13% of retired people. Among workers over retirement age, 37% were worse off compared with 7% of retired people. Some had few resources to weather a difficult period. Twenty-three percent of worse-off people had a net financial worth of less than £500. Ninety percent of retired respondents were usually not worried about their future financial situation, but over a third who had been working were somewhat worried. In summary, most adverse financial consequences of economic disruption were borne by people active in the job market, with the most severe consequences for people affected by the precarity of an increasingly insecure *gig* economy (casual or short term, insecure work). While this particularly affected younger people, older people who were still working, probably because of poverty in old age due to inadequate retirement pensions, were also affected.

In response to health concerns and financial pressures, governments introduced virus transmission control measures which led to social disruption for everyone, but with a few exceptions did not focus on the specific impacts on older people. Being more at risk from COVID-19, they were forced to isolate themselves further from social connections. Retirement from the job market meant they had already experienced more attenuated social networks, relying on friendship and kinship relations.

At some stages of mitigation measures, which varied in different countries depending on the progress of the virus and decisions made, government transmission control measures such as lockdowns were strict. At other stages, they were more relaxed. Older people needed to be clear about what measures affected them at any particular time to work out how they would respond. There were three types of measures. One was personal action to reduce transmission of the virus in daily life. Examples were frequent and effective hand-washing to prevent transmission from surfaces and products they handled and wearing masks in confined environments to avoid airborne transmission of the virus. While mask-wearing was unfamiliar in some countries, older people may also have experienced previous pandemics. Older people had to find masks, not easily available in the early stages of the pandemic or get people to make them or have the skills and resources to make their own. The second measure was *physical distancing*, avoiding sustained close contact with other people, particularly in confined environments, especially difficult for people who need physical assistance to achieve daily living tasks. The third was to receive needed medical and social care, which was disrupted by pressures on health and social care agencies of providing for the large number of people affected by COVID-19 and the consequent disruption of wider health and social care provision.

An Office for National Statistics study (2020, June) examined the effects of the first UK lockdown in April-May on older people, the government's first phase of strict transmission control measures. The study found that older people worried less about finances than younger people but were more concerned about access to essentials. Keeping in touch with friends and family remotely and doing activities such as gardening and reading helped them to cope. They are more likely to be looking out for their neighbours and feel supported by their local communities. People in their 60s were the least optimistic about when life would return to normal, with more than a quarter thinking it would take at least a year or would never return to normal.

An international survey found that community and home-based care arrangements were also disrupted with day centres and community facilities closing (Dawson et al., 2020). Governments were less able to maintain oversight than with hospitals and residential care, and some governments tried to move both patients and staff into residential settings with disruptive results, especially for older people suffering from dementia. Few countries, except for Australia, collected data on what was happening in community care provision. National measures to support community-based care were lacking. Another survey of the effects in nine countries of the pandemic on people with dementia concluded that, in many places, the basic human rights of people with dementia might have been compromised during the pandemic (Suárez-González et al., 2020). These rights included access to intensive care units, hospital admissions, healthcare and palliative care. The ban on visits (including spouses and care partners) to care homes across the world, kept people with dementia detached from essential affective bonds and provision of family care for many months.

Difficulties were not only present for patients in the community. The Care Quality Commission (2020) organised an independent study of in-patient experience during the pandemic in the UK. Feedback on patient-centred care, emotional support from staff and treatment generally was overwhelmingly positive, and 86% said they were always treated with respect and dignity. Most patients with COVID-19 said they were able to keep in contact with their family and friends, but patients aged 75+, especially those with sensory impairments, learning disabilities or mental health and neurological conditions were less able to do so. Patients with COVID-19, many of them elderly, reported that their home situation was not taken into account in planning discharge. Thirty-two percent said they were not told whom to contact with problems after leaving hospital and 29% said they did not receive necessary post-discharge care and support. Again, this reflects a focus on the hospital rather than the community.

One issue with virus transmission controls was the demand on water and sanitation provision. Unproblematic in Western industrialised countries, it could not be taken for granted in many countries across the world. Older people were affected because younger, fitter people are better able to travel to get water, and to gain access to washing and other hygiene requirements. Older and disabled people might not be able to use communal provision for washing, sanitation and hygiene (Helpage International, 2020).

As stay-at-home and physical distancing measures to control virus transmission were implemented, efforts were made in some countries to target older people because of the higher risk. An international survey of information in 27 countries found that, despite knowing about the much higher risk, older people in their 70s or older were no more likely to comply with these measures than younger groups in their 50s (Daoust, 2020). This seems to have been because their practical circumstances made compliance with restrictions too difficult.

For example, in March 2020, the UK government advised people at high risk of contracting COVID-19 to stay home and avoid face-to-face contact. A survey in the UK showed that 20% did not self-isolate strictly, and the proportion fell to less than 50% by July (Steptoe & Steel, 2020). This high-risk group had twice the level of depression and anxiety compared with average risk people. Satisfaction with life, happiness, sense of purpose, sleep and general quality of life were impaired. Loneliness was much more common in the high-risk group, although there was little difference in levels of contact compared with average-risk people. People in the high-risk group were more likely to have been hospitalised with COVID-19, to have experienced death among family and friends and to be worried about obtaining food and other essentials.

The other side of caring was also affected. Older people make a significant contribution to caring for family members and neighbours, and in volunteering in community activities. A survey of carers found that 42% experienced no change in their caring activities, 23% increased and 35% either decreased or stopped their caring activities (Chatzi et al., 2020). Women were more likely than men to continue the same level of caring. Carers aged 80 years or over were less likely to stop or reduce care, probably because they had no choice. Carers without paid jobs, the least wealthy or who were self-isolating were more likely to maintain their caring; again, no choice. During the outbreak, 11% of men and 12% of women became new carers for someone outside their household, mostly people in the 50–59 age group. People in lower wealth groups, who were vulnerable to contracting COVID-19 or who had functional limitations, were less likely to start new caring responsibilities. Among people who were volunteering before the pandemic, 18% reduced activity and 43% stopped completely. Only 9% increased volunteering activity.

The biggest deteriorations in mental health affected the youngest adults and younger retired older people. This pattern is clearer still and extends to the oldest adults when looking at changes in life satisfaction since before the pandemic. Rates of high life satisfaction had fallen by most in May 2020 compared to 2018–19 (15%) for under-30s and over-65s (though satisfaction levels remained highest for younger pensioners).

End-of-life care

End-of-life care is a range of services provided to people as they approach the end of their lives. It includes palliative medicine, specialised medical and nursing care that responds to the healthcare needs of people in the dying phases of their lives. Palliative care is a multiprofessional service, involving several healthcare professions including social work and social care provision. End-of-life care includes specialised management of pain and other symptoms, together with arrangements to meet psychological, social and spiritual needs.

Since the COVID-19 pandemic would lead to increases in the number of people dying, end-of-life care needs were expected to increase and increased palliative care provision would probably be required. An extensive global survey of 458 end-of-life care services – 277 from the UK, 85 from other European countries and 95 from the rest of the world, found that 81% cared for patients with COVID-19 (Oluyase et al., 2020). Seventy-seven percent had staff with COVID-19, 48% reported shortages of personal protective equipment (PPE) to ensure staff safety from infection, 40% staff shortages, 24% medicine shortages and 14% shortages of other equipment. Of the services surveyed, 91% changed how they practised, mainly shifting to increased community and hospital care with fewer admissions to inpatient palliative care. Factors associated with increased PPE shortages were charity rather than public management and inpatient palliative care units rather than other settings. UK services experienced a higher likelihood of staff shortages. Staff described increased workloads, concerns for sick colleagues, time spent trying to get essential equipment and a feeling that they were not regarded as a frontline service.

An international study that conducted a directed documentary and content analysis of 21 guidance documents addressing COVID-19 healthcare issues affecting nursing homes identified poor coverage of end-of-life care issues (Gilissen et al., 2020). Documents focused primarily on infection prevention and control, including only a few sentences on palliative care topics. Palliative care themes most frequently mentioned were end-of-life visits, advance care planning documentation, and clinical decision-making towards the end-of-life, this latter material focused on hospital transfers. Topics such as symptom management, staff education and support, referral to specialist services or hospice and family support were neglected.

Poor practice followed the poor guidance. A Swedish study of 1,346 deaths from COVID-19, for example, found that people dying in care homes were on average more than six years older than those who died in hospital and were more likely to be women (Strang et al., 2020). Care home deaths were significantly more likely to be of people who could not express their will and were less likely to have relatives present at the time of death, but were more likely to have staff present although these still only represented 54% of cases. Significantly fewer end-of-life discussions had been held than in 2019 and significantly more died without someone being present.

While there has been press comment, often alarmist, on adverse mental health consequences of family members not being able to grieve because arrangements for attendance at funerals was restricted, many adverse bereavement reactions occur after several months or years and so problems may not yet be apparent (Parkes & Prigerson, 2010; Sowden et al., 2020). A systematic survey of the limited research on the impact of funeral practices on bereaved relatives' mental health, grief and bereavement suggests that there is no consistent pattern of adverse reactions (Burrell & Selman, 2020). Some evidence suggests that relatives' involvement in planning for funeral rituals and opportunities to say *goodbye* in meaningful ways are the most important factors, but transmission control restrictions have meant that provision for this in care homes and hospitals seriously disrupted these arrangements.

Care homes (long-term care facilities)

In almost all countries, a high proportion of deaths linked to COVID-19, were among care home residents. On average 46% of all COVID-19 deaths are care home residents (based on 21 countries), ranging from 0.01% in South Korea to over 4% (that is, one in 25 residents in care homes died) in Belgium, Ireland, Spain, the UK and the USA. This share correlates with COVID-19 deaths in populations living outside care homes. This means that deaths in care homes probably derive from the extent of community transmission. Where death rates in the community are high, that death rate transfers into care homes (Comas-Herrera et al., 2020).

What preparation would have been expected in care homes? A Welsh study pointed out that even in normal times care home populations experience more respiratory disease outbreaks than the general population (Emmerson et al., 2020). Health and social care authorities should therefore have expected a high incidence of morbidity and mortality in care homes and made preparations accordingly. But it was not so. Most European countries, for example, did not have surveillance systems able to monitor respiratory diseases systematically and consistently and provide timely reporting at local or national level to inform interventions (European Centre for Disease Prevention and Control, 2020a). General healthcare and hospital services were prioritised with little thought given to the fragmented and separate systems for social care in many countries.

The international aid charity, Médecins Sans Frontières (MSF), working in several countries, found substantial failings in preparation for medical emergencies. Its report on the situation in Spain, where it worked with nearly 500 nursing homes, identified structural failings in the residential care system (Médecins Sans Frontières, 2020). These facilities lacked health and care resources which had a direct impact on the health of the residents when the responsibility for emergency health resources and life or death fell on structures designed for social situations (housing/residence). This led to medical care being neglected, high mortality and a decrease in the quality of social care. Many older people died isolated and alone (Médecins Sans Frontières, 2020, p. 5).

Spain was not alone in its lack of preparation. MSF also reported on its work in Belgium, where its activities shifted from hospitals to LCTFs in early April, visiting 174 care homes. There was a lack of knowledge of basic hygiene rules and safety and treatment protocols, as well as shortages of staff and protective equipment. Retirement homes were asked to operate like hospitals but were not given the protective means and necessary personnel to do so (Thornton, 2020).

Daly (2020) studied the UK policy responses on care homes in England from the first coronavirus action plan published on 3 March 2020 until the announcement of a care home financial support package on 13–15 May. The initial aim of guidance on reducing transmission in care homes issued on the 13th of March was to deny entry to staff and visitors with suspected COVID-19, thus increasing the social isolation of the residents and staff. The Coronavirus Act 2020 *eased* the duty on local authorities to meet care-related need and neither the Act nor any guidance enabled or encouraged homes to reduce capacity. Care homes were consequently perversely incentivised to maintain crowded facilities by the need to maintain income, much of which, particularly in the richer south of the country, is from residents' payments.

A core element of government strategy was to free National Health Service (NHS) capacity by rapid discharge to the community, with care homes mentioned as a downstream, low-risk receiving location as a way of solving problems for the NHS (Daly, 2020). Some 25,000 patients were discharged to care homes, and on 2nd April, the government explicitly stated that negative tests would not be required before transfer. This policy was changed on the 15th of April when, for the first time applying a testing regime to care homes, the government required testing before admission. A shortage of available testing capacity meant that very little testing of residents or staff took place, which meant that safety required incarcerating residents in their rooms, especially if they developed symptoms, and introducing stringent physical distancing within homes continued.

The challenges identified by Médecins Sans Frontières (2020) in its study of Spain's care homes are typical of the problems elsewhere. They included:

- The absence of forward and contingency planning in both public and private organisations
- High occupancy and poor infrastructure, which meant that quarantine and distancing measures were not possible
- Lack of training in using PPE
- Inability to respond to loss of personnel on sick leave
- Limitations in the availability of diagnostic tests and inability to act on the results
- Strict isolation measures taken indiscriminately due the scarcity and limited credibility of diagnostic tests
- No protocol and staffing for end-of-life care
- No psychosocial care for residents and staff (Médecins Sans Frontières, 2020, p. 7)

MSF reported a refusal to accept referrals for hospital treatment so that "… homes were forced to keep patients with a very severe prognosis. In this situation, the virus spread rapidly, affecting residents and workers who, without adequate means to protect themselves, became ill…" (Médecins Sans Frontières, 2020, p. 7).

Mortality was not, however, universal in care homes. A Scottish study of 189 care homes with 5,843 beds found that 37%, mostly those for older people, experienced a COVID-19 outbreak (Burton et al., 2020). There were 852 confirmed cases and 419 COVID-related deaths, 95.7% of which occurred in the resident's care home, and 3.8% after transfer from the care home to hospital. A quarter of COVID-related deaths occurred in 2.6%, and half in 6.9% of the care homes. Care home size was strongly associated with an outbreak, the bigger the care home, the more deaths that occurred.

A systematic scoping study of the importance of social connection in long-term care found that the most-studied aspects of social connections were social support, social engagement, loneliness and social networks (Bethell et al., 2020). Reported mental health outcomes were: depression; responsive behaviours; mood, affect and emotions; anxiety; medication use; cognitive decline; death anxiety; boredom; suicidal thoughts; psychiatric morbidity; and daily crying. All of these could be expected by care homes adversely affected by transmission control restrictions applied in care homes.

In many countries, the social care workforce was not able to respond to help with residents' social connections. One issue in the UK derived from the low pay of social care staff working in care homes and staff shortages which became more problematic as staff were self-isolating because of infection in someone they had contact with or were sick themselves with COVID-related illness. The situation was compounded both because they caught the virus and because of the stress of the work. The result of these pressures on the system was that some staff had jobs in different care homes, or agency staff working in several homes were employed. A London study found that the risk of infection was significantly greater among staff who worked in more than one home, a risk even greater than for those who had extensive contact with residents in a single home (Ladhani et al., 2020).

The National Audit Office, the UK's independent watchdog on government efficiency, undertook several relevant enquiries. An initial report on structural problems replicated some of MSF's findings in Spain (National Audit Office, 2020a). It noted failures over many decades to integrate aspects of health and social care. Daly's (2020) study of the social care response pointed to separate funding and management structures, and the political and cultural value attached to health services as a public good, but not to the de-politicised social care system which had a high proportion of private provision and limited pooling of risk. Other problems identified by the National Audit Office were that lack of preparedness led to the reliance on national and international external suppliers who were also under pressure, financial pressures due to one-off short-term funding fixes that focused on immediate needs over the previous decade, and prioritising health services rather than local government social care, leading to a lack of forward planning for sustainable services.

A later report on PPE provision for protecting staff from infection as they worked noted some of the consequences of these structural issues (National Audit Office, 2020b). It found that the government department redeveloped its plans in 2018 to prioritise financial savings. Before the pandemic, responsibility for managing PPE supply and stockpiles was spread across multiple public bodies and private sector contractors. Government's stockpiles of PPE were intended for an influenza pandemic and were inadequate for the COVID-19 coronavirus pandemic. Government attempted to use its stockpiles to meet demand for PPE but faced distribution problems and a lack of information on local requirements. Guidance to staff on the use of PPE was confusing. After its publication on 10 January 2020, the guidance was changed 30 times by 31 July. Social care staff, and health staff to a lesser extent, were concerned that the frequency of changes made it confusing and that the measures outlined were not sufficient to protect workers properly. Even when labelled as being for social care, much of the guidance was explicitly for healthcare settings and had not been tailored for social care settings. The adult social care sector received about 331 million items of PPE from central government between March and July (14% of the total PPE distributed and 10% of their estimated need). This compared with 1.9 billion items sent to NHS trusts (81% of PPE distributed and 80% of estimated need). Employers reported 126 deaths and 8,152 diagnosed cases of COVID-19 among health and care workers as being linked to occupational exposure.

Institutionalised ageism and the response to COVID-19

Chapter 1 pointed out that responses to health emergencies always illuminate underlying values and political ideologies: cultural attitudes and policy predispositions stand revealed. The reason for much of the troubles in services for COVID in older people is ageism, hidden prejudice in many people's cultural assumptions and social norms that see young people as more important because they are the future. This connects with neoliberal policy choices that prioritise maintaining the economy above the health, social relations and even the lives of older people. The Médecins Sans Frontières (2020) report on nursing homes in Spain describes an extreme situation, but the prejudices lying behind it were replicated across the world. Showing institutional lack of coordination and lack of leadership, governments prioritised the healthcare response in hospitals which left behind the elderly in the nursing homes, even though they were the most vulnerable group with the highest mortality (Médecins Sans Frontières, 2020, p. 9).

Ageism is clearly apparent in the experience of older people and the community social care provision that most supports their quality of life during the COVID-19 pandemic. Young people, their medical treatment, their work and the freedom to live their lives was a greater concern than the security of older people's care. Governments knew little about the infrastructure of social provision that supports the resilience of older people's lives in the community and had not planned to maintain it in a healthcare emergency.

Advised mainly by doctors and public health professionals, governments prioritised hospital services and social restrictions to prevent virus transmission for the benefit of the young and thought little about the psychological and social consequences for older people affected by lack of care and social isolation. Care homes had been poorly funded over the years and were staffed by poorly paid, devalued employees unable to deliver services with PPE that would enable them to work safely. Sick and elderly people were clustered together in these often over-crowded buildings which were difficult to adapt so that residents were protected from respiratory infections, even though older people are most likely to suffer such infections, and financial pressures and the needs of hospitals meant that full capacity was a more important priority than safe and appropriate care.

Strict infection control measures aimed at protecting younger people in the community, meant that residents, even those with dementia, were cut off from family and friends. In some countries, residents with COVID-19 were refused treatment in hospital or discharged to care homes that were unable to cope with caring for them safely. Discharge support and care outside hospitals was unsatisfactory. Neoliberal economic policies ramped up rates of infection by governments balancing economic activity against the need for public health infection control measures. Community social care provision was closed down or made inaccessible by public health measures and community involvement in volunteering and caring was lost. Although end-of-life and bereavement care was obviously needed because of increasing COVID-19 deaths, little guidance was offered. Palliative care services came under pressure and were de-prioritised in favour of hospital treatment including the distribution and provision of PPE.

The European Union Fundamental Rights Agency (FRA) carried out studies on the human rights implications for older people of European countries' COVID-19 pandemic policies, relating to the EU Charter of Fundamental Rights. It found widespread evidence of discrimination against older people in medical, political and social decisions and practices (EU Agency for Fundamental Rights, 2020).

Age discrimination in overt policies is not the only issue; academic priorities are also in question. Technical requirements in healthcare and social research often exclude older people, and so even though they are known to be susceptible, their needs are not the first priority in research. For example, Lithander et al. (2020) pointed out that older people and those with comorbidities are usually not included in intervention studies since there may be confounding factors, but in the case of COVID-19, this was the group that required treatment and preventive measures such as vaccination. Daoust (2020), reviewing publications about older people's compliance with transmission control measures, found that even though older people were known to have an increased risk of morbidity and mortality, no special efforts were made in the early research to identify factors specific to older people.

Yet providing good care is not difficult. Bethell et al.'s (2020) care home study identified 12 interventions helpful in improving social connections for residents, most of them easy to arrange. They were: managing pain; addressing vision and hearing loss; promoting sleep at night rather than in the day; building opportunities for creative expression; exercise; maintaining religious and cultural practice; gardening, indoors or outside; visiting with pets; using technology to improve communication; encouraging reminiscence about events, people and places; and addressing communication impairments; and increasing non-verbal communication. Some of these could be achieved by addressing the fundamental aspects of the care home regime, while others were a matter of choice for some residents. Research had not been conducted in the context of disease outbreaks, and strategies to ameliorate the consequences of infection control restrictions relied on a healthy sustained workforce. But nothing was done over years to ensure that such a workforce was facilitated, prepared, supported and trained. Or funded properly.

In conclusion, the impact of ageism, historical policy neglect and omission from pandemic preparedness led to many unnecessary deaths of older people with many of those deaths occurring in the context of loss of human dignity and breaches of basic human rights.

BOX 10.1

REFLECTIVE QUESTIONS

1. How should policy and practice be developed to balance the needs of medical treatment and long-term social care?
2. Thinking about older people that you know, how would you provide for their social needs in their own homes in everyday life in a way that could be adapted to improve social connection in healthcare emergencies?
3. What initiatives would help to change attitudes and experiences in life that lead people to give a low priority to older people's health and social needs?

References

Bethell, J., Aelick, K., Babineau, J., Bretzlaff, M., Edwards, C., . . . McGilton, K. (2020, November). Social connection in long-term care homes: A scoping review of published research on the mental health impacts and potential strategies during COVID-19. *Journal of the American Medical Directors Association*. https://doi.org/10.1016/j.jamda.2020.11.025

Burrell, A., & Selman, L. E. (2020). How do funeral practices impact bereaved relatives' mental health, grief and bereavement? A mixed methods review with implications for COVID-19. *OMEGA-Journal of Death and Dying*. https://doi.org/10.1177/0030222820941296

Burton, J. K., Bayne, G., Evans, C., Garbe, F., Gorman, D., ... Guthrie, B. (2020, October). Evolution and impact of COVID-19 outbreaks in care homes: Population analysis in 189 care homes in one geographic region. *Lancet Healthy Longevity*, 1(1), E21–E31. https://doi.org/10.1016/S2666-7568(20)30012-X

Care Quality Commission. (2020, November). *Inpatient experience during the COVID-19 pandemic: National report*. London: CQC.

Chatzi, G., deGessa, G., Nazroo, J. (2020, September). *Changes in older people's experiences of providing care and of volunteering curing the Covid-19 pandemic*. London: English Longitudinal Study of Ageing, ELSA Covid-19 Substudy. https://www.elsa-project.ac.uk/covid-19

Chen, T., Wu, D., Chen, H., Yan, W., Yang, D., . . . Ning., Q. (2020, March). Clinical characteristics of 113 deceased patients with coronavirus disease 2019: Retrospective study. *British Medical Journal*, 368. https://www.bmj.com/content/368/bmj.m1091

Comas-Herrera, A., Zalakaín, J., Litwin, C., Hsu, A. T., Lane, N., & Fernández, J. L. (2020, October). *Mortality associated with COVID-19 outbreaks in care homes: Early international evidence*. London: International Long-Term Care Policy Network. https://ltccovid.org/2020/04/12/mortality-associated-with-covid-19-outbreaks-in-care-homes-early-international-evidence/

Crawford, R., & Karjalainen, H. (2020, September). *Financial consequences of the coronavirus pandemic for older people*. London: English Longitudinal Study of Ageing, ELSA Covid-19 Substudy. https://www.elsa-project.ac.uk/covid-19

Daly, M. (2020). COVID-19 and care homes in England: What happened and why? *Social Policy & Administration*, 54(7), 985–98.

Daoust, J.-F. (2020). Elderly people and responses to COVID-19 in 27 Countries. *Public Library of Science ONE*, 15(7). https://doi.org/10.1371/journal.pone.0235590

Dawson, W. D., Ashcroft, E., Lorenz-Dant, K., & Comas-Herrera, A. (2020, May) *Impact of the COVID-19 outbreak on community-based care services: A review of initial international policy reponses*. London: International Long-Term Care Policy Network. https://ltccovid.org/wp-content/uploads/2020/05/Community-Based-Care-Report-19-May.pdf

Emmerson, C., Adamson, J., Turner, D., Gravenor, M. B., Salmon, J., . . . Williams, C. J. (2020, August). Risk factors for outbreaks of COVID-19 in care homes following hospital discharge: A national cohort analysis. *Available at SSRN 3677861*. https://www.medrxiv.org/content/10.1101/2020.08.24.20168955v1

European Centre for Disease Control and Prevention (2020a, May). *Surveillance of COVID-19 in long-term care facilities in the EU/EEA*. Stockholm: ECDC.

European Centre for Disease Control and Prevention (2020b, July). *Guidance on the provision of support for medically and socially vulnerable populations in EU/EEA countries and the United Kingdom during the COVID-19 pandemic*. Stockholm: ECDC. https://www.ecdc.europa.eu/en/publications-data/guidance-medically-and-socially-vulnerable-populations-covid-19

European Union Agency for Fundamental Rights (2020, June). *Coronavirus pandemic in the EU – Fundamental rights implications*. Luxembourg: Publications Office of the European Union.

Gardiner, L., Gustafson, M., Brewer, M., Handscomb, K., Henehan, K., Judge, L., & Rahman, F. (2020, October). *An intergenerational audit for the UK, 2020*. London: Resolution Foundation. https://www.resolutionfoundation.org/publications/intergenerational-audit-uk-2020/

Gilissen, J., Pivodic, L., Unroe, K. T., & Van den Block, L. (2020, August). International COVID-19 palliative care guidance for nursing homes leaves key themes unaddressed. *Journal of Pain and Symptom Management,* 60(2), E56–E69. https://doi.org/10.1016/j.jpainsymman.2020.04.151

Helpage International (2020). *Principles of WASH in response to COVID-19*. https://www.helpage.org/resources/publications/

Ladhani, S. N., Chow, J. Y., Janarthanan, R., Fok, J., Crawley-Boevey, E., . . . Ramsay, M. E. (2020, October). Increased risk of SARS-CoV-2 infection in staff working across different care homes: enhanced CoVID-19 outbreak investigations in London care homes. *Journal of Infection*, 81(4), 621–24.

Lithander, F. E., Neumann, S., Tenison, E., Lloyd, K., Welsh, T. J., ... Henderson, E. J. (2020). COVID-19 in older people: A rapid clinical review. *Age and Ageing,* 49(4), 501–15.

Mallapaty, S. (2020, September). The coronavirus is most deadly if you are old and male. *Nature,* 585, 16–17.

Médecins Sans Frontières (2020, August). *Too little, too late: The unacceptable neglect of the elderly in care homes during the COVID-19 pandemic in Spain*. https://www.msf.org/covid-19-urgent-measures-needed-spains-care-homes

National Audit Office (2020a, June). *Readying the NHS and adult social care in England for COVID-19*. London: NAO.

National Audit Office (2020b, November). *The supply of personal protective equipment during the COVID-19 pandemic*. London: NAO.

Office for National Statistics (2020, June). *Coronavirus and the social impacts on older people in Great Britain: 3 April to 10 May 2020*. London: Office for National Statistics.

Oluyase, A. O., Hocaoglu, M., Cripps, R., Maddocks, M., Walshe, C., . . . Higginson, I. J. (2020, November). The challenges of caring for people dying from COVID-19: A multinational, observational study of palliative and hospice services (CovPall). *medRxiv*. https://www.medrxiv.org/content/10.1101/2020.10.30.20221465v1

Parkes, C. M., & Prigerson, H. G. (2010). *Bereavement: Studies in adult life*. London: Penguin.

Promislow, D. E. (2020, April). A geroscience perspective on COVID-19 mortality. *Journals of Gerontology: Biological Sciences,* 75(9), E30–3. http://doi:10.1093/gerona/glaa094

Propper, C., Stockton, I., & Stoye, G. (2020). *COVID-19 and disruptions to the health and social care of older people in England*. London: Institute of Economic Studies.

Sowden, R., Sowden, R., Selman, L. & Borgstrom, E. (2020). "Praying for your loved one wearing masks and gloves is what night-mares feels like." What do newspapers tell us about experiences of grief, bereavement and death from COVID-19? *Elizabeth Blackwell Institute Focus Week: COVID-19*, 26 September 2020. http://oro.open.ac.uk/73834/

Strang, P., Bergström, J., Martinsson, L., & Lundström, S. (2020, October). Dying From COVID-19: Loneliness, end-of-life discussions, and support for patients and their families in nursing homes and hospitals. A National Register study. *Journal of Pain and Symptom Management*, 60(4), e2–e13. https://doi.org/10.1016/j.jpainsymman.2020.07.020

Steptoe, A., & Steel, N. (2020, September). *The experience of older people instructed to shield or self-isolate during the Covid-19 pandemic*. London: English Longitudinal Study of Ageing, ELSA Covid-19 Substudy. https://www.elsa-project.ac.uk/covid-19

Suárez-González, A., Livingston. G., Low, L. F., Cahill, S., Hennelly, N., . . . Comas-Herrera, A. (2020, August). *Impact and mortality of COVID-19 on people living with dementia: cross-country report*. London: International Long-Term Care Policy Network. https://ltccovid.org/2020/08/19/impact-and-mortality-of-covid-19-on-people-living-with-dementia-cross-country-report/

Thornton, J. (2020). Covid-19: Care homes in Belgium and Spain had "alarming living conditions," says MSF report. *British Medical Journal*, 370, m3271. https://doi.org/10.1136/bmj.m3271

Wu, Z., & McGoogan, J. M. (2020, April). Characteristics of and important lessons from the coronavirus disease 2019 (COVID-19) outbreak in China: Summary of a report of 72,314 cases from the Chinese Center for Disease Control and Prevention. *Journal of the American Medical Association*, 323(13), 1239–42.

11

IMPACTS OF GLOBAL PANDEMICS ON PEOPLE ON THE MOVE

Justin S. Lee and Carmen Monico

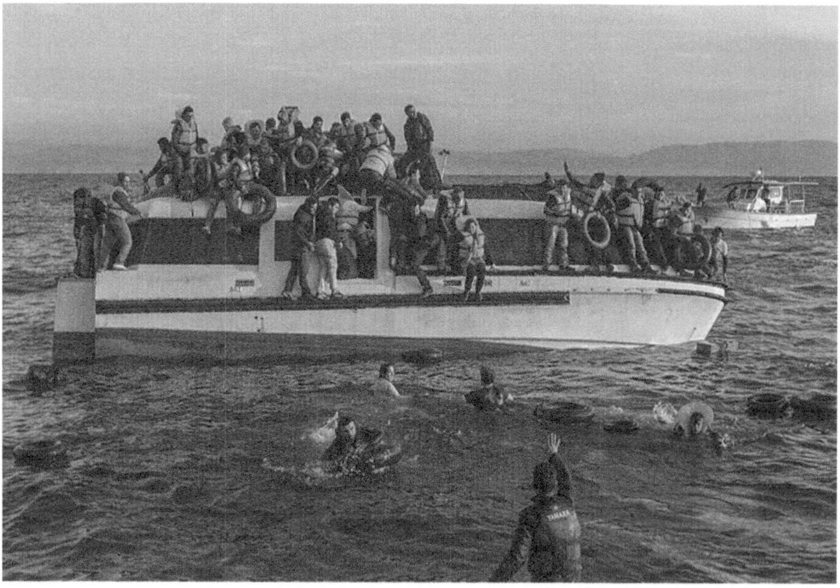

FIGURE 11.0 Syrian refugees flock to the Greek island of Lesbos

Source: Photograph by Georgios Giannopoulos

DOI: 10.4324/9781003111214-13

Many terms are used to describe people on the move in a global context, in both forced and voluntary situations. The COVID-19 pandemic multiplied risks for people who had already escaped dangerous situations and lived in precarious conditions, further compounding adverse effects on physical and mental health, and breaches of their basic human rights and dignity, discussed in Chapter 4. With the spread of COVID-19, countries at various times established strict rules about managing the pandemic and many governments ignored lost livelihoods during emergency responses focussing their attention only on the broader economies and much needed and urgent healthcare services. The survival of the most vulnerable people globally was threatened. Responses and planning paid less attention to the well-being of migrants, refugees and other displaced people. These factors impacted heavily on people forced to flee their homes in several unique ways. Not every person is the same nor described in the same way, so let us first unravel some of these terms as outlined in Box 11.1.

BOX 11.1

PEOPLE ON THE MOVE

Forced migrants are individuals and families who have "... lost their means of livelihoods and at times [lack] access to adequate living standards including housing, food, water and sanitation, education and access to health services" (OECD, 2020).

An *internally displaced person* is a person or groups of people who have been forced to leave their homes in order "... to avoid the effects of armed conflict, situations of generalized violence, violations of human rights or natural or human-made disasters, and who have not crossed an internationally recognized state border" (United Nations High Commissioner for Refugees, 2004). There were 50.8 million internally displaced persons in the world as of the end of 2019 (IDMC, 2020).

A *Refugee* is a person who has crossed a border from their country of origin due to a "well-founded fear of persecution" on the basis of race, social group, political opinion, religion, or national origin, and are unable or unwilling to receive protection from their country of origin as laid out in the United Nations Convention Relating to Status of Refugees of 1951(Geneva Convention) and the 1967 Protocols. According to the *United Nations High Commissioner for Refugees* (UNHCR), there were 26 million refugees as of June 2020, half under the age of 18 (UNHCR, 2020a).

An *asylum seeker* is a person who potentially meets the criteria of a refugee but has yet to be processed. There are approximately 4.2 million asylum seekers worldwide awaiting a status decision (UNHCR, 2020b). Each country

(*Continued*)

BOX 11.1 (*Continued*)

PEOPLE ON THE MOVE

maintains their own set of policies and procedures when it comes to processing asylum claims.

A *stateless person,* according to the 1954 *United Nations Convention Relating to the Status of Stateless Persons,* is not considered a national (citizen) under the law of a particular state, and without legal status. There are likely many millions of stateless people across the globe, often as a result of political exclusion due to ethnic or religious intolerance (UNHCR, 2020b).

Undocumented migrants, also known as unauthorised migrants or illegal migrants comprise a diverse group of people who have entered or remained in a country outside of the regulatory norms (UNESCO, 2008). This broad term refers to a range of circumstances from visa overstays to unsuccessful asylum seekers to victims of human trafficking. These migrants are especially vulnerable to exploitation and lack of access to many basic human needs.

Although the impact of the pandemic on each person and family was unique, there are commonalities that make people on the move especially vulnerable to health risks and long-term socioeconomic consequences for which social workers need to be prepared as structural disadvantage is likely to be felt far into the future. In this chapter, we focus on the impact of COVID-19 on mobile populations, among the most affected people globally.

The impact of the COVID-19 pandemic on migrants and mobile populations

The COVID-19 pandemic is not the first health emergency faced by people on the move. Globalisation poses risks for the rapid spread of infectious diseases, which has increased alongside international travel and the desperate conditions that impel people to leave their homes and seek asylum elsewhere. Chapter 3 explored lessons learned from past pandemics, however, many of these lessons were not applied to the well-being of migrants and other vulnerable groups during the COVID-19 pandemic.

One earlier acknowledgement of vulnerability to communicable disease concerned HIV/AIDS. In 2001, the UN General Assembly adopted the *Declaration of Commitment on HIV/AIDS* that acknowledged the vulnerability of refugees and internally displaced people to HIV exposure and transmission during and after humanitarian emergencies. Through forced migration, refugees are uprooted from homes and communities, lose livelihoods, family and other social networks.

These combine with other factors, such as limited access to healthcare and education including reproductive and sexual health, prolonged displacement, complex trauma caused by conflict, violence and exploitation, substance use and other health-related needs. Together, these factors increase the risk of acquiring HIV and other communicable diseases during all phases of migration. This is why global responses bring together governments, international organisations and civil society around the world to respond to such crises. To promote the health of refugees and internally displaced peoples, the UNHCR advocates for access to healthcare, respect for confidentiality and privacy, provision of voluntary counselling, and health information and education (UNHCR, undated). Lockdowns and border closures imposed during the COVID-19 pandemic, while addressing health concerns, also inhibited the distribution of antiretrovirals for HIV/AIDS and other essential medications, increased costs and access for people on the move.

As we entered the COVID-19 pandemic, close to 80 million people had been displaced by war, political persecution, conflict, organised crime, natural disasters, and climate change. The UNHCR Global Trends for 2019 reported 79.5 million people had been forcibly displaced due to persecution, conflict, violence, human rights violations or social disturbances (UNHCR, 2019). Twenty-six million people were considered refugees (a formal legal status granted to forced migrants who have crossed and international border), 45.7 million were internally displaced (forced to leave their homes but remained within the borders of their home country) and 4.2 million were asylum seekers (people who have been forced across an international border but are awaiting formal refugee legal status). In addition, 40% of the 79.5 million were children and about half of those displaced worldwide are in two regions: the Americas and South Asia (UNHCR, 2020d). Refugees living in developing countries (90%) lacked basic services like clean water, sanitation, let alone masks or handwashing facilities. One hundred and thirty-four countries in affected regions hosted refugees with confirmed COVID-19 transmission in these populations.

Chapter 2 provided examples of the overcrowded conditions in camps and detention and holding centres, which was a significant contributing factor in the pandemic spread. Adjustments to a *new normal* have been impossible in refugee and displaced camps where people live in unsanitary and overcrowded conditions with inadequate healthcare services, as well as the lack of personal protective equipment, hygiene products, sanitiser and even soap. Infection rates in camps and detention centres were still multiplying throughout 2020.

Pandemic preparedness and coordinated pandemic responses were limited in many countries and generally did not consider the needs and risks to people living in refugee camps, shelters or detention centres, or migrants resettled and living in lower socioeconomic, urban communities. The majority of migrant and mobile populations are separated families, largely women parenting children, unaccompanied children, persons with disabilities, and older people as well as ethnic and gender minorities whose specific needs are neglected (Karlsson & Jönsson, 2020). Underlying the threat of infection and death, the marginalisation, stigmatisation and discrimination they faced aggravated risks to health and safety. Concerns were high for unaccompanied and displaced children due to heightened risks of abuse and exploitation and further disadvantage through the death of parents, kin or caregivers or forced separation from them. Children and women became more vulnerable to abuse and violence during lockdowns and crowded jail-like conditions. Border closures and other restrictions of movement resulted in delayed delivery of humanitarian aid to refugee camps and more opportunities for corruption, which further threatened livelihoods and the well-being of people due to limited access to food, cash transfers, and medical assistance (ICRC, 2020). Many aid workers returned to their countries as nations closed borders and went into lockdown, creating further problems.

The global pandemic required an unprecedented response to mitigate risks to the entire global population and people forcibly displaced from their homes and countries were still entitled to their human rights. The UN's Universal Declaration of Human Rights was introduced in 1948 on the heels of World War II. The 30 articles give an overview of the rights to which every human is entitled including the right to own property, claim asylum, receive an education, express their opinion, earn compensation for labour, be free of discrimination on the basis of race, sex, religion, national origin, or ideology, among many more (UN General Assembly, 1948). Article 25 of the declaration specifically identifies the right to a standard of living that includes food, clothing, housing, medical care, and social services. This includes the right to security in situations brought on by circumstances beyond the control of the individual. As social workers, we have an obligation to uphold the basic human rights of all people, especially when governments and societies attempt to prioritise one group over another.

The following five case studies from Syria, Greece, Bangladesh, India and the US illustrate the challenges when inequality and discrimination, and competing values and resources hampered the response to people on the move during the COVID-19 pandemic and the breaches of human rights and dignity, leaving them more vulnerable than ever.

Case study 1: Syrian refugees

In March 2020, UN officials identified three main sites at high risk due to overcrowded and unsanitary conditions: refugees in the Greek island camps, Rohingya refugees in Bangladesh and the other, a camp in north-western Syria with more than one million displaced people.

Since the beginning of the Syrian civil war in 2011, 13.5 million of the 21 million Syrian citizens have been forcibly displaced and discriminated against (Smajlovic & Murphy, 2020). Roughly half were internally displaced while the others sought refuge predominantly in Turkey, Greece, Lebanon, Jordan, Iraq, and Egypt. 93.7% of Syrians, currently the largest forcibly displaced population in the world, live in urban rather than camp settings. The vast majority live below the overall poverty line (less than US $3.84 per day) (UNHCR, 2020e). Access to basic necessities such as food, shelter, education, employment, and healthcare were already problematic and worsened in pandemic conditions. In Egypt, for example, at least 130,000 registered Syrians lost their livelihoods and faced eviction and food shortages (ACAPS, 2020). Lebanon and Jordan, hosts to hundreds of thousands of Syrians, rely heavily on humanitarian aid, a situation made worse by the explosion in Lebanon in August 2020 which destroyed the busy port area of the city causing significant loss of life and property, and pushed Lebanon into heightened political and economic crisis. In Turkey, organisations that supported refugees resorted to managing demand through triage by telephone and introducing gatekeeping measures that placed barriers to linking people with increasingly scarce resources (Nisanci et al., 2020).

Escalating conflict in the Idlib province of Syria forced a further one million people into a camp from December 2019 (UNHCR, 2020e). The WHO provided the first coronavirus test kits to those displaced in the Idlib region and identified cases of COVID-19. Substandard living conditions and limited access to healthcare contributed to disproportionately high numbers of cases and deaths due to coronavirus (Rosen, 2020). Common to all people on the move, many deaths were likely to be undiagnosed cases of COVID-19 due to limited testing and access to treatment. The capacity to isolate, survive poverty and their exclusion from the same rights and services as other people were and continue to be common experiences.

Case study 2: the Greek refugee crisis

Greece, Spain, and Italy are on the Central Mediterranean Migration Route from North Africa, along which many adults and children have lost their lives at sea while seeking refuge (UNICEF, 2017). Greece is the locale of a significant refugee crisis, where social and economic unrest escalated xenophobia and discrimination at individual and structural levels during the pandemic.

At the start of the pandemic, the European Commission financially supported the new, conservative Greek administration to protect the estimated 121,000 migrants and asylum seekers already in camps, over half of whom are women and children. Greece reached a *breaking point* in the refugee crisis after Turkey, a country that hosted 3.6 million Syrian refugees, announced in February 2020 that it would no longer prevent refugee transit into the European Union (IRC, 2020). In 2019 alone, the Greek Council for Refugees reported receiving 77,289 asylum applications, mostly from Afghanistan, Syria, Pakistan, Iraq, and other conflict zone countries. The overcrowded conditions in Greek refugee camps made physical distancing impossible, alongside inadequate healthcare and poor sanitation including limited access to water, which escalated the risk of exponential spread. From mid-April to June 2020, Greek authorities relocated 3,000 refugees to the mainland but as of the 9th of June, over 31,000 refugees remained on the five Aegean Islands, housing five times the original camp capacity.

In August, a health warning came for the safety of 19,500 refugees living in Moria, the largest camp on the island of Lesbos, with a capacity of 2,800 people, facing dire overcrowded and unsanitary conditions. Queuing for food made physical distancing impossible. The UN and human rights groups raised grave concerns about the conditions for 40,000 people living in reception centres with a capacity of only 6,000 (IRC, 2020). Local politics and the increased stress placed on local citizens due to the decline in tourism, an industry vital to the economy of the Greek islands, escalated discrimination and heightened risks for refugees and asylum seekers in Greece. Locals helping refugees were subjected to harassment within communities and refugees, doing what they could to survive, escalated tensions further.

In early September 2020, a series of fires broke out in Moria, destroying the camp and ousting people from already substandard conditions. The camp's official capacity was 2,800 but was housing nearly 13,000 refugees. The tensions between far-right groups and refugees hit a boiling point as new COVID-19 restrictions were imposed on the camp after 35 people tested positive (Labropoulou et al., 2020). Although it was unclear how the fires started, the result was desperate refugees left with nothing and without a clear path forward. Since the fire, about 2800 people left the island but more than 7,000 people continue to live in Mavrovouni, a camp hastily established as an emergency site for those left homeless following the fire (The Guardian, 2020). The conditions at Mavrovouni raised further concerns about unexploded ammunition as it was built on a disused firing range (Libal et al., 2021). The Greek government were strongly criticised for their neglect of people under their protection.

Case study 3: Rohingya refugees in Bangladesh

The next case study explores the plight of Rohingya refugees, a Muslim, ethnic minority from Myanmar, one of the most discriminated against minority groups in the world subject to what has been described as a *slow burning genocide* since 1978 (Zarni & Cowley, 2014, p. 683). The challenges faced by the Rohingya can be traced back to at least 1948 when they were partially excluded by law from citizenship rights in their own country, which was further limited in 1962 following a military junta (CFR, 2020). In 1978, the Myanmar military evicted 200,000 Rohingya from their homes, committed widespread human rights violations which caused an influx into Bangladesh. In 1990, following a failed democratic election, 250,000 Rohingya fled, then many again in 1997 (ACAPS, 2017). The pattern of discrimination, violence, and expulsions has worsened since 2012, and more so during the pandemic.

At least one million Rohingyas who fled violence and persecution in Myanmar were in Bangladeshi camps at the onset of the COVID-19 pandemic. These camps had a density population four times that of New York City, where physical distancing, lockdown, handwashing and other measures were impossible due to lack of space and supplies. Although the UN was constructing isolation shelters and quarantine facilities around the camps since late March 2020, international volunteers who were providing basic primary care in the camps were evacuated. The role of refugee volunteers had become critical and conditions worsened for the Rohingya. Monsoonal weather heightened risks of the rapid spread of disease within the camps.

Simulations of the potential impact of COVID-19 on the largest expansion site, Kutupalong-Balukhali, which had a largely young and female population, suggested that the spread of the disease would supersede any preparedness planning and prevention activities (Truelove et al., 2020). Given pre-existing comorbidities (poverty, lack of protective equipment, limited facilities, and health access), the high-spread scenario predicted high mortality numbers (Truelove et al., 2020). In addition to the myriad of risk factors, the internet ban imposed in September 2019 made access to accurate information extremely difficult, leading to rumours and fears of being abducted or killed in isolation centres if healthcare was sought (Barua & Karia, 2020). Although rumours lacked specific evidence, fears led many people to believe them based on decades of experience with persecution and human rights violations.

Prior to the onset of the pandemic, plans were established between the Bangladesh and Myanmar governments to begin the process of repatriation (returning refugees to Myanmar). Human rights groups voiced concerns citing the lack of evidence that Myanmar had addressed the systems in place that led to decades of persecution and violence (Human Rights Watch, 2019). While repatriation is problematic, the one million refugees in Bangladeshi camps face extreme deprivation of basic needs like sanitation and healthcare. The Rohingya have experienced a long-standing history of persecution, forced migration into impoverished neighbouring countries where discrimination continued, and now highly concentrated numbers of people live in confined spaces with scarce food and contaminated water, lack of access to healthcare or basic sanitation making this group incredibly vulnerable to the COVID-19 pandemic.

Case study 4: migrants displaced in India

The social and economic impact of the COVID-19 pandemic affected migration and refugee systems in all host countries. Alongside extreme climate events and other disasters, people on the move and internally displaced persons including migrant workers risked high exposure in dire circumstances which leads us to the situation in India.

India, home to 1.3 billion people, is not a signatory of the 1951 UN Convention Relating to the Status of Refugees. Instead, India follows the Foreigners Act of 1946, which covers tourists, migrant workers, forced migrants, asylum seekers, refugees, and stateless persons together with enormous latitude in how each is treated (World Population Review, 2020). The way India supports refugees is largely based on relationships with the home country, leading to a wide range of inequities (Athray, 2020). There were over 40,000 refugees registered with

UNHCR in India, who were hit hard by the pandemic. More than two million people, including internally displaced people, asylum seekers, and stateless persons, were vulnerable due to their status with varied and limited rights (Hussain & Sharma, 2020). Floods, dam and mining development projects, and border conflicts left millions of people internally displaced from their homes and vulnerable to extreme poverty prior to the significant adverse consequences of the COVID-19 health emergency. Johns Hopkins University (2020) reported nearly nine and a half million confirmed cases and more than 137,000 deaths making India one of the fastest growing rates of COVID-19. Although India began surveillance early, testing rates have been low and confirmed cases continued to rise exponentially (Bharali, Kumar & Selvaraj, 2020). UNICEF published a report that estimated the number of children living in extreme poverty could grow from 240 million to 360 million in South Asia by the end of 2020. Food insecurity, health programs on hold, limited access to education, increased domestic violence, and suicide were only a few of the indirect consequences of coronavirus on women and children in South Asia (UNICEF, 2020).

Migrant workers who travelled from far flung villages to find work in cities were suddenly left without a job or means to get home when a three-week lockdown was announced on the 24th of March with little warning. Tens of thousands of migrant workers and their families had no choice but to walk. The journeys were perilous, on highways and railroad tracks. Families, including children, walked hundreds and some thousands of kilometres, and hundreds lost their lives (Pandey, 2020).

Case study 5: detention, family separation, and deportation at the US-Mexico border

People in prisons and prison-like conditions were at high risk of uncontrollable outbreaks given overcrowded, unsanitary conditions in these facilities. The US has the most people per capita in detention centres (which are prison-like environments) in the world and 2.3 million people in prison, with a disproportionate number of African Americans, minority groups and socioeconomically disadvantaged, conditions which worsened under the Trump administration. In one facility alone, the Federal Terminal Island prison in San Pedro, 600 inmates and 14 staff members tested positive for COVID-19 and six people were dead by the 5th of May 2020 (Trevizo, 2020). Immigrants in detention centres across the US faced similar conditions and were under significant threat of COVID-19 spread. The pandemic further jeopardised the safe repatriation or resettlement in a third country, a practice already politicised and even more challenging as it was often forcefully enacted in violation of the *principle of non-refoulement* (ICRC, 2020). The principle of non-refoulement under international law guarantees "… that no one should be returned to a country where they would face torture, cruel, inhuman or degrading treatment or punishment and other irreparable harm. This principle applies to all migrants at all times, irrespective of migration status" (OHCHR, n.d.).

Detention, family separation and deportation at the US–Mexico border, exemplified how political opportunism during the COVID-19 pandemic severely affected children and their families from the Central American Northern Triangle who crossed the US–Mexico border to seek asylum and found themselves in detention or shelters, families forcibly separated, and eventually deported to unsafe countries (Trevizo, 2020). In 2019, over 43,000 immigrants were held in over 100 US Immigration Customs Enforcement (ICE) run facilities. By August 2020, more than 7,000 minors who travelled alone or were forcibly separated from their families at the US–Mexico border were placed in Office of Refugee Resettlement (ORR) shelters and ICE family detention centres after being declared unaccompanied minors.

Prior to and during the pandemic, families were placed in detention centres where crowded and unsanitary conditions increased the risk of infection, parents deported without their children (later placed under ORR custody), or entire families sent to Mexico whether or not that was their home country. Mounting evidence regarding the continued practice of family separation through force, fraud and coercion triggered legal claims and judicial orders, mostly aimed at improving immigrant conditions and releasing minors, particularly in emergency health conditions (Kassie & Marcolini, 2020; Rotabi & Monico, 2020). These acts breached human rights and especially the Rights of the Child (CRC) further traumatising victims of this system.

Although the Trump administration's 2019 *zero tolerance policy* was short-lived, it was followed by new practices that undermined the Flores Settlement Agreement, which restricted detention of minors to 20 days and ordered their placement in child-friendly facilities. The same year, Customs and Border Protection (CBP) began expediting the screening of asylum seekers including children and applied the Migrant Protection Protocols, to return applicants to Mexico to await their migration proceedings. On the 20th of March 2020, the Centers for Disease Control and Prevention (CDC) invoked the 1944 Surgeon General's power issuing an order that returns all foreign nationals without entry authorisation to their contiguous or home countries. A combination of these and other executive actions resulted in a drastic drop in border apprehensions and new asylum applications, and the expansion of detention and deportation of asylum seekers through expedited proceedings or during annual immigration follow up appointments.

The ICE became a spreader of COVID-19 within and outside US borders. Despite limiting access to testing for detainees, 3,000 cases of COVID-19 were confirmed among immigrants under custody. Human rights groups and the media documented cases of immigrants suspected or tested positive for COVID-19 moved from one detention centre to another, presumably to place them in isolation. Others were deported to their countries of origin or to third countries while infected. At least 200 deportation flights to eleven countries were confirmed to have transported migrants sick with COVID-19 (Kassie & Marcolini, 2020). Besides overcrowding making physical distancing impossible, immigrant detention facilities were unsanitary and offered no protections. Furthermore, the agencies responsible for the detained migrants' well-being contributed to their suffering, retraumatisation, and the spread of the virus across international borders. Since the fall of the Trump administration, President Biden is reversing many of Trump's policy decisions made against migrants especially the separation of children from their families and how to manage unaccompanied minors arriving at the border (Krogstad & Gonzalez-Barrera, 2021).

Where to from here?

Governments across the globe have failed to act for the health and safety of people residing within their borders, entitled to basic rights independent of their country of origin or status, especially during a global health crisis. There have been far too few examples of culturally sensitive strategies in the design and delivery of services to migrant and mobile populations and the exclusion of social workers in planning (Smajlovic & Murphy, 2020). Few efforts have addressed discrimination or supported the efforts of the people themselves or governments heeding their concerns. This is particularly challenging in places like Lesbos where friction and tensions have been dangerous for refugees and asylum seekers for a long time. Multi-pronged approaches and models that take environmental factors into account, including population density and mobility, have greater potential to prevent outbreaks and combat COVID-19 more effectively (OECD, 2020). However, some locations were more vulnerable than others due to a combination of contextual factors.

With widely varied approaches to pandemic management, levels of preparedness, second and third waves, and the promise of vaccinations in an ambiguous future, discriminated against groups were at greater risk due to limited access to support. Mobile populations were mostly excluded at all national planning and are likely to be last in line in vaccination distribution. In May of 2020, Orcutt and colleagues published a correspondence in the Lancet calling for three action items at the intersection of the pandemic and migration:

1. urgent universal access to health systems
2. inclusion of migrant and refugee populations in health responses and
3. responsible, transparent, and migrant-inclusive public information strategies (Orcutt et al., 2020)

Under-resourced international and national non-profit organisations to their credit continued to work at meeting unmet need and supporting state efforts by filling the public sector gap while advocating for necessary social investments and funding for public health programs.

As healthcare systems across the world attempted to meet the challenges presented by COVID-19, a light has been shone on the inequality of health outcomes based on legal status, a disproportionate share of the disease burden, and systemic barriers that preclude immigrants and refugees from their right to health, and breaches of the rights of children among others. Exclusion stems from a lack of documentation (e.g. born in a refugee camp without a birth certificate or forced to flee without documentation) to bureaucratic obstacles and outright discrimination (Chuah et al., 2018; Hacker et al., 2015). Both beneficiaries and healthcare providers are often unaware of the entitlements in place, which vary greatly from country to country.

Although migrants are a heterogeneous group with varied vulnerabilities, the process of migration in and of itself is a social determinant of health. Chronic non-communicable diseases such as cancer, chronic respiratory diseases, cardiovascular diseases, and diabetes make up 60% of global causes of death with 80% occurring in low and middle-income countries. Since many immigrants and refugees come from these countries, they will likely experience an additional layer of risk and have worse outcomes from COVID-19 (WHO, 2018). Labour migrants tend to experience poorer working conditions, higher risk jobs, lower pay, few legal protections, and limited access to health systems, resulting in increased use of emergency care and poorer health outcomes. The COVID-19 global pandemic should serve as a wakeup call to align legal protections and the right to health and to reduce these inequities.

Immigrant and refugee populations often find themselves struggling to meet competing basic needs of food, shelter, and safety, and as a result, require special treatment during a pandemic. We argue that integrating migrant populations into health systems and reducing barriers to care through offering legal protections, health literacy education in culturally and linguistically accessible ways, and increasing cultural awareness, sensitivity and cross-cultural efficacy of providers. Lockdowns to contain disease would be more successful if people are provided with the means to protect and feed themselves, provided with the necessary equipment such as PPE and soap, and are included rather than excluded from the rights other people enjoy. Forced migrants are disproportionately impacted by the economic and health consequences of a global pandemic and require specialised support to recover (OECD, 2020). Social workers have a specialised set of skills and an ethical obligation to advocate for the human right of health, equal access to resources, support for mental health needs, and fighting for economic justice on behalf of immigrant and refugee populations.

Implications for social work

Social work is a discipline actively engaged with people on the move in all scenarios and has the potential to make significant contributions at the intersection of health and migration at the macro, mezzo, and micro levels. The profession is guided by ethical shared principles and values of "… social justice, human rights, collective responsibility and respect for diversities …" (IFSW, 2014). Social workers across the globe therefore have professional obligations to meet the challenges of this latest global public health crisis and into the future, particularly the consequences for vulnerable people forced from their homes. Smajlovic and Murphy (2020) critiqued social work's attention to this field, particularly in the US for exerting insufficient pressure on the plight of people on the move and in social work education and suggested a range of interventions from micro through to macro practice.

This public health emergency has illuminated the precariousness and instability of circumstances faced by people on the move and brought with it the realisation that even in privileged parts of the world, pandemics, recessions, persecution, extreme climate events, floods, fires, hurricanes, earthquakes, volcanic eruptions and so on can make all people vulnerable to displacement. It is not about the *other* but about resources and access to those resources without discrimination. A global pandemic has long been predicted and social work as a profession needs to be actively advocating to include people on the move in preparedness planning to ensure they have food and other supplies to survive essential period of lockdown, have sufficient protective equipment, equal access to healthcare, and adequate and safe housing. Most of all, the forced separation of families as a matter of state policy is one of the greatest breaches of human and child rights.

At this macro level, interventions should include global advocacy related to migration policy reform. This requires developing partnerships with forced migrant communities and supporting their grassroots activist activities. Governments' social service supports are imperative during lockdowns and social workers can advocate a strong social response on behalf of forced migrants. According to OECD (2020), policy options can include engaging refugee communities in health sector strategies and programming, adjusting border restrictions in a way that respects human rights as well as refugee law (including non-refoulement), and building health system resilience with a focus on fragile contexts of forced migration. As social work professionals, we must continue to develop cultural sensitivity, awareness and cross-cultural efficacy in working with forced migrant communities. The field of social worker must prepare future social work professionals to address systemic barriers to healthcare access.

At the micro level, social workers should be brokers of needed resources between people on the move, families, and communities with needed services as well as attending to trauma. When gaps are identified in these communities and needed services, social workers can raise awareness and work toward filling the gaps. These may include providing culturally and linguistically appropriate information and improving health literacy, linking forced migrants with legal services, and case management services in tracing and reuniting children and adolescents who have been separated from families. In many cases, remote case management will be necessary and may fill a long-standing gap in services that existed before the pandemic (IFSW, 2020).

In times of crisis, social workers must also maintain a longer view of the systems at play. The decisions that are made as a result of this pandemic provide a chance to work as a global community to address the intersection of these two challenges. As Guterres (2020) said, "the COVID-19 crisis is an opportunity to reimagine human mobility .... No country can fight the pandemic or manage migration alone". In addition to fighting the pandemic and addressing human mobility issues, long-term economic hardship will likely impact forced migrants disproportionately and should be the target of social work intervention. Moreno et al. (2020) identified ways in which the mental health system of care should take advantage of the global pandemic to make important changes in order to reach the most vulnerable populations. Such changes include increased community outreach and education, adjusting settings to prevent the spread of infectious disease, and increasing access to mental health services for healthcare workers and those impacted by the virus. The clinical arm of social work practice should be involved in the research and policy changes enacted to increase mental healthcare access and reduced disparities based on criteria like migration status.

BOX 11.2

REFLECTIVE QUESTIONS

1. Select one of the case studies. Imagine you are a person who has been forced to leave their country, endured extreme hardships on your journey and found yourself in a camp or detention centre in this foreign country. You do not speak the language. You have heard rumours of a new disease that is killing people. Consider the following in the context of the circumstances of your migration and the sociopolitical context of the host country:
   - What health, legal and social challenges might you face including having your basic needs for sustenance and security met?
   - How might you address these challenges considering the resources at your disposal?
2. Consider the forced separation of children from their families at the US–Mexico border under the Trump administration.
   - What are the developmental, psychological and social impact on children?
   - What rights have been violated?
   - What actions might social workers take to redress the impact of these policies in macro and micro practice?
3. The case studies have highlighted some of the competing values and ethics at play when considering policies aimed at providing access to resources equitably across the entire population of a country. Imagine you are a social worker working for an international organisation in this context. How do you make sense of these competing values and ethics? Unpack these to understand the dilemmas and conflicts in resource poor environments alongside social work values and ethics.

References

ACAPS. (2017, December). *Review: Rohingya influx since 1978.* https://reliefweb.int/sites/reliefweb.int/files/resources/20171211_acaps_rohingya_historical_review_0.pdf

ACAPS. (2020, June 23). *Egypt.* https://www.acaps.org/country/egypt/crisis/syrian-refugees

Athray, D. (2020, July 7). *The plight of refugees in India during COVID-19.* https://www.orfonline.org/expert-speak/the-plight-of-refugees-in-india-during-covid19-69287/

Barua, A., & Karia, R. H., 2020. Challenges faced by Rohingya refugees in the COVID-19 pandemic. *Annals of Global Health*, 86(1), 129. http://doi.org/10.5334/aogh.3052

Bharali, I., Kumar, P., & Selvaraj, S. (2020, July 02). *How well is India responding to COVID-19?* https://www.brookings.edu/blog/future-development/2020/07/02/how-well-is-india-responding-to-covid-19/

CFR. (2020). *The Rohingya crisis.* Council on Foreign Relations. https://www.cfr.org/backgrounder/rohingya-crisis

Chuah, F., Tan, S. T., Yeo, J., & Legido-Quigley, H. (2018). The health needs and access barriers among refugees and asylum-seekers in Malaysia: A qualitative study. *International Journal for Equity in Health*, 17(1), 1–15.

Guterres, A. (2020, June 3). *The COVID-19 crisis is an opportunity to reimagine human mobility.* https://www.un.org/en/coronavirus/covid-19-crisis-opportunity-reimagine-human-mobility

Hacker, K., Anies, M., Folb, B. L., & Zallman, L. (2015). Barriers to healthcare for undocumented immigrants: A literature review. *Risk Management and Healthcare Policy*, 8, 175–183. https://doi.org/10.2147/RMHP.S70173

HROHC. (n.d.) *The principle of non-refoulement under international human rights law.* https://www.ohchr.org/Documents/Issues/Migration/GlobalCompactMigration/ThePrincipleNon-RefoulementUnderInternationalHumanRightsLaw.pdf

Human Rights Watch. (2019, August 20). *Myanmar/Bangladesh: Halt Rohingya returns.* https://www.hrw.org/news/2019/08/20/myanmar/bangladesh-halt-rohingya-returns

Hussain, Z., & Sharma, G. (2020, July 19). Floods in India, Nepal displace nearly four million people, at least 189 dead. *Reuters.* https://www.reuters.com/article/us-india-floods/floods-in-india-nepal-displace-nearly-four-million-people-at-least-189-dead-idUSKCN24K06S

ICRC. (2020). *Annual report.* International Committee of the Red Cross. https://www.icrc.org/en/document/annual-report-2020

IDMC. (2020). *2020 Global report on internal displacement.* https://www.internal-displacement.org/global-report/grid2020/

IFSW. (2014). *What is social work?* https://www.ifsw.org/what-is-social-work/global-definition-of-social-work/

IFSW. (2020, July 1). *The social work response to covid-19 – six months on: Championing changes in services and preparing for long-term consequences.* https://www.ifsw.org/the-social-work-response-to-covid-19-six-months-on-championing-changes-in-services-and-preparing-for-long-term-consequences/

IRC. (2020, March 03). *As Greece reaches breaking point, the International Rescue Committee urges Europe to step in.* https://www.rescue.org/press-release/greece-reaches-breaking-point-international-rescue-committee-urges-europe-step

Johns Hopkins University. (2020). *Coronavirus Resource Center: India.* https://coronavirus.jhu.edu/region/india

Karlsson, S. G. & Jönsson, J. H. (2020). Forced migration, older refugees and displacement: Implications for social work as a human rights profession. *Journal of Human Rights and Social Work*, 5(3), 212–222.

Kassie, E., & Marcolini, B. (2020, July 10). 'It was like a time bomb': How ICE helped spread the coronavirus. *New York Times*. https://www.nytimes.com/2020/07/10/us/ice-coronavirusdeportation.html?referringSource=articleShare&fbclid=IwAR1BIj4tak-nqjslk4lRoTd6hfb4BMGq9yGFk43I-nH1WcvvCxRdaIjWyiAI

Krogstad, J. M., & Gonzalez-Barrera, A. (2021, March 22). Key facts about U.S. immigration policies and Biden's proposed changes. *Pew Research Center*. https://www.pewresearch.org/fact-tank/2021/03/22/key-facts-about-u-s-immigration-policies-and-bidens-proposed-changes/

Labropoulou, E., Liakos, C., Halasz, S., & Qiblawi, T. (September 10, 2020). Fire ravages Europe's largest migrant camp on Lesbos. *CNN*. https://www.cnn.com/2020/09/09/europe/greece-lesbos-fires-intl/index.html

Libal, K., Harding, S., Popescu, M., Berthold, S. M., & Felten, G. (2021). Human rights of forced migrants during the COVID-19 pandemic: An opportunity for mobilization and solidarity. *Journal of Human Rights and Social Work*. doi:10.1007/s41134-021-00162-4

Moreno, C., Wykes, T., Galderisi, S., Nordentoft, M., Crossley, N., Jones, N., Cannon, M., Correll, C. U., Byrne, L., Carr, S., Chen, E. Y. H., Gorwood, P., Johnson, S., Kärkkäinen, H., Krystal, J. H., Lee, J., Lieberman, J., López-Jaramillo, C., Männikkö, M., Phillips, …, Arango, C. (2020). How mental healthcare should change as a consequence of the COVID-19 pandemic. *The Lancet: Psychiatry*, 7(9), 813–824.

Nisanci, A., Kahraman, R., Alcelik, Y., & Kiris, U. (2020). Working with refugees during COVID-19: Social worker voices from Turkey. *International Social Work*. https://doi.org/10.1177/0020872820940032

OECD. (2020, June 15). *The impact of coronavirus (COVID-19) on forcibly displaced persons in developing countries*. http://www.oecd.org/coronavirus/policy-responses/the-impact-of-coronavirus-covid-19-on-forcibly-displaced-persons-in-developing-countries-88ad26de/

OHCHR. (n.d.) *The principle of non-refoulment under international human rights law*. https://www.ohchr.org/Documents/Issues/Migration/GlobalCompactMigration/ThePrincipleNon-RefoulementUnderInternationalHumanRightsLaw.pdf

Orcutt, M., Patel, P., Burns, R., Hiam, L., Aldridge, R., Devakumar, D., Kumar, B., Spiegal, P., & Abubakar, I. (2020). Global call to action for inclusion of migrants and refugees in the COVID-19 response. *The Lancet*, 395(10235), 1482–1483.

Pandey, V. (May 19, 2020). Coronavirus lockdown: The Indian migrants dying to get home. BBC. https://www.bbc.com/news/world-asia-india-52672764

Rosen, K. R. (2020, July 10). 3 million Syrians will lose aid as first COVID-19 case is reported in Idlib. *Newsweek*. https://www.newsweek.com/syria-idlib-coronavirus-aid-1516858

Rotabi, K. & Monico, C. (2020, July 3). 20 Facts that you should know about current immigration policies and procedures including child separations, loss of children in the system, and asylum seeking. *National Association of Social Workers: California News*. https://naswcanews.org/feature-20-facts-that-you-should-know-about-current-immigration-policies-and-procedures-including-child-separations-loss-of-children-in-the-system-and-asylum-seeking/?fbclid=IwAR0-NuyhCQPHEfZiMtjvUDib27ruIhKVKbGt9WuwnAcw0GmjIuJKGTFyl6k

Smajlovic, A., & Murphy, A. L. (2020). Invisible no more: Social work, human rights, and the Syrian refugee crisis. *Journal of Human Rights and Social Work*, 5(2), 139–144.

The Guardian. (2020, December 2). Aftermath of Moria refugee campfire – photo essay. *The Guardian*. https://www.theguardian.com/artanddesign/2020/dec/02/aftermath-moria-refugee-camp-fire-photo-essay

Trevizo, P. (2020, May 11). COVID-19 cases at one Texas immigration detention center soared in a matter of days. Now, town leaders want answers. https://www.propublica.org/article/covid-19-cases-at-one-texas-immigration-detention-center-soared-in-a-matter-of-days-now-town-leaders-want-answer

Truelove, S., Abrahim, O., Altare, C., Lauer, S. A., Grantz, K. H., Azman, A. S., & Spiegel, P. (2020). The potential impact of COVID-19 in refugee camps in Bangladesh and beyond: A modeling study. *PLoS Medicine*, 17(6), 1–15.

UN General Assembly. (1948). *Universal Declaration of Human Rights (217 [III] A)*. Paris.

UNESCO. (2008). *People on the move: Handbook of selected terms and concepts*. https://unesdoc.unesco.org/ark:/48223/pf0000163621

UNHCR. (2019). *Global trends: Forced displacement in 2019*. https://www.unhcr.org/en-au/statistics/unhcrstats/5ee200e37/unhcr-global-trends-2019.html

UNHCR. (2020a, June 18). *Figures at a glance*. United Nations High Commissioner for Refugees. https://www.unhcr.org/en-us/figures-at-a-glance.html

UNHCR. (2020b). *Asylum-seekers*. United Nations High Commissioner for Refugees. https://www.unhcr.org/en-us/asylum-seekers.html

UNHCR. (2020d). *Refugee statistics*. United Nations High Commissioner for Refugees. https://www.unrefugees.org/refugee-facts/statistics/

UNHCR. (2020e, June 30). *Syria refugee crisis explained*. United Nations High Commissioner for Refugees. https://www.unrefugees.org/news/syria-refugee-crisis-explained/

UNICEF. (2017, February). *A deadly journey for children: The Central Mediterranean migration route*. https://www.unicef.org/publications/index_94905.html

UNICEF. (2020, June). *Lives upended: How COVID-19 threatens the futures of 600 million South Asian children*. https://www.unicef.org/rosa/sites/unicef.org.rosa/files/2020-06/UNICEF%20Upended%20Lives%20Report%20-%20June%202020.pdf

United Nations High Commissioner for Refugees. (2004). *Guiding principles on internal displacement*. https://www.unhcr.org/en-us/43ce1cff2

WHO. (2018). *Health of refugees and migrants: Regional situation analysis, practices, experiences, lessons learned and ways forward*. https://www.who.int/migrants/publications/EURO-report.pdf

World Population Review. (2020). *India population 2020 (Live)*. https://worldpopulationreview.com/countries/india-population

Zarni, M., & Cowley, A. (2014). The slow burning genocide of Myanmar's Rohingya. *Pacific Rim Law and Policy Journal*, 23(3), 683–754.

12

MENTAL HEALTH SOCIAL WORK IN HONG KONG DURING THE COVID-19 PANDEMIC

Ching-Wen Chang and Marcus Chiu

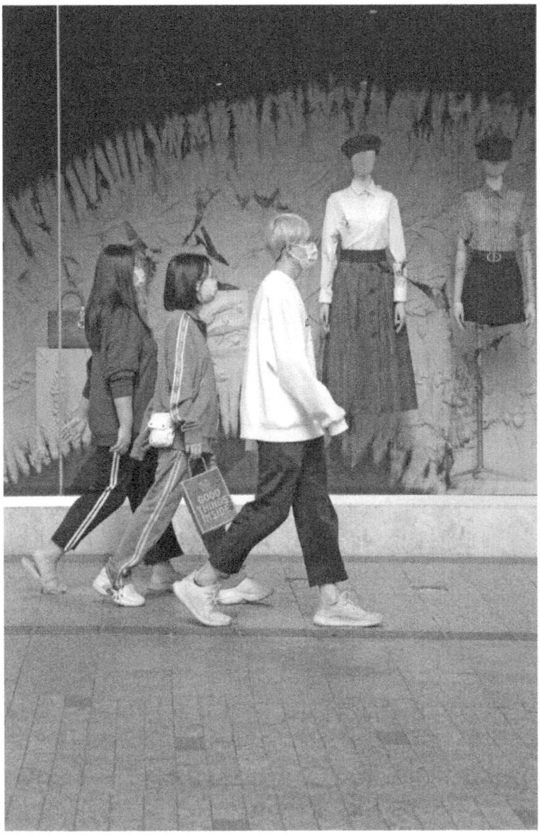

FIGURE 12.0 Life changed during the COVID-19 pandemic

Source: Photograph by Stephen Finkel

DOI: 10.4324/9781003111214-14

Mental health services in Hong Kong were established prior to the COVID-19 pandemic. Conventional welfare-based mental health social work is provided mainly through different medical settings, hospital-based medical social work and psychiatric outpatient clinics. In 2010, the Hong Kong Social Welfare Department established Integrated Centres for Community Mental Well-being (ICCMWs) to provide a one stop, accessible and integrated community mental health support service. A total of 24 ICCMWs are set up in all 18 districts in Hong Kong (Hong Kong Hospital Authority & Hong Kong Social Welfare Department, 2016; Hong Kong Social Welfare Department, 2021). The target populations are those people with mental health issues or suspected mental illness, their family members and individuals with an interest in promoting their mental well-being (Hong Kong Hospital Authority & Hong Kong Social Welfare Department, 2016). Mental health services cut across different age groups and are handled by different health and social service units – District Elderly Centres, Integrated Family Services Centres, Integrated Children and Youth Centres and ICCMWs, depending on the nature of the clientele and the intensity of the mental health issues.

Social workers are the main service providers in ICCMWs. For individuals with mental disorders, mental health social workers in ICCMWs provide social and rehabilitation services aimed at developing clients' physical, mental and social capabilities to reach their full potential. The ultimate objective is to help individuals with mental illness re-integrate into the community. Mental health social workers also provide services to support family members in caring for individuals with mental illness. For the general population, ICCMW social workers provide services to promote mental well-being through outreach education activities.

The state of mental health in Hong Kong during the pandemic

The first confirmed case of COVID-19 in Hong Kong was announced on 23 January 2020. Due to the fear of virus spread, physical distancing practices were implemented across Hong Kong. A variety of measures, including quarantine for people entering Hong Kong, school suspensions, work from home arrangements, and the closure of non-essential businesses were adopted to reduce the risk of the virus spread. In February, there was a shortage of surgical masks, food, toilet paper, and other daily necessities which caused hardship for many people. At the beginning of the COVID-19 outbreak, worry about contracting the virus, not being able to work from home, and not having enough surgical masks caused emotional distress at the individual level. Social isolation and disruptions to daily routines were also major contributors to mental health issues (Choi, Hui & Wan, 2020).

As the city has one of the world's highest property prices, the home space of many Hong Kongers is small and compact. The lack of personal space makes physical distancing almost impossible within the family. It not only raises the risk of group contagion within the family, but confined spaces also increases the risk of family conflicts, particularly for double-income parents with children schooling from home especially children with special educational needs, families who care for elderly people with cognitive impairment and people with chronic illness (Lau, Chan & Ng, 2020).

Because of the preventive measures for infection, business hours for beverage, food consumption and entertainment were shortened, travel and holidays almost came to a complete halt, and retail businesses were hardest hit. When special subsidies from the government to businesses ceased, many employees were asked to be on no-pay leave. As a result, the unemployment rate rose dramatically and hit a 16-year high with a rate of 6.6% in the final quarter of 2020 (Yau & Tsang, 2021). The worry about unemployment and joblessness became a strong contributing factor for mental health issues.

A survey conducted in late April 2020 in Hong Kong indicated that the prevalence rates of adults with depression was 19.8% and the anxiety rates was 14.0%. The prevalence rate of having both depression and anxiety was 12.4%. In addition, 25.4% of the respondents reported that their mental health had deteriorated since the COVID-19 pandemic began (Choi, Hui & Wan, 2020). Another biannual survey with more than 1300 respondents found 23% of respondents showed moderate to severe depression. The rate was the highest in the decade with a 30% increase compared to the rate two years ago. Moreover, 65% of the participants followed prevention advice and reduced their social contacts with others. People from a lower working class with less education and income demonstrated a higher stress and depression level, and furthermore, the general picture was that women had significantly poorer mental health than the male subjects (Chan, 2021).

The people of Hong Kong are familiar with the measures they must take to guard against disease due to prior experience with health emergencies including SARS in 2003 and H1N1 in 2009. While saying this, the impact of COVID-19 on mental health cannot be underestimated because it has lasted much longer and killed more people than either SARS or H1N1. Interestingly, the findings of a survey indicated that individuals who had not lived in Hong Kong during the 2003 SARS outbreak were more likely to have depression. Potentially, people in Hong Kong who experienced SARS in 2003 might be more psychologically prepared to fight the current virus outbreak and be more knowledgeable about what they should do to protect themselves. On the other hand, for those who did not live in Hong Kong during 2003 SARS outbreak, the first experience of a pandemic was an extremely stressful and unprepared for event (Choi, Hui & Wan, 2020). Results of the survey also revealed that individuals who were more worried about being infected by COVID-19 were more bothered by not having enough surgical masks, were more bothered by not being able to work from home, and were more likely to have depression, anxiety, or combined depression and anxiety (Choi, Hui & Wan, 2020).

Coexisting political stressors

Hong Kong was a British colony from 1841 to 1997. On 1 July 1997, Hong Kong was returned to China and became a special administrative region. Under the 1984 agreement between China and Britain, Hong Kong should have its own political system and a high degree of autonomy in all matters except for foreign relations and military defence. The joint declaration of China and Britain also specified that Hong Kong maintains its capitalist economic system and the rights and freedoms of Hong Kong people should be guaranteed for at least 50 years after the 1997 handover.

From 26 September to 15 December 2014, the Occupy Central Movement, a civil disobedience campaign, occurred in Hong Kong. There was an ongoing protest led by students against the decision regarding reforms to Hong Kong electoral system issued by China's Standing Committee of the National People's Congress. However, government officials in Hong Kong and in Beijing denounced the occupancy of the central area of Hong Kong as *illegal* and police tactics against the protesters led more citizens to join.

Starting in June 2019, a series of large-scale demonstrations proceeded in Hong Kong to express concern over the Extradition Bill which would allow the transfer of fugitives to jurisdictions where Hong Kong lacks an extradition deal, including mainland China, Taiwan and Macau, and later in response to the Hong Kong National Security Law in June 2020. Due to concerns about undermining Hong Kong's autonomy and its people's civil rights, a series of protests were organised. From June 2019 to January 2020, there was serious ongoing and large-scale social unrest with escalating levels of violence, assault, arson and vandalism. Subsequent arrests and court convictions severely impacted Hong Kong citizens' mental health in a time of uncertainty and a diminishing sense of safety (Ng, 2020).

A large-scale longitudinal survey conducted on adults found that during the anti-extradition bill movement in 2019, 11.2% of participants reported probable depression. It was estimated that the prevalence of suspected Post-Traumatic Stress Disorder (PTSD) was 12.8%. In addition, one out of five adults reported either probable major depression or suspected PTSD. The prevalence of probable depression during the 2019 social unrest was substantially higher, compared to around 2% in 2009–2014 before the 2014 Occupy Central Movement, and 6.5% in 2017 after the Occupy Central Movement. The investigation of risk factors found that heavy social media use of two or more hours per day was associated with depression and PTSD. However, family support was a protective factor for depression (Ni et al., 2020). Civil unrest coincided with the COVID-19 pandemic, causing a double jeopardy for the mental health of people in Hong Kong.

Mental health social work during the COVID-19 pandemic

In the early stage of the COVID-19 pandemic, mental health services provided by ICCMW social workers were seriously disrupted due to the requirement for physical distancing. When mental health sites were closed, the majority of mental health services shifted from face-to-face to online delivery. However, the online mode may have compromised the efficacy of some services that relied on human interaction and resonance. For many mental health workers, an online alternative was a new option of which they had little experience and accumulated wisdom even though they were more than willing to try and err. Some situations like the conduct of preliminary psychiatric assessments with unwilling clients or clients who had no access to online means meant it was difficult to determine how these and other crisis interventions could be carried out. The more viable scope of online services included, but were not limited to, information giving, educating clients on self-care during the pandemic and developing strategies to cope with social isolation. In-house facilities were resumed where possible, depending on the current state of the pandemic, to provide clients with opportunities to stay connected. In addition, an online educational kit, such as videos for self-care, were provided for clients.

Since many service users were already disadvantaged before the pandemic, delivering necessities such as surgical masks and used smartphones to enable access to online services and coaching clients how to use the devices, were the main foci of service providers. However, check-up services and emotional support were provided by telephone for those who were not able to access or use mobile devices. As the pandemic was proving difficult to control and became long-lasting, providing emotional support was emphasised in mental health services. In addition to assisting clients' self-care, listening to clients' concerns and supporting clients to manage their fears, worries and pandemic-related stress were a major focus for hotlines.

From January to the end of December 2020, there were four major waves of virus spread periods, each lasting between one and three months and, hence, limiting face-to-face services able to be provided during those periods. In between these waves, there were days when zero COVID-19 cases were identified. During COVID-19, limited services were provided at three levels of prevention for health and mental health issues (Constantino & Privitera, 2011; Perlmutter, Vayda & Woodburn, 1976). Increasing psychological resistance to mental health issues related to COVID-19 was one of the important strategies in primary prevention. At the primary intervention level, mental health social workers supported their existing clients to self-care providing information and tangible support. Secondary prevention focussed on reducing the negative impacts of disease and mental health issues that had already manifested. When disease or mental health challenges occurred, secondary prevention aimed to detect and treat disease and mental health problems as early as possible. Also, at the secondary level, mental health social workers provided emotional and psychological support to relieve COVID-19 related anxiety and depression.

Tertiary prevention aimed to alleviate the effects of ongoing illness and complex mental health issues that have long-term impacts, enhance individuals' abilities to function, increase their life expectancy and improve their quality of life as much as possible. At this tertiary prevention level, mental health social workers provided ongoing, longer-term assistance to help those people with pre-existing, complex mental health issues cope with the impact of anxiety and depression. Although conceptually, mental health social work can take part in all three levels of prevention, services on the ground had to be selective and focussed because a *Jack-of-all-trades* approach could easily become master of none. In other words, the services would not be able to deliver any service well if they were stretched too far. It is good practice for services to establish their best practice at the three levels of intervention and share what they are good at with service users and community agencies so that service users can choose which service to contact and what to ask for.

In terms of mental health services for the general population, interventions at the primary prevention level were lacking during COVID-19 due to pandemic management constraints. Before the COVID-19 pandemic, mental health services for the general population were provided mainly through community outreach for mental health promotion education and risk identification. Conducting outreach activities in the community was no longer feasible during the COVID-19 outbreak, and so, some mental health social workers stopped delivering services to the general population while others provided online education programs for mental health enhancement. However, how to engage the general population in the use of online services and how to evaluate the outcomes of these services were certainly challenges for the social work profession in the mental health field during this unusual time.

Challenges for mental health social workers during the COVID-19 pandemic

The first and foremost challenge for mental health social workers was to identify groups in the community who were directly or indirectly vulnerable to the negative impact of the pandemic. Pre-existing users of mental health services with psychiatric diagnoses were already known to be vulnerable to general and specific stress related to the pandemic which would further complicate their mental health status. Exaggerated fears and, in some cases, delusional beliefs about contracting the virus had negative mental health outcomes. Injections can be associated with persecutory and involuntary mental health treatment which may have affected people's willingness to receive vaccination against COVID-19. In some cases, clients were at risk of relapse if they were unable to cope with a prolonged stressful environment.

Apart from mental health service users, there are particular groups in the community who suffer more than others. Understaffed private nursing homes used to augment their service by allowing family caregivers to visit and assist with care. During the pandemic, visitors were refused entry to curb community spread which has had a devastating effect on the frail elderly in nursing homes. Family caregivers who were refused visits for months held burning concerns for their loved ones and felt absolutely helpless because they could not do anything at all from outside the nursing home. News of virus transmission to nursing home residents created many fears for family caregivers, affecting their own well-being as well as the devasting impact on older people.

Mental health social workers were also at-risk while doing their work. This was particularly so when medical settings became highly vulnerable places for everyone, especially professional staff. Social workers whose offices were in a clinic or hospital worried whether surgical masks alone were good enough to protect them and their own family members. On the other hand, there were concerns that the efficacy of interventions may have been compromised when they were allowed to work from a home office. In reality, to cope with COVID-19 related anxiety and to protect their own family members, few workers in the human services left home.

As the implementation of online modes of service delivery became unavoidable, learning how to conduct administrative functions smoothly and how to deliver clinical services were urgently needed. Coaching at the institutional level and service sector level was necessary. Equipment and capacity building were necessary supports which should be built into service policy and strategies to realise the goals set for online service delivery.

Although Hong Kong people had experienced SARS and H1N1 pandemic, mental health social workers still faced great challenges during the COVID-19 pandemic. In 2003, mental health social work in the community was still in the development stage in Hong Kong and ICCMWs were not yet established. Hence, very limited services were provided by mental health social workers during the 2003 SARS pandemic, apart from one or two teams of government social workers who were stationed at sites to provide tangible, psychological support. While the 2003 SARS pandemic was resolved in six months, the COVID-19 pandemic has lasted for more than a year and had yet to be resolved at the time of writing this chapter. The conditions for the pandemic and measures announced by the government for virus control has changed over time which led to constant readjustments in service provision. As a result, a major challenge for mental health social workers in Hong Kong was the lack of empirical evidence to support the development of a framework for service provision to guide them through the constantly changing conditions. Social workers had to rely instead on their flexibility, creativity, and responsiveness.

Since ICCMWs are government-funded, usually the service orientation is indisputably guided by the government's vision (Hong Kong Social Welfare Department, 2017). However, during the COVID-19 pandemic, the guidance was mostly practical (for example, opening hours, preventive measures, reporting of cases etc.), and guidance on mental health practices from government was generally unavailable. Social workers were therefore left to rely on their flexibility and skills to deliver the service with the best fit. Although the responses were very much coloured by the implicit problem-based and remedial orientation, it was still the role and challenge for the profession to extend interventions beyond treatment and symptom control to further develop their capacity to intervene.

Although technology was widely used to provide mental health services during the COVID-19 pandemic, many people with pre-existing mental illness, particularly older people, did not have access to smartphones or computers. A recent telephone survey conducted by a local non-governmental organisation in Hong Kong found that among 552 older adult respondents living in the community, only 63% had a smartphone, and 57% had internet access at home

(Wong et al., 2020). As a result, those people without a smartphone or internet access received limited service provision.

Although Hong Kongers have experienced multiple stressors including the COVID-19 pandemic and the series of unsettled political conditions, the most recent related to the passing of the Hong Kong National Security Law in June 2020, little attention has been paid to the impact of political unrest on mental health in terms of service provision. Because of physical distancing practices, protests were discontinued. However, when protests did occur, people wore masks to protect themselves as best they could. The public's attention shifted due to the virus outbreak. However, the impact of social unrest potentially makes mental health issues more complicated. As the efforts of mental health social workers were mainly on handling COVID-19 related issues, education on how to address the impact of political conflict on mental health was lacking and perhaps to do so became perilous in Hong Kong in the context of a tightened political control, and so the distress from political conflicts remained unaddressed.

Lessons learned from the COVID-19 pandemic thus far

Five key lessons for social work practice can be gleaned from experiences in Hong Kong thus far.

Lesson 1: using a strengths perspective to build new normal life

It was critical to help clients establish new and changed daily routines for mental health promotion. A social work focus was on supporting clients' strengths by incorporating those strengths into practice and building rewarding activities into daily planning to build resilience and coping. In daily life planning, helping clients enhance stress management, build on their existing coping skills and supporting new ones, disseminating information and helping people understand that information, were warranted interventions. Although the progress of the pandemic is unpredictable, it is important to help clients develop life goals, maintain working towards their life goals, and to recognise and celebrate what they can achieve during the pandemic.

Lesson 2: strengthening service coordination

COVID-19 related mental health issues were not only confined to personal life adjustment, family issues such as managing the care of children due to school shutdowns, family conflicts due to competing political positions, and potential and actual unemployment each contributed to worsening mental health. As mental health service needs increased, linking clients to organisations that addressed family or financial issues is indicated. In recognition of the lack of experience handling a long-term pandemic and its consequences, information exchanges and sharing practice experiences among organisations providing mental health services is needed. These exchanges along with empirical data would help service providers develop service models for mitigating the impact of health emergencies on mental health and better prepare them for the next pandemic.

Lesson 3: mobilising peer support to address mental health issues

Helping clients connect to social networks made up of community members and peers were critical interventions as disruptions to daily life routines and social connections were known stressors. As face-to-face services provided by social workers became limited, helping clients develop peer networks was an effective strategy to strengthen social supports and to prevent deterioration of mental health from social disconnection. The development of regular peer support facilitated by peer-led online activities would be helpful into the future, particularly during periods of isolation. Involving and supporting volunteers to provide one-on-one emotional support is an important a measure for mental health promotion.

Lesson 4: strengthening primary prevention for mental health in the general population during crisis

While depression and anxiety rates increased during the COVID-19 pandemic are likely to continue in the aftermath, primary prevention for the general population was extremely limited in community mental health services due to the urgency of other demands and COVID-19 restrictions. Services for identifying people with mental health needs and helping high-risk populations including parents who were home schooling their children during the pandemic, those with financial hardship, and the elderly were particularly in need of support to enhance their coping capacities. As not all Hong Kong social workers fully understood or were aware of the three levels of health and mental health prevention, social work education should include concepts of prevention and response to better prepare social workers to promote mental health and well-being in the aftermath of COVID-19 and in future crises.

Lesson 5: enhancing capability in crisis intervention in social work education

Social work education in Hong Kong emphasises crisis intervention at the casework level. Crisis intervention, particularly in the context of natural disasters, pandemics, and political conflict has certain limitations. Moreover, crisis intervention at the community level is lacking. Education on how to mobilise community resources to help individuals and families be more resilient in various crisis situations has become critical in addressing mental health issues during the pandemics. Most importantly, during crisis situations, such as pandemics and social unrest, an emphasis on empowering clients in social work practice would be crucial for building resilience and in mental health promotion.

BOX 12.1

REFLECTIVE QUESTIONS

1. What can be done to promote mental health well-being for the general population during pandemics?
2. How could mental health social workers engage vulnerable populations, such as the elderly and people in low socioeconomic circumstances with less access to resources, during pandemics?
3. How could social workers mobilise community resources to help individuals and families be more resilient in various crisis situations?
4. What do mental health social workers need to consider in preparation for the next health emergency?

References

Chan, K. (2021, January 21). Biannual survey on depression in Hong Kong (港人抑鬱指數創新高, 抑鬱市民兩年增三成, 因政治環境疫情感無力). Hong Kong 01. https://www.hk01.com/%E7%A4%BE%E6%9C%83%E6%96%B0%E8%81%9E/577396/%E6%B8%AF%E4%BA%BA%E6%8A%91%E9%AC%B1%E6%8C%87%E6%95%B8%E5%89%B5%E6%96%B0%E9%AB%98-%E6%8A%91%E9%AC%B1%E5%B8%82%E6%B0%91%E5%85%A9%E5%B9%B4%E5%A2%9E%E4%B8%89%E6%88%90-%E5%9B%A0%E6%94%BF%E6%B2%BB%E7%92%B0%E5%A2%83%E7%96%AB%E6%83%85%E6%84%9F%E7%84%A1%E5%8A%9B

Choi, E., Hui, B., & Wan, E. (2020). Depression and anxiety in Hong Kong during COVID-19. *International Journal of Environmental Research and Public Health*, 17(10), 3740. https://doi.org/10.3390/ijerph17103740

Constantino, R. E., & Privitera, M. R. (2011). Prevention terminology: Primary, secondary, tertiary, and an evolution of terms. In M. R. Priviera (Ed.), *Workplace violence in mental and general healthcare settings* (pp. 15–22). Boston: Jones and Bartlett Publishers.

Hong Kong Hospital Authority & Hong Kong Social Welfare Department. (2016). Service framework for personalized care for adults with severe mental illness in Hong Kong. https://www.ha.org.hk/haho/ho/icp/ServiceFramework_Adults_with_SMI_ENG.pd

Hong Kong Social Welfare Department. (2017). Annual report 2016–2017. https://www.swd.gov.hk/en/index/site_pubpress/page_swdarep/

Hong Kong Social Welfare Department (2021, January 29). Integrated community centre for mental wellness. https://www.swd.gov.hk/en/index/site_pubsvc/page_rehab/sub_listofserv/id_supportcom/id_iccmw/

Lau, B. H. P., Chan, C. L. W., & Ng, S. (2020). Resilience of Hong Kong people in the COVID-19 pandemic: Lessons learned from a survey at the peak of the pandemic in Spring 2020. *Asia Pacific Journal of Social Work and Development*, 1–10. https://doi.org/10.1080/02185385.2020.1778516

Ng, R. M. K. (2020). Mental health crisis in Hong Kong. *Psychiatric Times*, 37(1). https://www.psychiatrictimes.com/view/mental-health-crisis-hong-kong

Ni, M.Y., Yao, X. I., Leung, K., Yau, C., Leung, C., Lun, P., Flores, F. P., Chang, W. C., Cowling, B. J., & Leung, G. M. (2020). Depression and post-traumatic stress during major social unrest in Hong Kong: A 10-year prospective cohort study. *Lancet (London, England)*, 395(10220), 273–284.

Perlmutter, F. D., Vayda, A. M., & Woodburn, P. K. (1976). An instrument for differentiating programs in prevention - Primary, secondary and tertiary. *American Journal of Orthopsychiatry*, 46(3), 533–541.

Wong, S.Y. S., Zhang, D., Sit, R. W. S., Yip, B. H. K., Chung, R.Y, Wong, C. K. M., … Mercer, S.W. (2020). Impact of COVID-19 on loneliness, mental health, and health service utilisation: A prospective cohort study of older adults with multimorbidity in primary care. *British Journal of General Practice,* 70(700), E817–E824. https://doi.org/10.3399/bjgp20X713021

Yau, C., & Tsang, D. (2021, January 19). Hong Kong fourth wave: Jobless rate hits new 16-year high of 6.6 per cent with city deep in coronavirus fight. South China Morning Post. https://www.scmp.com/news/hong-kong/hong-kong-economy/article/3118331/hong-kong-fourth-wave-jobless-rate-hits-new-16

13

URBAN HOMELESSNESS

Housing and health equity during health emergencies

Elizabeth Bowen and Nicole Capozziello

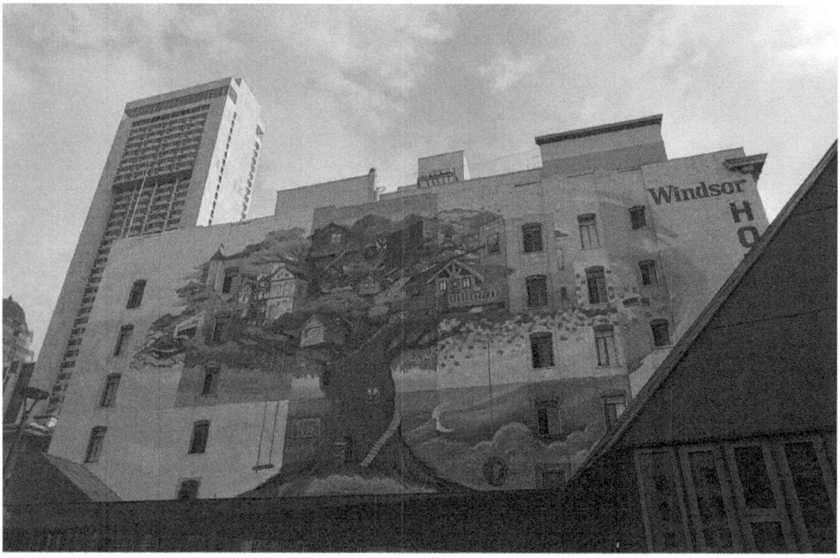

FIGURE 13.0 *Everyone Deserves a Home* mural, San Francisco

Source: Photograph by Elizabeth Bowen

DOI: 10.4324/9781003111214-15

Advocates for fair, safe, affordable, and accessible housing – including social workers – have adopted the phrase *housing is health*. It follows that a lack of safe and stable housing invites vulnerability to a variety of health conditions and even death. Such has proven to be the case for persons experiencing or at risk of homelessness during the COVID-19 pandemic. This chapter will review the ways in which COVID-19 and homelessness are mutually reinforcing and describe the response to homelessness in the United States (US) during the COVID-19 pandemic. We also provide critical reflections on the shortcomings of this response and suggest alternative ways of addressing homelessness and pandemics as intersecting and urgent public health crises.

Background and definitions

In this chapter, we use the word *homelessness* and related terms (e.g. *people experiencing homelessness*; *unhoused persons*) to refer broadly to people in a variety of unsafe and unstable housing situations. Although the US federal government uses strict criteria to define homelessness with regard to eligibility for various assistance programs, we believe it is important to capture the range of conditions that people may experience. This includes staying outdoors or in other places not intended for residential occupancy (e.g. cars, abandoned buildings), as well as in shelters, short-term housing programs, couch-surfing (frequently moving between the residences of other people), and doubling up (staying temporarily with friends, family, or associates).

Because people move frequently between these circumstances and because people may not interact with service providers or even identify as homeless themselves, it is difficult to accurately estimate the true number of people experiencing homelessness in the United States. The US Department of Housing and Urban Development (HUD) provides an official count of the total persons experiencing homelessness on a single night, which was 567,715 in 2019 (National Alliance to End Homelessness [NAEH], 2020a). However, given the challenges in locating unhoused people and the fact that this estimate is based on a definition of homelessness that does not include doubling up or couch-surfing, the actual number of people experiencing homelessness on a given night is much higher. In addition, countless others are at high risk of homelessness, such as those going through the process of eviction or people being discharged from jails or prisons with limited resources – two populations that have increased during the COVID-19 pandemic.

COVID-19 and homelessness: mutually reinforcing problems

We view homelessness and the COVID-19 pandemic as mutually reinforcing: the state of being homeless increases vulnerability to COVID-19, and the COVID-19 pandemic enhances vulnerability to homelessness. In this section, we highlight factors and pathways that contribute to this intersecting vulnerability, including: the link between homelessness and health disparities; demographic factors; the conditions in which unhoused people live; incarceration; and trauma.

Homelessness and health disparities

In the US and in most countries where research on health and homelessness has been conducted, individuals experiencing homelessness are disproportionately affected by a range of chronic health and mental health conditions. Homeless individuals experience elevated prevalence of mental health disorders (Fazel, Geddes & Kushel, 2014; Henwood et al., 2018); substance use disorders (Roncarati et al., 2018; Thompson et al., 2013); cardiovascular disease (Baggett, Liauw & Hwang, 2018); infectious diseases including HIV/AIDS, Hepatitis C, and tuberculosis (Fazel, Geddes & Kushel, 2014); and cancer (Baggett et al., 2015). In addition to increased prevalence, homeless populations also frequently report greater severity related to these conditions (Baggett et al., 2015; Baggett, Liauw & Hwang, 2018; Henwood et al., 2018).

This disproportionate burden of health problems is concerning during the COVID-19 pandemic due to the potential for a variety of chronic conditions to complicate and worsen the course of COVID-19, leading to drastically higher mortality rates (Banerjee et al., 2020). Although cardiovascular disease and diabetes have arguably received the greatest attention as factors contributing to COVID-19 risk, other conditions that affect homeless populations, such as substance use disorders, also enhance COVID-19 vulnerability (López-Pelayo et al., 2020; Mehra et al., 2020). At the same time, the circumstances of the pandemic have made it more difficult to maintain continuity of care for people with chronic physical and behavioural health conditions, potentially worsening outcomes (López-Pelayo et al., 2020; Wagle et al., 2020).

Demographic vulnerability

Overall, the homeless population in the US is disproportionally male, aging, and composed of people of colour including Black Americans, Native Americans, Pacific Islanders, and Americans identifying as Hispanic or Latino/a (NAEH, 2020a). Although the reasons for this are multifaceted, systemic racism and its intersection with socioeconomic disadvantage is a major underlying factor. With research indicating that COVID-19 prevalence, severity, and mortality are elevated in men, older adults, and people of colour (particularly Black Americans), the demographic profile of US homelessness suggests a magnified risk for COVID-19 (Golestaneh et al., 2020). A particular concern is that many homeless people essentially age faster, developing geriatric conditions years before their counterparts who have stable housing (Brown et al., 2017).

Living conditions

Stable housing is widely recognised as a key social determinant of health (Thornton et al., 2016). Without stable housing, it is difficult for people to do basic activities that are critical for staying healthy, such as eating nutritious food and managing medications. During a pandemic of a disease that carries a high risk of airborne transmission, the living conditions of people who are homeless present heightened concerns. Physical distancing is a challenge and likely an impossibility for many homeless people – particularly in dense urban areas – including those who are unsheltered and staying on the street as well as people using emergency shelters or doubled up with friends or family. Similarly, basic hygiene practices such as frequent handwashing may not be accessible.

Furthermore, the conditions instigated by pandemic, in terms of shutdowns and stay-at-home orders enacted in many US states and municipalities, pose a unique threat to the day-to-day survival of unhoused people. Many people experiencing homelessness rely on institutions such as public libraries, stores, and coffeeshops as safe places to sleep, get water, use the bathroom, make social connections, and meet other basic needs (Giesler, 2019). With many of these places closed or operating on reduced hours and/or under new guidelines in response to the pandemic, unhoused people have fewer reliable and safe places to go to meet their survival needs.

Incarceration

Incarceration presents an acute source of COVID-19 vulnerability. The US is the highest incarcerator in the world per capita, and incarceration rates are particularly high among Black men and women who are also disproportionately likely to be homeless (Sawyer & Wagner, 2020). Homelessness itself serves as a risk factor for incarceration as unsheltered homeless people are frequently criminalised for actions including sleeping outdoors, loitering, or begging in public, as well as substance-related charges (Bauman et al., 2014; Greenberg & Rosenheck, 2008). As jails and prisons quickly emerged as hotspots for COVID-19 transmission in the US and elsewhere, unhoused people were rendered more vulnerable to COVID-19 through their direct contacts with the criminal justice system, as well as through indirect contact via close proximity to persons recently released from jail or prison (Akiyama, Spaulding & Rich, 2020).

Trauma

The overall health of people who are homeless is often shaped by histories of severe trauma. Traumatic life events frequently play a role in people becoming homeless, and trauma is perpetuated by the high rates of physical and sexual violence that homeless individuals experience, along with state-sanctioned violence in the form of criminalisation and incarceration (Bauman et al., 2014). One study conducted in Vancouver, Canada, found that homeless adults reported an average of 3.9 adverse childhood experiences (such as physical or sexual abuse and parental incarceration) on a standardised measure, and that the number of such experiences was associated with the likelihood of various physical and behavioural health problems in adulthood (Patterson, Moniruzzaman & Somers, 2014).

Trauma histories may complicate efforts to prevent and treat COVID-19 in homeless populations, as homeless people who have endured trauma may not trust or feel safe with outreach workers and health care personnel who seek to administer testing, treatment, or emergency housing programs during the pandemic. Collin-Vézina, Brend and Beeman (2020) argue that principles of trauma-informed care – such as enhancing safety and providing opportunities for meaningful collaboration – should be integrated into COVID-19 responses with and for vulnerable children and families, a notion that we believe should extend to engagement with people experiencing homelessness during the pandemic.

The US response to COVID-19 and homelessness

In the following section, we describe the US response to homelessness during the COVID-19 pandemic in 2020. We begin by highlighting how people experiencing homelessness and service providers were impacted by this unprecedented situation. Next, we discuss responses at federal, state, and local levels, followed by a case study of the Project Roomkey/Project Homekey program in the state of California. We conclude with early evaluations of the overall homelessness response and the unique roles and perspectives of social workers.

Onset of the pandemic

As COVID-19 and information about it began to spread in March 2020, the US Centers for Disease Control and Prevention (CDC) released recommendations meant to guide the public, including physical distancing, urging people to stay at home as much as possible, and suggesting quarantine if exposed to the disease (Culhane et al., 2020). For homeless people and the organisations that serve them, these orders were challenging – if not impossible – to follow. Providers quickly realised that in addition to the usual risks their clients faced, many could find themselves in life-or-death scenarios. An analysis by Culhane and colleagues (2020) predicted that due to their intersecting vulnerabilities and lack of services, homeless individuals infected with COVID-19 would be twice as likely to be hospitalised, two to four times as likely to require critical care, and two to three times as likely to die, when compared to the general population. They stated that to avoid such outcomes, an additional $11.5 billion for shelter alone was needed for 2020.

In March 2020, NAEH captured the concerns of 785 direct service providers, organisation leaders, advocates, and those with lived homelessness experience from across the country. In a survey, these respondents expressed worries about the lack of shelter space, limitations in capacity and services due to safety guidelines, a dearth of supplies, and challenges because of reduced supportive services (NAEH, 2020b). To meet these needs, NAEH called for leadership from local, state, and federal partners, expansion of temporary shelter options, increased investment in staff, funding to provide rapid rehousing, and improvement of health and safety within existing programs.

The federal government's response

The response to the COVID-19 pandemic, both in its immediate onset and throughout, was a patchwork effort by federal, state, and local governments, as well as private and public organisations. This is reflective of how homelessness is generally approached in the US. In March 2020, the US Congress passed the Coronavirus Aid, Relief, and Economic Security (CARES) Act. While providing small business loans, aid to unemployed Americans, and other funding, this act also included $4 billion in Emergency Services Grants for Homeless Assistance, defined as street outreach, rapid rehousing, homelessness prevention, shelter operations, and administration. Of that amount, up to $2 billion was set aside to be given to current grant recipients, with HUD allocating the remaining amount to state, local, and territorial governments based on need.

This influx of funding, while still far short of the investment needed to end homelessness, provided local governments across the country with opportunities for improvement and innovation. To help service organisations strategically use this federal funding, a coalition of organisations – the Center on Budget and Policy Priorities, National Low Income Housing Coalition, National Health Care for the Homeless Council, Center on Budget and Policy Priorities, and Urban Institute – came together to create the Framework for an Equitable COVID-19 Homelessness Response (The National Alliance to End Homelessness, 2020c). The framework's resources and tools focussed on five action areas–unsheltered people, shelters, housing, diversion and prevention, and strengthening systems for the future–with recommendations for how to implement and strengthen immediate and future responses to each, as well as how to strategically make use of related funding streams.

Recognising that the increase in unemployment could make many Americans unable to pay their rent or mortgage, the CARES Act also included a moratorium on evictions and foreclosures for many properties for 120 days starting on 18 March 2020. The CDC then extended this national eviction moratorium, drawing on a 1944 public health law created to curb the spread of a pandemic. In their Agency Order, the CDC disallowed landlords from evicting tenants who didn't pay rent until at least 31 December 2020.

Forthcoming research will show the extent to which the orders helped to prevent or slow incidents of homelessness, or perhaps failed to do so. Many advocates and researchers have predicted that these protections will have limited benefits, as "they do little to address a renter's underlying financial distress, and do nothing to help prevent even more renters from falling behind" (Walter, 2020). In an analysis of Americans' checking accounts, economist Peter Ganong found that unemployed Americans, and the overall US economy, were "living off the exhaust fumes of the CARES Act heading into the fall", leaving many Americans struggling to pay rent and afford day-to-day necessities (Badger & Bui, 2020). Early analyses also indicated that evictions continued to be filed in many US cities, such as Houston, Texas and Phoenix, Arizona, despite the CDC moratorium (Eviction Lab, 2020).

State and local responses

Cities and states' responses for addressing COVID-19 and its impacts varied greatly, and each place's treatment of individuals experiencing homelessness, or those at risk of homelessness, was no exception. While individual states had numerous options, including extending their own eviction moratoriums, barring utility shut offs, and offering rent relief programs, most did not consistently offer such aid or protection, placing many of the nation's 43 million rental households in precarity (Walter, 2020).

When it came to approaching those already experiencing homelessness, many state governors and city mayors publicly recognised homeless people as a population at risk and in need during the COVID-19 pandemic, sometimes backing up this commitment with policy. In Virginia, for example, the governor announced $2.5 million in funding for temporary housing, including hotel and medical vouchers (Office of the Governor, 2020). Another example is Connecticut, which in June 2020 rolled out a comprehensive plan to mitigate housing issues (NBC Connecticut, 2020). This plan included allocating $4 million in rapid rehousing funds for security deposits and initial rent for people to exit homelessness to housing, and providing $1.8 million in funding for housing for people being released from prison, an oft-neglected population in both policy and practice.

Case study: Project Roomkey/Project Homekey

Perhaps no state was as vigorous in its homelessness response during COVID-19 than California, where, as of 2019, an estimated 27% of the entire US homeless population lived (Gabriel & Ciudad-Real, 2020). Perhaps most concerning, between 2017 and 2018, homelessness in California increased by 16.4%, far outpacing the national increase of 2.7%. In April 2020, Governor Gavin Newsom spearheaded an innovative program that paired social services and the hospitality industry, called Project Roomkey. For the initiative, the state secured Federal Emergency Management Agency funding, at 75% cost share reimbursement, to rent isolation rooms in hotels and motels for people experiencing homelessness. Project Roomkey had an initial goal of securing 15,000 rooms with the purposes of protecting the medically vulnerable, reducing the shelter population to allow for physical distancing, and slowing the spread of COVID-19 (Office of Governor Gavin Newsom, 2020a). Although this number was far short of housing California's more than 150,000 homeless people (US Interagency Council on Homelessness [USICH], 2019), the project was still regarded as ambitious.

The $100 million program prioritised three groups within the homeless population: 1) individuals who were asymptomatic but at high risk (such as those over 65 or with underlying health conditions); 2) individuals exposed to COVID-19 and requiring isolation; and 3) individuals suffering from

COVID-19 but who did not require hospitalisation (Office of Governor Gavin Newsom, 2020a). The vision was for support teams in California counties to identify shelter clients or encampment residents in particular need and then transport them to hotels for intake. These local teams also worked to identify hotels and negotiate agreements, coordinate wraparound services (such as custodial, laundry, security, and support staff) at each site, and keep the records necessary for federal reimbursement.

In August 2020, Project Roomkey wrapped up. Governor Newsom stated that it had housed more than 22,300 homeless individuals, and had met the goal of acquiring over 16,000 hotel rooms (Office of Governor Gavin Newsom, 2020c). However, implementation and follow-through of the program varied greatly by county and, according to *The Los Angeles Times*, had not reached 50% occupancy statewide in June (Smith & Oreskes, 2020). Key challenges that contributed to the program's shortfall on local levels were: initially securing hotels to participate in the program, hotels being located far from the usual areas of homeless services, quickly identifying individuals to participate, and offering the flexibility homeless people needed (Zahniser & Alpert Reyes, 2020). In addition, some local programs ended abruptly, returning people to precarious health and safety situations (Paoli & Sparling, 2020).

In July 2020, Governor Newsom announced Project Homekey, the next phase in the state's response to protecting Californians experiencing homelessness who are particularly vulnerable to COVID-19 (California Department of Housing and Community Development, 2020). Under the $600 million Project Homekey program, the state buys and converts properties, such as hotels and vacant apartment buildings, into permanent housing for Californians experiencing or at risk of homelessness (Office of Governor Gavin Newsom, 2020b).

Evaluations of the US homelessness response during the pandemic

A report by USICH evaluating homelessness service efforts and outcomes from 1 January through 30 June 2020, stated that COVID-19 cases and fatalities had been significantly lower than original projections. According to data from the CDC, among the homeless population there had been 4,845 positive COVID-19 cases and 130 deaths as of June 30th (USICH, 2020). However, a report by the Howard Center for Investigative Journalism, looking at just six cities and counties with significant homeless populations, found 153 deaths (Bohannon et al., 2020). Considering the difficulties in estimating and tracking the number of people who are homeless in the US at any given time, it is not surprising that data measuring the impact of the coronavirus on this population is unreliable.

The extent to which the federal funding was actually allocated was another point of concern. The Howard Center found that, as of early August 2020, HUD had given communities under one-third of the $4 billion provided by the

CARES Act (Surma, 2020). Homeless service providers were only able to access funds after HUD had finalised grant agreements, which they had done for only about 29% of the funds. As a result of lag and uncertainty, many municipalities and organisations found themselves unable to meet needs and fulfil promises, such as that of transitioning vulnerable people into permanent housing.

These issues were representative of the American political climate at the time, showing the existing tension between approaches that offer housing assistance conditionally and those meant to make housing access easier, such as the Housing First model which emphasises helping homeless people obtain permanent housing and supportive services as quickly as possible (Padgett, Henwood & Tsemberis, 2016). Shortly after beginning his appointment in December of 2019, Robert Marbut, a former housing consultant and the then-head of USICH, criticised existing American housing policy including Housing First, blaming it for the US' high rates of homelessness. As a result, during the pandemic, Marbut advocated for meeting the population's needs through group shelters, as opposed to hotels and motels, a position criticised by his three predecessors. "What I've seen is those services [hotels and motels] are organised and that people are so much more able, in a less chaotic environment, to engage in services", said Laura Zeilinger, former USICH Executive Director during the Obama administration and Washington, DC's current Director of Department of Human Services (Surma, 2020).

Role of social workers in responding to COVID-19 and homelessness

American social workers in a range of practice settings, from schools to post-incarceration reentry programs, have long confronted the intersecting issues that have historically surrounded housing, including housing affordability, racial discrimination in lending and housing access, and homelessness. Both prior to and during the pandemic, social workers have worked in direct service roles as providers and advocates for those experiencing homelessness, as well as in organisational leadership and public policy capacities. Social workers are also all too aware of homelessness as a symptom of the US' lack of prioritisation of an effective and equitable social safety net, particularly from the 1980s onwards. As Canadian social work scholars Wu and Karabanow (2020) put it, "the real enemies are not the different types of hazards … the real enemies are the long-time existing societal vulnerabilities, such as poverty, discrimination, stigma, and marginalization, that corrode citizens' coping capacities and convert various hazards into catastrophic disaster events. Homeless populations suffer from these vulnerabilities during non-emergency settings. During disaster cycles, vulnerabilities worsen already traumatized situations".

An example of social work advocacy on homelessness and housing during the COVID-19 pandemic is a 2020 opinion piece authored by social work researchers Thomas Hugh Byrne and Benjamin F. Henwood and real estate scholar Anthony

W. Orlando. They write, "as scholars of social work and real estate, we have opined for years that homelessness is a public health emergency and deserves to be treated as such. Instead, policymakers have bowed to the status quo, allowing local regulations, bureaucratic delays and NIMBY [Not in My Back Yard] vetoes to stymie their efforts to acquire sites and build affordably" (Byrne, Henwood & Orlando, 2020). They note with hope, however, that the federal government's emergency response to the coronavirus, and the associated funding available, positions the US – for the first time in its history – to meet the homelessness crisis with the response it has always deserved.

Discussion

Beneath the fragmented but hurried efforts to address homelessness in the United States during the COVID-19 pandemic lies a critical truth: that people living in unsheltered and unsafe conditions – particularly in a country of vast wealth and resources – is a perpetual emergency. As such, we believe that homelessness requires urgent attention, irrespective of COVID-19, future pandemics, or other public health threats. In this discussion section, we describe alternative solutions and directions for addressing homelessness and health equity and articulate directions for ongoing social work practice.

Homelessness and health equity: long-term solutions

COVID-19 taught the US a lesson that it should have already learned: that the outbreak of infectious disease is too late to begin addressing homelessness as a pressing and solvable problem. People who are homeless are generally more vulnerable to infectious diseases, as decades of research on tuberculosis, HIV/AIDS and Hepatitis B and C demonstrates (Fazel, Geddes & Kushel, 2014). Thus, the intersection of homelessness and infectious disease poses a constant risk to the health of unhoused people, as well as to the health of the broader communities in which people experiencing homelessness live, work, and engage.

We are wary, though, of presenting public health as the singular rationale for addressing homelessness. We believe that housing is a human right – and with this approach, a public health rationale remains salient, but not required. Human beings have a right to housing that is safe, stable, and affordable. It is our belief that the welfare of society at large would be better off if this right was reflected in US housing policy. Treating housing as a human right implies that housing assistance should be an entitlement benefit, for example, a benefit that all eligible persons are entitled to receive. In contrast to other benefits such as food assistance, housing assistance – including rental subsidies, public housing, and permanent supportive housing for persons experiencing homelessness – has never been designated an entitlement at the federal level in the US. As a result, Scally et al. (2018) estimate that only one in five US households that is eligible for federal rental assistance actually receives it. Codifying housing as a human right, as

Canada did in 2019, and guaranteeing entitlement to a range of forms of housing assistance is a long-term solution that would be an investment in the health of the millions of Americans who are and will be vulnerable to homelessness before, during, and after the COVID-19 crisis.

The COVID-19 pandemic is also a potent reminder that achieving health equity for people who are homeless will require more than just housing access. One macro-level policy solution to rampant poverty is universal basic income, which shifts the focus from self-responsibility to recognising the dignity and value of every human being. In the US, universal basic income would ultimately redirect government spending away from the current ineffective and insufficient responses of the criminal justice system and emergency services. A stable financial base is the necessary foundation from which people can establish stability and, importantly, engage with the services that enable a transition to and maintenance of permanent housing.

Furthermore, access to mental health and substance use treatment, as well as comprehensive medical care, should be treated as a right of all people, including those experiencing homelessness. Along with many other shifts, the COVID-19 pandemic forced a reworking of how treatment services of all kinds are delivered. For instance, the widespread use of telehealth eliminated some of the barriers that have posed significant challenges to both service providers and their clients. Not having to travel to service sites, as well as not having to meet in person, provided flexibility at a lower cost. In Seattle, Washington, an investment of only $12,000 in technology devices enabled clients based in a hotel sheltering program to attend appointments with their mental health specialists and doctors (Garg & Fields, 2020). In addition, in response to the pandemic, most American insurance companies eased their stringent restrictions around telehealth, expanding options and making it more easily billable.

In some areas, substance use treatment was approached more expansively during the pandemic, showcasing the potential of embracing a harm reduction model. In San Francisco, California, service providers gave homeless people with substance use disorders small, measured doses of alcohol and nicotine to curb potentially deadly withdrawal symptoms and encourage them to stay in quarantine in hotel housing (Garg & Fields, 2020). Nationally, the US Drug Enforcement Administration made it easier for doctors to prescribe opioid treatments such as buprenorphine. While in New York City, methadone, another opioid treatment, was allowed to be delivered directly to homeless isolation sites (Garg & Fields, 2020). In sum, the pandemic provided opportunities for service providers to test innovative solutions, some of which they had been sceptical of working with their clients. We believe that many of these service innovations are commendable and warrant further implementation and dissemination, well beyond the context of the COVID-19 pandemic.

Lastly, with the pandemic came increased attention about how we go about public life. For the thousands of Americans experiencing homelessness, the distinction between private and public life that many people take for granted simply has not existed – and never has this reality been laid so bare as during the pandemic. While others sought protection indoors, homeless people remained in a variety of unstable settings, including on the streets and in encampments, where they remained vulnerable to the virus as well as the criminalisation that comes with being unhoused. Visiting the US in 2017, Philip Alston, United Nations Special Rapporteur on extreme poverty and human rights, noted the reverberating and cyclical ways that the US punishes people for simply not having shelter: "sleeping rough, sitting in public places, panhandling, public urination (in cities that provide almost zero public toilets) and myriad other offenses have been devised to attack the 'blight' of homelessness" (Alston, 2017). He went on to write, "homelessness on this scale is far from inevitable and again reflects political choices to see law enforcement rather than low cost housing, medical treatment, psychological counselling, and job training as the solutions". We concur that health equity will not be achieved without ending the criminalisation of homelessness and reallocating resources accordingly.

Directions for micro, organisational, and structural social work practice

As Farkas and Romaniuk (2020) note, social workers have an ethical imperative to continue providing competent services to vulnerable individuals and groups, even and perhaps especially during public health emergencies. At a micro level, we acknowledge and commend the countless social workers in direct practice roles across the globe who have taken considerable risks to continue providing services to people experiencing homelessness during the COVID-19 pandemic (Wasilewska-Ostrowska, 2020; Wu & Karabanow, 2020). From an organisational perspective, we believe that social workers have a mandate to leverage organisational resources and policies to minimise potential harm to both social service workforces and clientele during and beyond the pandemic. In addition, we believe it is the duty of social workers to *never waste a crisis* and use the COVID-19 pandemic to advocate for structural change to advance housing and health equity at a macro level. Social workers in various settings can take direct and indirect steps to advocate for local, state, and federal policies that expand housing assistance, ensure housing as a human right, and provide access to the trauma-informed services and resources required as a foundation for health equity.

Conclusion

As in past epidemics and public health crises, COVID-19 has presented particular vulnerabilities to people who are homeless or at risk of becoming homeless, further threatening what is, for many, an already precarious existence. When and if the

COVID-19 pandemic wanes, we urge social workers not to lose sight of the urgent need for advocacy to protect both public health and human rights. After all, as Shah (2016) has warned, the sparks that will ignite the next pandemic are already lurking somewhere in our cells, cities, and forests. Given this reality, we urge social workers and their allies and partners to advocate for policy choices that will reverse the seeming inevitability of homelessness, with the ultimate vision that homelessness would become a rarity instead of a common occurrence throughout the world.

BOX 13.1

REFLECTIVE QUESTIONS

1. What factors (structural, familial, individual, and otherwise) make homeless people more vulnerable to COVID-19, and what factors lead to a rise in homelessness in global health emergencies such as COVID-19?
2. The authors show that the COVID-19 pandemic forced many service providers to quickly experiment with different methods of service delivery for people experiencing homelessness, including telehealth and expanded substance use treatment.
   - What barriers have social workers faced when trying to implement more accessible and innovative treatment approaches for this population in the past?
   - What other novel interventions could surface as a result of increased funding and attention on homelessness in light of the pandemic?
3. In the US, advocates struggle not only with securing policy adoption and funding for addressing homelessness but also with generating support from the public. For example, neighbourhood residents may oppose the building of a shelter or service site, business owners and others may discriminate against homeless people, and, as shown during COVID-19, hotels might resist participating in funded housing programs. However, many advocates are cautiously hopeful that the pandemic has created opportunities to help more people obtain housing, as well as to shift the narrative on homelessness from an individual failing to one of collective responsibility.
   - What valuable and unique training, perspectives, and connections do social workers have to offer when it comes to engaging with communities and organisations that may have competing interests and beliefs?
   - How might social workers use these strengths to engage with, gather support from, and work together with others on solutions for homelessness?

References

Akiyama, M. J., Spaulding, A. C., & Rich, J. D. (2020). Flattening the curve for incarcerated populations – COVID-19 in jails and prisons. *New England Journal of Medicine*, 382(22), 2075–2077.

Alston, P. (2017). *Statement on Visit to the USA, by Professor Philip Alston, United Nations Special Rapporteur on extreme poverty and human rights*. https://www.ohchr.org/EN/NewsEvents/Pages/DisplayNews.aspx?NewsID=22533

Badger, E., & Bui, Q. (2020, October 16). Jobless workers built up some savings. Then the $600 checks stopped. *The New York Times*. https://www.nytimes.com/2020/10/16/upshot/stimulus-checks-unemployment.html

Baggett, T. P., Chang, Y., Porneala, B. C., Bharel, M., Singer, D. E., & Rigotti, N. A. (2015). Disparities in cancer incidence, stage, and mortality at Boston Health Care for the Homeless Program. *American Journal of Preventive Medicine*, 49(5), 694–702.

Baggett, T. P., Liauw, S., & Hwang, S. (2018). Cardiovascular disease and homelessness. *Journal of the American College of Cardiology*, 71(22), 2585–2597.

Banerjee, A., Pasea, L., Harris, S., Gonzalez-Izquierdo, A., Torralbo, A., Shallcross, L., Noursadeghi, M., Pillay, D., Sebire, N., Holmes, C., Pagel, C., Wong, W.K., Langenberg, C., Williams, B., Denaxas, S., & Hemingway, H. (2020). Estimating excess 1-year mortality associated with the COVID-19 pandemic according to underlying conditions and age: A population-based cohort study. *The Lancet*, 395(10238), 1725.

Bauman, T., Rosen, J., Tars, E., Foscarinis, M., Fernandez, J., Robin, C., & Nicholes, H. (2014). *No safe place: The criminalization of homelessness in US cities*. Washington, DC: National Law Center on Homelessness and Poverty.

Bohannon, M., Surma, K., Fast, A., Abdaladze, N., Lupo, M., Fields, J., Garg, S., & for the Howard Center for Investigative Journalism (2020, August 24). COVID-19 is a 'crisis within a crisis' for homeless people. *Cronkite News*. https://cronkitenews.azpbs.org/howardcenter/covid-homeless/stories/homeless.html

Brown, R. T., Hemati, K., Riley, E. D., Lee, C. T., Ponath, C., Tieu, L., Guzman, D., & Kushel, M. B. (2017). Geriatric conditions in a population-based sample of older homeless adults. *The Gerontologist*, 57(4), 757–766.

Byrne, T.H., Henwood, B.F., & Orlando, A.W. (2020, August 2). What the pandemic taught us about the homeless – and what we shouldn't forget. *The Hill*. https://thehill.com/opinion/finance/509666-what-the-pandemic-taught-us-about-the-homeless-and-what-we-shouldnt-forget

California Department of Housing and Community Development. (2020). *Homekey*. https://hcd.ca.gov/grants-funding/active-funding/homekey.shtml

Collin-Vézina, D., Brend, D., & Beeman, I. (2020). When it counts the most: Trauma-informed care and the COVID-19 global pandemic. *Developmental Child Welfare*. https://doi.org/10.1177%2F2516103220942530

Culhane, D., Treglia, D., Steif, K., Kuhn, R., & Byrne, T. (2020). *Estimated emergency and observational/quarantine capacity need for the US homeless population related to COVID-19 exposure by county; projected hospitalizations, intensive care units and mortality*. https://works.bepress.com/dennis_culhane/237/

Eviction Lab. (2020). *A looming eviction crisis?* https://evictionlab.org/eviction-tracking/

Farkas, K. J., & Romaniuk, J. R. (2020). Social work, ethics and vulnerable groups in the time of coronavirus and COVID-19. *Society Register*, 4(2), 67–82.

Fazel, S., Geddes, J. R., & Kushel, M. (2014). The health of homeless people in high-income countries: Descriptive epidemiology, health consequences, and clinical and policy recommendations. *The Lancet*, 384(9953), 1529–1540.

Gabriel, I., & Ciudad-Real, V. (2020). *State of homelessness in California fact sheet.* Homelessness Policy Research Institute. https://socialinnovation.usc.edu/wp-content/uploads/2020/02/Homelessness-in-CA-Fact-Sheet-v3.pdf

Garg, S., Fields, J., & for the Howard Center for Investigative Journalism. (2020, August 28). COVID-19 work-arounds are silver linings for homeless programs. *Cronkite News*. https://cronkitenews.azpbs.org/2020/08/28/coronavirus-homeless-work-arounds-turn-into-silver-linings/?fbclid=IwAR0M8xTH4ME69p-E_oG6S10z8yR4Ity9e2e3m7EA_Ps0AGXKQJkMNyu3yUg

Giesler, M. A. (2019). The collaboration between homeless shelters and public libraries in addressing homelessness: A multiple case study. *Journal of Library Administration*, 59(1), 18–44.

Golestaneh, L., Neugarten, J., Fisher, M., Billett, H. H., Gil, M. R., Johns, T., Yunes, M., Mokrzycki, A. H., Coco, M., Norris, K.C., Perez, H. R., Scott, S., Kim, R. S., & Bellin. E. (2020). The association of race and COVID-19 mortality. *EClinicalMedicine*, 25, 100455. https://doi.org/10.1016/j.eclinm.2020.100455

Greenberg, G. A., & Rosenheck, R. A. (2008). Jail incarceration, homelessness, and mental health: A national study. *Psychiatric Services*, 59(2), 170–177.

Henwood, B. F., Lahey, J., Rhoades, H., Winetrobe, H., & Wenzel, S. L. (2018). Examining the health status of homeless adults entering permanent supportive housing. *Journal of Public Health*, 40(2), 415–418.

López-Pelayo, H., Aubin, H. J., Drummond, C., Dom, G., Pascual, F., Rehm, J., Saitz, R., Scafato, E., & Gual, A. (2020). "The post-COVID era": Challenges in the treatment of substance use disorder (SUD) after the pandemic. *BMC Medicine*, 18(1), 1–8.

Mehra, M. R., Desai, S. S., Kuy, S., Henry, T. D., & Patel, A. N. (2020). Cardiovascular disease, drug therapy, and mortality in COVID-19. *New England Journal of Medicine*, 382, e102. https://doi.org/10.1056/NEJMoa2007621

National Alliance to End Homelessness. (2020a). *State of homelessness: 2020 edition.* https://endhomelessness.org/homelessness-in-america/homelessness-statistics/state-of-homelessness-2020/

National Alliance to End Homelessness. (2020b, March 30). *Protecting people experiencing homelessness from COVID-19.* https://endhomelessness.org/wp-content/uploads/2020/03/COVID-19-Survey-Final-Report.pdf

National Alliance to End Homelessness, (2020c). *Framework for an Equitable COVID-19 Homelessness Response* (Version 4). Center on Budget and Policy Priorities, National Low Income Coalition, National Health Care, & for the Homeless Council. https://housingequityframework.org/

NBC Connecticut. (2020, June 29). *State announces financial aid for renters, homeowners affected by COVID-19.* https://www.nbcconnecticut.com/news/coronavirus/state-announces-financial-aid-for-renters-homeowners-affected-by-covid-19/2295100/

Office of Governor Gavin Newsom. (2020a, April 3). *At newly converted motel, Governor Newsom launches Project Roomkey: A first-in-the-nation initiative to secure hotel & motel rooms to protect homeless individuals from COVID-19.* https://www.gov.ca.gov/2020/04/03/at-newly-converted-motel-governor-newsom-launches-project-roomkey-a-first-in-the-nation-initiative-to-secure-hotel-motel-rooms-to-protect-homeless-individuals-from-covid-19/

Office of Governor Gavin Newsom. (2020b, October 9). *Governor Newsom announces release of $147 million in fourth round of Homekey awards.* https://www.gov.ca.gov/2020/10/09/governor-newsom-announces-release-of-147-million-in-fourth-round-of-homekey-awards/

Office of Governor Gavin Newsom. (2020c, November 16). *Governor Newsom announces emergency allocation of $62 million to local governments to protect people living in Project Roomkey hotels.* https://www.gov.ca.gov/2020/11/16/governor-newsom-announces-emergency-allocation-of-62-million-to-local-governments-to-protect-people-living-in-project-roomkey-hotels/

Office of the Governor. (2020, April 3). *Governor Northam announces emergency funding to shelter Virginia's homeless population.* https://www.governor.virginia.gov/newsroom/all-releases/2020/april/headline-855925-en.html

Padgett, D., Henwood, B. F., & Tsemberis, S. J. (2016). *Housing first: Ending homelessness, transforming systems, and changing lives.* New York, NY: Oxford University Press.

Paoli, T., & Sparling, N. (2020, September 21). An update on Project Roomkey in Tuolumne County. *The New York Times.* https://www.nytimes.com/2020/09/21/us/project-roomkey-tuolumne-county.html

Patterson, M. L., Moniruzzaman, A., & Somers, J. M. (2014). Setting the stage for chronic health problems: Cumulative childhood adversity among homeless adults with mental illness in Vancouver, British Columbia. *BMC Public Health*, 14, 350. https://doi.org/10.1186/1471-2458-14-350

Roncarati, J., Baggett, T., O'Connell, J., Hwang, S., Cook, E., Krieger, N., & Sorensen, G. (2018). Mortality among unsheltered homeless adults in Boston, Massachusetts, 2000-2009. *JAMA Internal Medicine*, 178(9), 1242–1248.

Sawyer, W., & Wagner, P. (2020). *Mass incarceration: The whole pie 2020.* https://www.prisonpolicy.org/reports/pie2020.html

Scally, C. P., Batko, S., Popkin, S. J., & DuBois, N. (2018). *The case for more, not less: Shortfalls in federal housing assistance and gaps in evidence for proposed policy changes.* Urban Institute. https://www.urban.org/research/publication/case-more-not-less-shortfalls-federal-housing-assistance-and-gaps-evidence-proposed-policy-changes

Shah, S. (2016). *Pandemic: Tracking contagions from cholera to Ebola and beyond.* New York, NY: Farrar, Straus and Giroux.

Smith, D., & Oreskes, B. (2020, September 22). Program to house homeless people in hotels is ending after falling short of goal. *Los Angeles Times.* https://www.latimes.com/california/story/2020-09-22/homeless-people-hotels-project-roomkey-phasing-out

Surma, K., & for the Howard Center for Investigative Journalism (2020, August 25). Months later, communities still await federal homeless aid. *Cronkite News.* https://cronkitenews.azpbs.org/howardcenter/covid-homeless/stories/federal-response.html

Thompson, R. G., Wall, M. M., Greenstein, E., Grant, B. F., & Hasin, D. S. (2013). Substance-use disorders and poverty as prospective predictors of first-time homelessness in the United States. *American Journal of Public Health*, 103(S2), S282–S288.

Thornton, R. L., Glover, C. M., Cené, C. W., Glik, D. C., Henderson, J. A., & Williams, D. R. (2016). Evaluating strategies for reducing health disparities by addressing the social determinants of health. *Health Affairs*, 35(8), 1416–1423.

US Interagency Council on Homelessness. (2019, January). *Homeless in California statistics.* https://www.usich.gov/homelessness-statistics/ca/

US Interagency Council on Homelessness. (2020, July 6). *USICH and SARS-CoV-21 – The federal response for families and individuals experiencing homelessness.* https://www.usich.gov/resources/uploads/asset_library/USICH_Covid_19_First_Six_Month_Report_FINAL.pdf

Wagle, A., Isakadze, N.; Eatz, T., Blumenthal, R., & Martin, S. S. (2020). *Continuing preventive care during the COVID-19 pandemic: Discussion of recent ASPC recommendations.* American College of Cardiology. https://www.acc.org/latest-in-cardiology/articles/2020/07/13/08/24/continuing-preventive-care-during-the-covid-19-pandemic

Walter, C. (2020, October 23). *We avoided a rent payment cliff, but we aren't in the clear by any stretch.* National Multifamily Housing Council. https://www.nmhc.org/news/nmhc-news/2020/we-avoided-a-rent-payment-cliff-but-we-arent-in-the-clear-by-any-stretch/

Wasilewska-Ostrowska, K. M. (2020). Social work with a person in the crisis of homelessness in the context of the COVID-19 pandemic in Poland: Problems and challenges. *International Social Work.* https://doi.org/10.1177/0020872820948944

Wu, H., & Karabanow, J. (2020). COVID-19 and beyond: Social work interventions for supporting homeless populations. *International Social Work.* https://doi.org/10.1177/0020872820949625

Zahniser, D., & Alpert Reyes, E. (2020, September 16). Why didn't these L.A. hotels house homeless people? A new report offers some answers. *The Los Angeles Times.* https://www.latimes.com/california/story/2020-09-16/hotels-not-participating-in-roomkey

14

THE NEW SOCIAL SERVICES

Organising community during ecosocial health crises

Joel Izlar

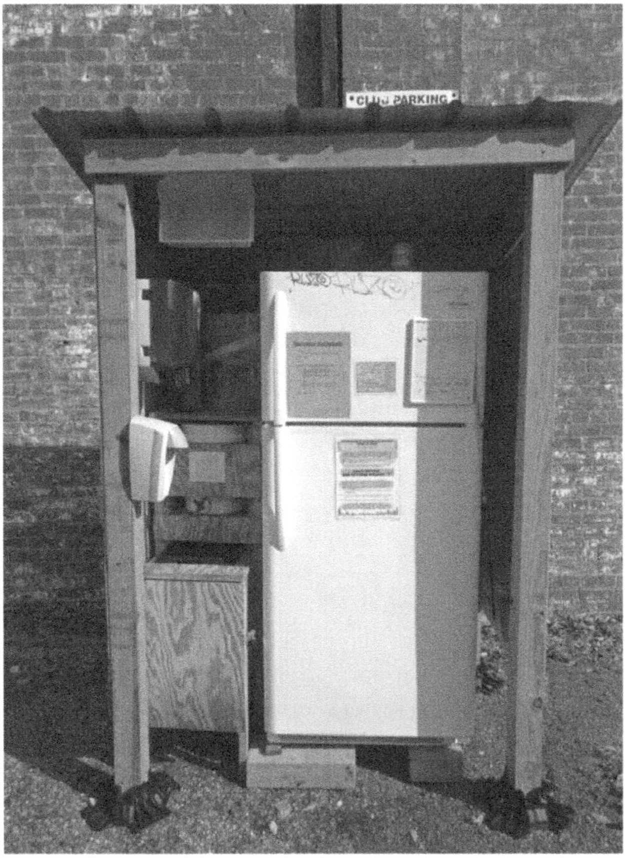

FIGURE 14.0 Community fridge, Athens, Georgia

Source: Photograph by Joel Izlar

DOI: 10.4324/9781003111214-16

Health emergencies are ecosocial crises of well-being. While this has been obvious to many oppressed and marginalised people throughout the world, the COVID-19 pandemic has brought this understanding to the fore, wreaking havoc through intersecting health, social, cultural, economic, political and ecological factors causing spiritual stress, trauma, death and grief throughout the world (Kaifie et al., 2020; Broughton, 2005; Rulli et al., 2017; Tao et al., 2013). The pandemic has exposed environmental destruction, poverty and classism, racism and xenophobia, and emergent *eco-fascism* (Clissold et al., 2020; Garcia, 2020; Gomez et al., 2020; Human Rights Watch, 2020; Nguyen, 2020; Parolin et al., 2020; Villarreal, 2020; Weal, 2020; Yam, 2020). Lawton (2019, p. 24) describes eco-facism as a "fusion of white nationalism and environmentalism", the core tenets of which connect environmental problems to anti-immigration and racist sentiment. People have become disconnected from neighbours and communities. Many overwork for low wages, and food waste and pollution have worsened alongside other systemic inequalities and inequities built-in to our global state, social, cultural, and economic systems (Briggs, 2020; Cohen, 2020; Corkery & Yaffe-Bellany, 2020; Covert, 2020; Fuller, 2020; Izlar, 2020a; Jervis et al., 2020; Kassam, 2020; Ogen, 2020).

Inequalities and inequities present challenges to primary, secondary, and tertiary responses to pandemics and highlight how the COVID-19 crisis is deeply connected to the destruction of the natural world, and that the destruction of our natural world is rooted in social problems (Carrington, 2020; Zimmer, 2019). In other words, how we treat nature is a reflection of how we treat one another and other species. Ecosocial crises are exacerbated by *speciesism*, or "the unjustified disadvantageous consideration or treatment of those who are not classified as belonging to one or more particular species", a position which enables further environmental destruction by devaluing the importance of ecosystem diversity (Horta, 2009, p. 2). A good example is deforestation that leads to encroachment on natural habitats and livelihoods (Platto et al., 2020; Poudel, 2020). The interdependent ecological roots of our health and social problems must be addressed to break the cycle of compounding disadvantage.

Social workers were presented with opportunities during ecosocial crises to shift from an "anthropocentric focus to an eco-centric focus" to meet the needs of the most vulnerable which includes humans, other species and ecologies, while prefiguring a new, healthy, just, and peaceful society based on mutual support and community – the idea that our current actions should embody the future world (Powers, Schmitz & Beckwith Moritz, 2019). As ecosocial crises worsen, there will be more pandemics, unstable ecosystems, erratic economies and state institutions (Carrington, 2020; Tollefson, 2020; Vilenica et al., 2020). As well as ecological systems, eco-austerity policies will fail to protect and meet the needs of the vulnerable, marginalised, and oppressed, creating an endless feedback loop of destruction and precarity. Given these possibilities, social workers should be prepared to organise resilient community projects and counter-institutions which offer alternatives to failing or unstable infrastructures and ecosocial systems, and embrace practices that reflect the *shared realities* of social welfare and social work in the 21st century (Pentaraki, 2016, p. 2).

This chapter focusses on community work and organising within the US during the COVID-19 pandemic. Community workers and organisers can draw lessons from the experience to build future community projects and counter-institutions that concurrently operate as forms of ecosocial protest, meeting need through mutual aid, social services, community work, organising and direct action in ways that support resilience, and building hope. The differences between *community organising* and *organising community* are examined and the feminist model is suggested as more appropriate for organising community in ecosocial crises which are understood within a glocalised context. *Glocalisation* is a concept that describes both local and global forces of interaction where the actions of one community may immediately affect another (and vice versa). The concepts of mutual aid, social welfare, and *new social services* are discussed as ways of addressing multiple problems, and examples of community responses to COVID-19 are reviewed. This chapter closes with challenges to organising and implications for social work and thoughts for the future.

What is community organising?

Community organising is hard to define as it means different things to different people such as:

- canvassing neighbourhoods, knocking on doors and asking people to complete surveys
- participating in a public protest to shame a business into paying better wages
- attending a local government meeting to speak up about neighbourhood pollution
- building a local grassroots organisation to run multiple pressure campaigns for incremental change over time
- getting together for a potluck (a communal gathering to share various dishes) that meets several times a week to save money, prevent food waste and to get to know neighbours
- developing a mutual support group with those experiencing the same problems
- starting a breakfast program for youth left out of school programs
- opening a shelter for (and with) those who have been shut out of mainstream shelter systems
- running a community technology centre to protest electronic waste and to provide computers to people that need them
- volunteering at a community garden to harvest healthy food, protest the industrialised food system and get to know one another

To put simply, community organising is the act of people getting together to make positive change in their lives and the lives of others with a shared understanding that they are mutually dependent.

In the West, the most common understanding of community organising is the Alinsky tradition, named after the 20th-century American community organiser Saul Alinsky (Alinsky, 1971; Hamington, 2010; Slayton, 1988). In this model, organising local neighbourhood associations that target public sphere institutions through short-term pressure campaigns intends to build power and resilience through campaign successes over time. The model's strengths lie in its ability to publicly draw attention to wide-ranging structural issues that agitate for immediate change and create fervour and empowerment from *battles* and *wins* that feed back into organising. These actions should complement one another, creating a strong, centralised organisation that is able to *fight back* against and *speak truth* to structures of power making a more uplifted, empowered, and self-determined community. However, the model has been criticised for its masculinist tendencies and focus on conflict, its failure to address racism and sexism within its organising, its lack of a long-term vision, a failure to build local capacity and leadership, and the focus on individualism and self-interest (Eichler, 2007; Martinson & Su, 2012, p. 64; Ohmer & DeMasi, 2009).

The tradition of organising community is from the north American, feminist, private sphere, women-centred model of community organising (Stall & Stoecker, 1998). In contrast to the Alinsky model, no singular individual, organisation, or movement can be credited with its beginnings, lending itself to being more adaptable and inclusive. While its history likely predates the written record, it can be traced back to three movements.

- Black women who organised safe havens of community under the brutality of 19th-century slavery in the United States (Stall & Stoecker, 1998). Safe havens *recognise and resist domination* and provided safety, health, community, resilience, and survival (Stall & Stoecker, 1998, p. 736).
- Black women of the late 19th century, such as Ida B. Wells, who organised campaigns against sexual violence and lynching, and local community social services that formed as structures of resistance and social care.
- Privileged White women community workers of the late 19th and early 20th centuries, such as Jane Addams and Ellen Gates Starr of the Settlement House Movement organised ecosocial community projects that operated as social services and a means to organise community (Addams, 1910).

In this long history, other peoples, struggles and organising practices cannot be ignored, for example, organising by Indigenous women and non-neurotypical/neurodivergent people (Gilio-Whitaker, 2020; Nelson et al., 2006), Throughout the 20th and 21st centuries, this model has had progressive to radical orientations in organising and maintaining discourses related to "civil rights, gay liberation, transgender, reproductive rights, AIDS, harm reduction, and global justice movements" (Shepard, 2010, p. 36). At its best, these connections show that the model is reflective and meet the unique and nuanced needs and experiences of people and social climates such as moving beyond viewing women and others as *constituenc[ies] in organising* and transcending ideas of genderism and binarism to entirely new forms of social relations and existence in everyday life (Hyde, 2005, p. 361).

In organising community, rather than pressuring structures of power to change through short-term, public sphere campaigns through singular neighbourhood associations, co-power and resilience are built outside of structures of power through organic counter-institutions and community projects that meet need and function as forms of protest. The basis of organising community is through building new and nurturing existing private sphere relationships, inclusive networking and community building, consensus-based decision making, and the rejection of centralised leadership. The principles of care, direct democracy, mutuality, empowerment, popular education (meaning *of the people* and rooted in ideas of class struggles, oppression and transformation), direct action, and the full participation and inclusion of people are central to organising. Ideally, these practices provide safe and nurturing *free spaces* (i.e. intimate spaces where smaller groups of people can get to know each other), empower individuals, build skills and confidence, support (self)-understanding, positive self-esteem and confidence, and create a more critical worldview resulting in the "cultivation of individual and collective skills and resources for social and political action" through repetitive cycles of process and reflection (Stall & Stoecker, 1998, p. 741).

The "emergency of now"

Organising ecosocial communities in a glocalised context

Ecosocial problems are glocalised. These affects are intersectional, interdependent, and massively accelerated in the COVID-19 pandemic. The progress and consequences of the pandemic presented opportunities to make radical change while meeting need. Organising communities in these contexts had the potential to provide deeper connections to ourselves and our communities, and to provide a *global access* that connects us to our planet, other communities, ecologies, and the repercussions of our collective behaviours on one another and nature (Gamble & Weil, 2010, p. 6). Like the intimate *free space* of a living room, organising can build glocal *free spaces* that empower individuals and communities to meet organising goals through reflections upon the interconnectedness between ourselves and our planet, each other, and our behaviours and their repercussions. The COVID-19 pandemic has brought the world together in ways not experienced in generations and has shown that single-issue organising is now multi-issue organising and vice versa. Despite divisions and unrest, many communities reflect the interconnectedness of ecosocial problems and their causes, responding through *social services* as organising, and organising as social services.

Mutual aid, organising community, and the new social services

Like community organising, mutual aid is hard to characterise. Before the pandemic, mutual aid as it is currently popularly understood, was mostly practised within Western, radical leftist circles whose philosophical roots can be traced to European social anarchism (Izlar, 2019b; Kropotkin, 1902).

Mutual aid is:

- a theory and practice of organising community to implement anti-authoritarian forms of social welfare
- a *voluntary and complementary* exchange of goods, resources and/or services for mutual welfare or "people giv[ing] what they can and get[ting] what they need" (Shepard, 2014, p. 166)
- based upon the shared understanding that official systems of power often fail to effectively, quickly, equitably, and justly meet the needs of communities, and that these needs can be better addressed through direct action outside of official structures of power (Izlar, 2020b)
- a horizontal practice that differs from charity or pathologised helping as it seeks to maintain no moralistic, scientific, or professional hierarchy of giver over receiver, organiser over organised, or helper over helped. Even so, forms of hierarchy may develop in mutual aid projects through conscious and unconscious power differentials within groups (Izlar, 2019a, 2019b). Unaddressed power differentials open the possibility for mutual aid projects to quickly devolve into *radical charities* or affinity groups characterised by hyper-individualism, insularity, exclusivity, poor organisation, a short-term focus, and social category homogeneity

Many governments and private institutions bungled responses to the COVID-19 health emergency, most notably the US under Trump, which led to an unprecedented explosion of mutual aid organisations and networks with many examples throughout the world, see Chapter 2 (Mutual Aid Disaster Relief, 2020). Mutual aid has *gone public* and its principles accurately (and inaccurately) are popularised by mainstream politicians, celebrities, influencers, journalists, bloggers, websites and news outlets. In a sense, mutual aid is now understood in broader discourses as long ignored traditions are voiced, expanding its scope and challenging its Eurocentrism and whiteness. These developments are connected with the "broad-based universalising dialogue[s]" of the global justice movements and the new community organising which emphasises the fusion of public and private spheres, the building of community projects and counter-institutions, and the rejection of social hierarchies (Shepard, 2005, 2010, p. 36).

If there is anything that uniquely characterises social welfare today, it is the new public recognition and acceptance of community organising through the lens of ecosocially focussed, glocalised, solidaric mutual support, or broadly speaking, a *new social services* that is concurrently guided by the principles of anti-authoritarianism and collectivism as well as the unique and diverse traditions and understandings of mutual support and community by marginalised and oppressed peoples. People have stepped in where institutions have failed them. However, brief this public legitimacy by a White, cis-heteropatriarchal society may be, it will continue to be practised as it has always been especially in the face of new ecosocial crises. Given this, it is important to examine practices during COVID-19 in order to prepare for the future.

COVID-19 organising

Organising during the COVID-19 pandemic has been multifaceted, nuanced and diverse reflecting unique needs, cultures, realities, experiences, and demands of peoples and communities outlined in the following examples. In the US, a significant portion of organising has revolved around projects aimed at promoting health, well-being, social welfare, community, solidarity, resilience, resistance, and self-determination.

Indigenous organising

Indigenous peoples, specifically the Diné (Navajo), have been one of the country's hardest hit communities with 575 lives lost and over 11,400 people infected (Navajo Department of Health & Navajo Epidemiology Center, 2020). According to Begay (2020a), the pandemic and its related effects on the Diné have further contributed to a *blood memory*, which is,

> "An embodied remembrance passed down from generation to generation ... that we pass down in our familial lineages, experiences and memories. Sometimes they are good and joyful and sometimes they are traumatic and rooted in grief".

For the Diné and other Indigenous peoples in the US, the challenges of the pandemic have been opportunities to build upon collective community strengths to "decolonize from individualism and reconnect with ways of community care" through a grounding in spiritual traditions, medicine, and knowledge as well as the building of community in ways that reject individualism and rampant capitalism (Begay, 2020b). The ideas, principles and strategies by the Diné manifested as resilient community projects that operated as ways to meet need while connecting with traditions that protested ecosocial injustice and government failures to protect Indigenous lives, cultures, traditions, and self-determination.

Predominantly led and organised by women, projects traversed the 43,000 square kilometre *reservation*, a construct forced upon Indigenous people by the US government through genocide (Santilli, 2020). Projects filling the gap left by failures of power structures focussed on fundraising, collectively making their own PPE, delivering water, food and medicine, educating about COVID-19 in their own language, and providing internet access (Cheetham, 2020; Grantham-Philips, 2020; Sottile, 2020; Wagner & Grantham-Philips, 2020; Woods, 2020). Not without its challenges, these efforts harnessed strengths and protected the health and well-being of the community through building upon tradition and community organising to address ecosocial issues such as long-standing food and water access, digital inequality, access to PPE, education and other protective measures while strengthening human connection, belonging, self-determination and autonomy.

Pollution, waste, and organising indirect community

Throughout the pandemic, many governments imposed lockdowns that showed immediate albeit, in some cases, temporary impacts to *visible nature*. Skies in chronically polluted cities were clear for the first time in decades, air quality improved and birds inundated with the stress of noise pollution changed their songs (Ellis-Petersen et al., 2020; Derryberry et al., 2020; Landrigan, Bernstein & Binagwaho, 2020; Picheta, 2020). Studies found correlations with pollution and high mortality rates of COVID-19 highlighting the importance of understanding ecosocial interconnectedness between humans, health and the environment which in turn creates conditions in which viruses thrive while unjust structures fail to adequately respond (Ogen, 2020; Petroni et al., 2020). While the Earth was able to take a momentary breath, environmentalism was captured by eco-fascist narratives creating a dark side that shifted blame from ecosocial systems of oppression to humans. It has been argued that focussing on short-term positives such as momentary dips in pollution may divert attention away from long-term strategies to address ecosocial crises such as global warming (Hijazi, 2020). Narratives such as these also drew attention away from new ecosocial problems, such as medical waste created by non-recyclable and single-use PPE and food thrown out while the hardest hit communities faced hunger (Corkery & Yaffe-Bellany, 2020; Kassam, 2020).

The pandemic impacted on organising in other ways. It was harder to conduct face-to-face interaction, generally considered to be the most effective form of organising. Nonetheless, *indirect community* are ways to address issues and organise community that may translate to forms of *direct community*. Little Free Libraries, geocaching (leaving a needed item where a person can find it via GPS), tool libraries (community tool sheds), time banking (a public ledger to record volunteer time), and community fridges are some examples of community projects that can meet ecosocial needs and build community while creating points of contact.

Community fridges offer a good example of how community organising continued despite the necessary limitations imposed to contain the pandemic. Community fridges are simply refrigerators set up in locations convenient to local people that provide free food and other supplies that a community needs and are monitored for safety by groups of volunteers. Before the pandemic, mutual aid-branded food fridges were mostly practised in predominantly White, radical leftist circles. Like the broad concept of mutual aid itself, free food fridges have spread throughout the US to meet the food needs of communities while diverting food waste from landfills. Many free food fridges have moved beyond just supplying food and goods to reflect the creativity, culture, and sense of place and community, for example, through elaborate and intricate art on refrigerators, elements that can be linked to improved health and well-being (Short, 2020; Stuckey & Nobel, 2010).

While relatively new, the community fridge movement is moving beyond its traditional roots in whiteness as many community fridges in the US are by women of colour (Short, 2020). So far, indirect community and socially distanced connections have not stalled the ability to organise community. Creative connections are inspiring. The pandemic has exposed waste in the face of mass hunger and capitalist surplus, for example, access to healthy food especially related to racialised and class inequities and how communities are responding to these problems on their own terms. Many people are reconnecting with their neighbours through art and other means of indirect sharing and collaboration which supports community empowerment, reinforces a sense of community and connection with ecosocial issues.

Organising under digital surveillance

The pandemic has made it harder to conduct in-person interaction, so digital organisation has become a central way to make on the ground organising happen, particularly those projects that aim to meet need while organising structural change. Digital interaction has proven to be effective for organising indirect community projects such as the community fridge movement and providing funds raised directly to people in need. It avoids face-to-face interaction while still helping others and maintaining a sense of community and connection. Facebook, Twitter, Instagram, Zoom, TikTok, GoFundMe, Venmo, and other proprietary social media platforms have been used to quickly and efficiently organise many community projects. However, the use of these platforms may perpetuate the very systems of domination that these community projects seek to undermine, namely surveillance capitalism (a form of capitalism based upon the commodification of personal data), digital centralisation, community factionalisation, digital inequality, and ecological destruction caused by disposal of technological equipment.

Those privileged enough to have consistent, affordable, understandable, and regular access to information and communications technologies (ICTs) can participate in the digital organising of community which assumes, among other things, that they have a regular, safe location to shelter-in-place. Those people unable to participate due to language barriers or disability, or simply refuse to participate to avoid state surveillance or the potential of being stalked by someone, are left out. ICTs also negatively influence how we view our communities and our very selves. In addition to our social identities, roles and titles, we are defined by our posts, messages, likes, comments, shares, blogs, vlogs, links, follows and followers, and during health emergencies how we should be coping. The use of ICTs that are not digitally just and their use in tandem with online organising are new challenges to consider in the ecosocial organising of community.

The global surveillance disclosures that began in 2013 reveal large-scale, illegal surveillance of private citizens by corporations such as Facebook and Microsoft. The sharing of data with governments such as the US and the UK has accelerated during the pandemic with the use of tracing apps (Gellman & Poitras, 2013; Newman, 2020). This is cause for concern for organising community projects that seek to work outside and against systems of power, particularly those projects that are seen as a threat to the established order such as how the Black Panther Party's survival programs were viewed during the Black Power movement (Hoover, 1969). Big Tech suggests that these alternatives should be embraced, although they increasingly play a role in developing *algorithms of inequality* that refer to the role of large technology corporations in state surveillance that disproportionately targets Black, Indigenous peoples of colour and other marginalised groups,.

Taking this further, the *network effect* describes the social phenomenon where the value of a service comes from how many people are using that service, for example, how many of your friends use a certain social media platform influences whether or not you join that platform. Given the strength of this effect and the already stressed and fractured state of communities, it is difficult for many to imagine the use of non-proprietary and non-centralised alternatives to platforms such as Facebook or Instagram. However, social movements such as Black Lives Matter and aspects of the free fridge movement are showing that the use of non-proprietary programs such as Signal are needed to organise more justly and effectively (Nierenberg, 2020; Short, 2020). Decentralised alternatives on the Fediverse, a large, interconnected network of independent servers such as Mastodon and PeerTube that can be used for blogging, social networking, media hosting, streaming, etc. hold promise as ecotechnologies that can be used to glocally organise communities and place the infrastructures of that technology into the community that owns it.

This autonomy over communications and infrastructure has the potential to allow a community to fill the gaps of digital inequality that centralised and proprietary platforms foster through popular education and the creation of free spaces that draw people into organising. The use of such non-proprietary, decentralised ecotechnologies may also make an impact on the carbon emissions of the *dirty cloud* created by web services that use very little clean energy inherent in centralised technologies that have become overburdened during the pandemic (Condon, 2020; Walsh, 2014).

Implications and conclusion

This chapter will never be completed, as COVID-19 is not the last ecosocial crisis. Because there will be more crises, constraints and complications in organising to meet need while addressing the structural problems that cause them will resurface. A common thread in community work during the COVID-19 health emergency has been the creativity and hope found in the unforeseen challenges of meeting need while protesting injustice during seemingly insurmountable odds. Survival and self-determination are forms of resistance and community building ways to reconnect with tradition and culture while protesting state failures. Harnessing food waste to organise indirect community, meet need, and protest food waste and food racism, and the emergent use of non-proprietary technologies provide the means to connect with one another to organise social movements and indirect community projects. In other words, communities have come together in ways not seen in generations by organising community. This is why it is important for social workers to view community work as an essential aspect of social work and those doing community work as doing vital work. Social workers who are doing community work have increasingly come to identify with service users, and that service users have increasingly come to identify as *doing social work* blurring traditional distinctions between the professional and service user (Izlar, 2019a; Pentaraki, 2016). The COVID-19 ecosocial crisis has flattened hierarchies between helper and helped, organiser and organised, giver and receiver, and now, social worker and service user, as we are interdependent in shared catastrophe. This brings forth numerous implications for practice.

As a narrative of a new social services has achieved greater legitimacy in the public eye in pandemic conditions, and as more people who would traditionally be seen as service users are publicly recognised for *doing social work* in their own communities, the legitimacy and credentialed boundaries of mainstream social work that claims a sharp division between social worker and *client* is increasingly called into question, a challenging notion for many (Ferguson & Lavalette, 2013; Fronek & Chester, 2016). Within an ecosocial context, new questions are raised concerning credentialism and professional protectionism versus social justice. It also brings forth additional questions for those that practice mainstream social work as to *what constitutes social work itself* and how to include community work and community organising which have become legitimate forms of practice in the US and many parts of the world where governments have failed to meet the needs of people (Rothman, 2013; Fogel & Ersing, 2016). Under cycles of crises and healing, social work has an opportunity to be democratised and transformed into a vehicle for human and ecological growth and liberation.

While crises will not stop occurring, the bluntness of their initial impacts do, as do their periods of clean-up and healing which allow for deeper reflection. Burnout, loneliness, and fear are all too common in new social services work and especially disaster-response mutual aid projects which have notoriously short lifespans, some of which are already showing signs of dissolution (Gathright, 2020). This has added to the tensions caused by failing infrastructures, poor funding, fractured communities, hate and violence toward human difference and so on, which make it difficult to even consider where reflection starts and actions begin or vice versa. However, the organising that occurred during the pandemic should be a point of inspiration for what is possible regarding building new social services for a new ecosocial society. In a world of uncertainty, one thing is certain, the *new normal* is that we are likely not going back to the *old normal* which gives us the opportunity to make the new, better.

BOX 14.1

REFLECTIVE QUESTIONS

1. If you were to imagine a social work that meets need while addressing structural problems, how would it look to you?
2. In your view, how, and in what ways, do ecological problems relate to social problems? How can communities best address these interlinking challenges during ecosocial health emergencies and prevent future ones from happening? How do you see yourself in this work?
3. Think of a social problem or a group of people that you have worked with or would like to work with. Now, place this social problem or group within an ecosocial context. How do you see yourself working with these people to address these social problems in this new context?

References

Addams, J. (1910). *Twenty years at hull house.* New York: The McMillan Company.

Alinsky, S. D. (1971). *Rules for radicals: A practical primer for realistic radicals.* New York: Vintage Books.

Begay, J. (2020a, May 11). What Indian country remembers about survival: The community care at the heart of Indigenous response. *YES! Magazine.* https://www.yesmagazine.org/issue/coronavirus-community-power/2020/05/11/coronavirus-indian-country-survival-2/

Begay, J. (2020b, March 13). Decolonizing community care in response to COVID-19: Responding to the COVID-19 pandemic responsibly, Indigenously. *NDN Collective.* https://ndncollective.org/indigenizing-and-decolonizing-community-care-in-response-to-covid-19/

Briggs, H. (2020, October 13). Covid: Why bats are not to blame, say scientists. *BBC News.* https://www.bbc.com/news/science-environment-54246473/

Broughton, E. (2005). The Bhopal disaster and its aftermath: A review. *Environmental Health,* 4(1). https://doi.org/10.1186/1476-069X-4-6

Carrington, D. (2020, April 27). Halt destruction of nature or suffer even worse pandemics, say world's top scientists. *The Guardian.* https://www.theguardian.com/world/2020/apr/27/halt-destruction-nature-worse-pandemics-top-scientists/

Cohen, J. (2020). COVID-19 capitalism: The profit motive versus public health. *Public Health Ethics.* https://doi.org/10.1093/phe/phaa025

Covert, B. (2020, April 14). 'The reality is, it's incredibly hard'. *The Atlantic.* https://www.theatlantic.com/health/archive/2020/04/women-fighting-covid-19-are-underpaid-and-overworked/609934/

Cheetham, J. (2020, June 15). Navajo Nation: The people battling America's worst coronavirus outbreak. *BBC News.* https://www.bbc.com/news/world-us-canada-52941984/

Clissold, E., Nylander, D., Watson, C., & Ventriglio, A. (2020). Pandemics and prejudice. *International Journal of Social Psychiatry,* 66(5), 421–423.

Condon, S. (2020, March 25). How Netflix is adjusting network operations during the COVID-19 outbreak. *ZDNet.* https://www.zdnet.com/article/how-netflix-is-adjusting-network-operations-during-the-covid-19-outbreak/

Corkery, M., & Yaffe-Bellany, D. (2020, May 2). 'We had to do something': Trying to prevent massive food waste. *The New York Times*. https://www.nytimes.com/2020/05/02/business/coronavirus-food-waste-destroyed.html

Derryberry, E. P., Phillips, J. N., Derryberry, G. E., Blum, M. J., & Luther, D. (2020). Singing in a silent spring: Birds respond to a half-century soundscape reversion during the COVID-19 shutdown. *Science*, 370(6516), 575–579.

Eichler, M. (2007). *Consensus organizing: Building communities of mutual self-interest*. Thousand Oaks: SAGE.

Ellis-Petersen, H., Ratcliffe, R., Cowie, S., Daniels, S. P., & Kuo, L. (2020, April 11). 'It's positively alpine!': Disbelief in big cities as air pollution falls. *The Guardian*. https://www.theguardian.com/environment/2020/apr/11/positively-alpine-disbelief-air-pollution-falls-lockdown-coronavirus/

Ferguson, I., & Lavalette, M. (2013). Crisis, austerity and the future(s) of social work in the UK. *Critical and Radical Social Work*, 1(1), 95–110.

Fogel, S. J., & Ersing, R. (2016) Macro-focused social work dissertations: A preliminary look at the numbers. *Journal of Social Work Education*, 52(2), 170–7.

Fronek, P., & Chester, P. (2016). Moral outrage: Social workers in the third space. *Ethics and Social Welfare*, 10(2), 163–176.

Fuller, G. (2020, October 8). Covid-19 lockdowns have improved global air quality, data shows. *The Guardian*. https://www.theguardian.com/environment/2020/oct/08/covid-19-lockdowns-global-air-quality-india-london-uk/

Gamble, D. N., & Weil, M. (2010). *Community practice skills: Local to global perspectives*. New York: Columbia University Press.

Garcia, B. (2020, September 30). The danger of eco-fascism for Latinos and other ethnicities in times of coronavirus. *AL DÍA News*. https://aldianews.com/articles/culture/environment/danger-eco-fascism-latinos-and-other-ethnicities-times-coronavirus/

Gathright, J. (2020, September 17). D.C. mutual aid groups face dwindling funds and burnout months into the pandemic. *WAMU*. https://wamu.org/story/20/09/17/dc-mutual-aid-network-funding-groceries-hotline/

Gellman, B., & Poitras, L. (2013, June 7). U.S., British intelligence mining data from nine U.S. Internet companies in broad secret program. Washington Post. https://www.washingtonpost.com/investigations/us-intelligence-mining-data-from-nine-us-internet-companies-in-broad-secret-program/2013/06/06/3a0c0da8-cebf-11e2-8845-d970ccb04497_story.html

Gilio-Whitaker, D. (2020). *As long as grass grows: The indigenous fight for environmental justice, from colonization to standing rock*. New York: Beacon.

Gomez, A., Grantham-Philips, W., Hughes, T., Jervis, R., Plevin, R., …Nichols, M. (2020, October 21). 'An unbelievable chain of oppression': America's history of racism was a pre-existing condition for COVID-19. USA To*day*. https://www.usatoday.com/indepth/news/nation/2020/10/12/coronavirus-deaths-reveal-systemic-racism-united-states/5770952002/

Grantham-Philips, W. (2020, October 25). On the Navajo Nation, COVID-19 death toll is higher than any US state. Here's how you can support community relief. USA Today. https://www.msn.com/en-us/news/us/on-the-navajo-nation-covid-19-death-toll-is-higher-than-any-us-state-heres-how-you-can-support-community-relief/ar-BB1alWSa/

Hamington, M. (2010). Community organizing: Addams and Alinsky. In M. Hamington (ed.), *Feminist interpretations of Jane Addams* (pp. 255–274). University Park: Pennsylvania State University Press.

Hijazi, J. (2020, April 8). 'We're the virus.' How eco-fascism hurts climate action. *E&E News*. https://www.eenews.net/stories/1062814031/

Hoover, J. E. (1969). *Black Panthers' breakfast for children program*. https://genius.com/Federal-bureau-of-investigation-hoover-memo-on-black-panthers-breakfast-for-children-program-annotated.

Horta, O. (2009). What is speciesism? *Journal of Agricultural and Environmental Ethics*, 23(3), 243–266.

Human Rights Watch. (2020, May 12). Covid-19 fueling anti-Asian racism and xenophobia worldwide. https://www.hrw.org/news/2020/05/12/covid-19-fueling-anti-asian-racism-and-xenophobia-worldwide/

Hyde, C. (2005). Feminist community practice. In M. Weil (ed.), *The handbook of community practice* (1st ed., pp. 360–371). Thousand Oaks: SAGE.

Izlar, J. (2019a). Local–global linkages: Challenges in organizing functional communities for ecosocial justice. *Journal of Community Practice*, 27(3–4), 369–387.

Izlar, J. (2019b). Radical social welfare and anti-authoritarian mutual aid. *Critical and Radical Social Work*, 7(3), 349–366.

Izlar, J. (2020a, May 20). Coronavirus brings out the best and worst in us. *Flagpole Magazine*. https://flagpole.com/news/letters-to-the-editor/2020/05/20/coronavirus-brings-out-the-best-and-worst-in-us/

Izlar, J. (2020b). *What is mutual aid?* https://ssw.uga.edu/news/article/what-is-mutual-aid-by-joel-izlar/

Jervis, R., Plevin, R., Hughes, T., & Ornelas, O. (2020). Worked to death: Latino farmworkers have long been denied basic rights. COVID-19 showed how deadly racism could be. USA Today. https://www.usatoday.com/in-depth/news/nation/2020/10/21/covid-how-virus-racism-devastated-latino-farmworkerscalifornia/5978494002/

Kaifie, A., Schettgen, T., Bertram, J., Löhndorf, K., Waldschmidt, S., …Küpper, T. (2020). Informal e-waste recycling and plasma levels of non-dioxin-like polychlorinated biphenyls (NDL-PCBs) – A cross-sectional study at Agbogbloshie, Ghana. *Science of the Total Environment*. https://doi.org/10.1016/j.scitotenv.2020.138073

Kassam, A. (2020, June 8). 'More masks than jellyfish': Coronavirus waste ends up in ocean. *The Guardian*. https://www.theguardian.com/environment/2020/jun/08/more-masks-than-jellyfish-coronavirus-waste-ends-up-in-ocean/

Kropotkin, P. (1902). *Mutual aid: A factor of evolution*. https://theanarchistlibrary.org/library/petr-kropotkin-mutual-aid-a-factor-of-evolution.pdf

Landrigan, P. J., Bernstein, A., & Binagwaho, A. (2020). COVID-19 and clean air: An opportunity for radical change. *The Lancet Planetary Health*, 4(10),e447–e449. https://doi.org/10.1016/S2542-5196(20)30201-1

Lawton, G. (2019). The rise of real eco-fascism. *New Scientist*, 243(3243), 24. https://doi.org/10.1016/s0262-4079(19)31529-5

Martinson, M., & Su, C. (2012). Contrasting organising approaches: The "Alinsky Tradition" and Freirian organizing approaches. In M. Minkler (ed.), *Community organizing and community building for health and welfare* (3rd ed., pp. 59–77). New Brunswick: Rutgers University Press.

Mutual Aid Disaster Relief. (2020). *About*. https://mutualaiddisasterrelief.org/about/

Navajo Department of Health & Navajo Epidemiology Center. (2020). Navajo *Nation COVID-19 dashboard*. https://www.ndoh.navajo-nsn.gov/COVID-19/Data/

Nelson, G., Ochocka, J., Janzen, R., & Trainor, J. (2006). A longitudinal study of mental health consumer/survivor initiatives: Part 1 – literature review and overview of the study. *Journal of Community Psychology*, 34(3), 247–260.

Newman, L. H. (2020, November 1). Internet freedom has taken a hit during the Covid-19 pandemic. *Wired*. https://www.wired.com/story/internet-freedom-covid-19-2020/

Nguyen, F. (2020, October 29). The invisible struggle of the Asian American small-business owner. *Vox*. https://www.vox.com/21536943/asian-american-restuarant-racism-coronavirus/

Nierenberg, A. (2020, June 12). Signal downloads are way up since the protests began. *The New York Times*. https://www.nytimes.com/2020/06/11/style/signal-messaging-app-encryption-protests.html/

Ohmer, M. L., & DeMasi, K. (2009). *Consensus organizing: A community development workbook: A comprehensive guide to designing, implementing, and evaluating community change initiatives*. Thousand Oaks: SAGE.

Ogen, Y. (2020). Assessing nitrogen dioxide (NO_2) levels as a contributing factor to coronavirus (COVID-19) fatality. *Science of the Total Environment*, 138605. https://doi.org/10.1016/j.scitotenv.2020.138605

Parolin, Z., Curran, M., Matsudaira, Waldfogel, J., & Wimer, C. (2020). *Monthly poverty rates in the United States during the COVID-19 pandemic* [working paper]. Center on Poverty and Social Policy, School of Social Work, Columbia University and Teacher's College, Columbia University.

Pentaraki, M. (2016). 'I am in a constant state of insecurity trying to make ends meet, like our service users': Shared austerity reality between social workers and service users – towards a preliminary conceptualisation. *British Journal of Social Work*, 47(4), 1245–1261.

Petroni, M., Hill, D., Younes, L., Barkman, L., Howard, S., Howell, I. B., Mirowsky, J., & Collins, M. B. (2020). Hazardous air pollutant exposure as a contributing factor to COVID-19 mortality in the United States. *Environmental Research Letters*, 15(9), 0940a9. https://doi.org/10.1088/1748-9326/abaf86

Picheta, R. (2020, April 2020). People in India can see the Himalayas for the first time in 'decades,' as the lockdown eases air pollution. *CNN*. https://edition.cnn.com/travel/article/himalayas-visible-lockdown-india-scli-intl/index.html/

Platto, S., Zhou, J., Wang, Y., Wang, H., & Carafoli, E. (2020). Biodiversity loss and COVID-19 pandemic: The role of bats in the origin and the spreading of the disease. *Biochemical and Biophysical Research Communications*. https://doi.org/10.1016/j.bbrc.2020.10.028

Poudel, B. S. (2020). Ecological solutions to prevent future pandemics like COVID-19. *Banko Janakari*, 30(1), 1–2.

Powers, M., Schmitz, C., & Beckwith Moritz, M. (2019). Preparing social workers for ecosocial work practice and community building. *Journal of Community Practice*, 1–14.

Rothman, J. (2013) *Education for macro intervention: A survey of problems and prospects*. https://drive.google.com/file/d/1zp3O0mpHYSOmHGrzYcYY5DgONUy6rdC/view?usp=srng

Rulli, M. C., Santini, M., Hayman, D. T. S., & D'Odorico, P. (2017). The nexus between forest fragmentation in Africa and Ebola virus disease outbreaks. *Scientific Reports*, 7(1). https://doi.org/10.1038/srep41613

Santilli, M, (2020, May 15). In Navajo Nation, women are on the front lines of COVID-19. *Marie Claire*. https://www.marieclaire.com/politics/a32404944/navajo-nation-women-covid-19/

Shepard, B. (2005). Play, creativity, and the new community organizing. *Journal of Progressive Human Services*, 16(2), 47–69.

Shepard, B. (2010). Lessons for multi-issue organizing: From the women's movement to struggles for global justice. *Social Justice in Context*, 5(1), 36–55.

Shepard, B. (2014). *Community projects as social activism: From direct action to direct services*. Thousand Oaks: SAGE.

Short, A. M. (2020, October 6). Community fridges and mutual aid amid the pandemic. *The Bullet*. https://socialistproject.ca/2020/10/community-fridges-mutual-aid-amid-pandemic/

Slayton, R. A. (1988). *Back of the yards: The making of a local democracy*. Chicago: University of Chicago Press.

Sottile, C. (2020, October 16). Native American teachers, entrepreneurs seek new ways to close digital divide. *NBC News*. https://www.nbcnews.com/news/us-news/native-american-teachers-entrepreneurs-seek-new-ways-close-digital-divide-n1243746/

Stall, S., & Stoecker, R. (1998). Community organizing or organizing community? Gender and the crafts of empowerment. *Gender & Society*, 12(6), 729–756.

Stuckey, H. L., & Nobel, J. (2010). The connection between art, healing, and public health: A review of current literature. *American Journal of Public Health*, 100(2), 254–263.

Tao, J., Barry, T., Segawa, R., Neal, R., & Tuli, A. (2013). Pesticides exposure assessment of Kettleman City using the industrial source complex short-term model version 3. *Journal of Environmental Quality*, 42(2), 373–379. https://doi.org/10.2134/jeq2012.0347

Tollefson, J. (2020). Why deforestation and extinctions make pandemics more likely. *Nature*, *584*, 175–176.

Vilenica, A., McElroy, E., Ferreri, M., Arrigoitia, M. F., García-Lamarca, M., & Lancione, M. (2020). Covid-19 and housing struggles: The (re)makings of austerity, disaster capitalism, and the no return to normal. *Radical Housing Journal*, 2(1), 9–28.

Villarreal, A. (2020, August 17). 'If you don't have a home, what do you do?': Covid-19 highlights Texas homeless crisis. *The Guardian*. https://www.theguardian.com/us-news/2020/aug/17/texas-austin-covid-19-homeless-crisis/

Wagner, D., & Grantham-Philips, W. (2020, October 26). 'Still killing us': The federal government underfunded health care for Indigenous people for centuries. Now they're dying of COVID-19. USA Today. https://www.usatoday.com/in-depth/news/nation/2020/10/20/native-american-navajo-nation-coronavirus-deaths-underfunded-health-care/5883514002/

Walsh, B. (2014, April 2). Your data is dirty: The carbon price of cloud computing. *Time*. https://time.com/46777/your-data-is-dirty-the-carbon-price-of-cloud-computing/

Weal, S. (2020, October 27). Covid-19: Toddlers from UK's poorest families 'hit hardest by lockdown'. *The Guardian*. https://www.theguardian.com/society/2020/oct/27/covid-toddlers-from-uks-poorest-families-hit-hardest-by-lockdown/

Woods, A. (2020, September 29). The federal government promised Native American students computers and internet. Many are still waiting. *The Range*. https://www.tucsonweekly.com/TheRange/archives/2020/09/29/the-federal-government-promised-native-american-students-computers-and-internet-many-are-still-waiting/

Yam, H. (2020, October 15). After Trump's Covid-19 diagnosis, anti-Asian tweets and conspiracies rose 85%: Report. *NBC News*. https://www.nbcnews.com/news/asian-america/after-trump-s-covid-19-diagnosis-anti-asian-tweets-conspiracies-n1243441/

Zimmer, K. (2019, November 22). Deforestation is leading to more infectious diseases in humans. *National Geographic*. https://www.nationalgeographic.com/science/2019/11/deforestation-leading-to-more-infectious-diseases-in-humans/

15

CHALLENGES AND INNOVATIONS IN FIELD EDUCATION IN AUSTRALIA, NEW ZEALAND AND THE UNITED STATES

Lynne Briggs, Jane Maidment, Kathryn Hay, Kai Medina-Martinez, Renie Rondon-Jackson and Patricia Fronek

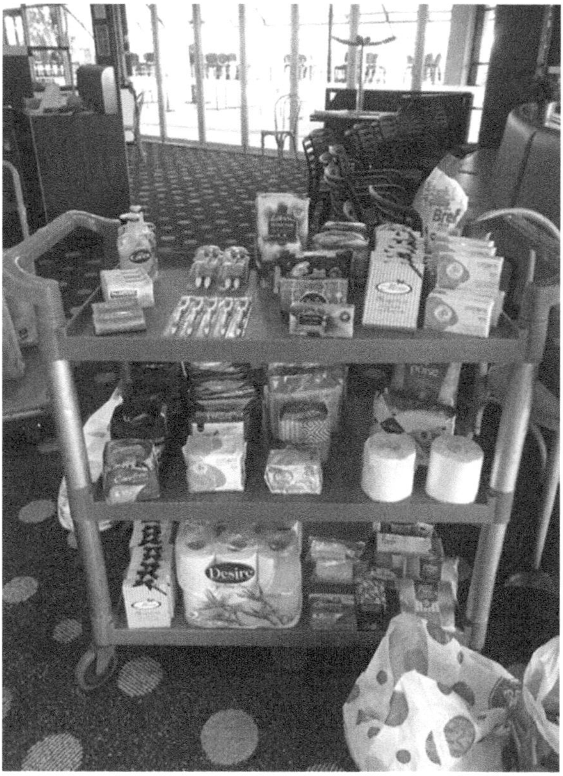

FIGURE 15.0 Stocking the university emergency food bank for international students excluded from COVID-19 Australian government support

Source: Photograph Hilary Gallagher

DOI: 10.4324/9781003111214-17

By March 2020, the COVID-19 pandemic had precipitated the greatest crisis in higher education since the Great Depression of the 1930s (Tija et al., 2020). Efforts to contain the virus, especially during lockdown or shelter-in-place orders, significantly impacted on higher education especially for students undertaking field education. A QS Quacquarelli Symonds (2020) survey of universities globally found that 50% of 400 university respondents moved courses online in response to COVID-19, 19% reported delayed starts, 17% changed application dates, 16% changed acceptance dates, 13% deferred 2020 offers, and 8% conducted their own English language tests. In the US, for example, most universities had moved to online delivery by March 2020. Enrolments declined at community colleges by 9.4% but rose by 3% at for-profit colleges in 2020 suggesting that students' access to material and social resources as well as access to alternative modes of delivery could play a role in students' capacity to pursue their education in pandemic conditions (National Student Clearinghouse Research Centre, 2020).

COVID-19 is not the first health emergency universities and students have faced. During the Severe Acute Respiratory Syndrome (SARS) pandemic in 2003 and the H1N1 (swine flu) pandemic in 2009, universities in affected regions learned the importance of leadership, communication with students, and keeping students safe. In Hong Kong, 17 medical students placed at the Prince of Wales Teaching Hospital were infected in the first two weeks of the outbreak. Wong, Gao and Tam et al. (2007) examined student anxiety and found high levels among the medical students, whereas anxiety was comparatively lower for students from other disciplines, especially for those not placed in hospital settings. These researchers suggested that while knowledge about the disease reduced anxiety and fear of discrimination, an inadequate understanding of SARS may have heightened anxiety. In China, during the HINI pandemic, female students were more fearful and at higher risk of post-traumatic stress if they had HINI symptoms or someone in their family had the disease (Xu et al., 2011). As the COVID-19 pandemic unfolded around the world in 2020, concerns emerged about student mental health, mainly related to health risks, online study, social isolation, and changed financial conditions (de Oliveira Araújo et al., 2020).

This chapter focuses on field education, an essential and compulsory aspect of social work education where students integrate their theoretical learnings with practice in agency settings. The impact of the pandemic on students undertaking field education was considerable, and the response varied. Issues in field education and the impact of COVID-19 on universities and students are examined, and how field education academics responded using examples from Australia, New Zealand and the United States.

Issues in field education

Before COVID-19, field education had changed little in terms of how it was delivered. A key issue for universities is that social work programs are required to follow the accrediting bodies' standards in each country. Failure to comply with recommended guidelines would jeopardise the accreditation of programs as well as compromising students.

Field education academics in social work programs report increasing competition and the subsequent difficulties they face when attempting to locate suitable placements, find social work supervisors, manage the logistics of placing large numbers of students, and resourcing those placements appropriately (Craik, 2019; Hay, 2018). Placements rely on the voluntary contributions of social workers in agencies to supervise students while in placement, professional functions that are undertaken without sufficient recognition of the significant impact this has on practitioners' usual workloads (Egan, 2005). The increasing pressure on practitioners to host students has resulted in a lack of alignment between the expectations of accrediting bodies and the capacity of agencies to deliver quality placements. Subsequently, this sometimes leads to diminished learning experiences for students (Bogo et al., 2017; Domakin, 2019).

A further issue is the increasing number of students who, through necessity, are employed and request part-time placements to avoid compromising their employment and undermining their capacity to meet placement requirements (McInnis, James & Hartley, 2000; Morley & Dunstan, 2013). These constraints have made it increasingly difficult for field education teams to place these students as agencies tend to prefer students to start and end placements around the same time. Although an increased number of schools are developing flexible placement arrangements such as part-time or after-hours placements in some settings and novel placements in new contexts. For example, in New Zealand, students are undertaking placement in cyber support assisting people affected by identity theft and other cybercrimes. In the US, public libraries have become placement agencies providing innovative ways to serve the homeless (Wahler et al., 2019).

Through field education, social work students learn professional skills by practising them in real-life settings in health and welfare agencies. Experiential learning in the field enables students to apply the knowledge taught in the classroom in real terms and provides opportunities to demonstrate their achievement of core competencies in professional skills. As Dewey (1933, 1938) and Smith (2001) noted, the idea that students learn from both classroom teaching and through practice experience is not new. While classroom education shapes the learning, reflection on practical experiences is an essential part of that learning. Fortune, Lee & Cavazos (2007) also argue that experience is a well-established social work education principle. Most accrediting bodies state that field placements must be in-person for a specified number of hours or days of supervised practice before the degree can be awarded. For these reasons, offering virtual field practice opportunities was not necessarily an option prior to COVID-19.

Several authors have noted that many social work programs have been particularly slow to adopt online delivery, perhaps resistant due to the interpersonal and in-person nature of social work practice alongside scepticism about whether the necessary skills can be effectively taught in a virtual classroom, a concern particularly relevant to field placement and other skill-based courses

(Lee, Hernandez & Marshall, 2019; McAllister, 2013; Smoyer, O'Brien & Rodriguez-Keyes, 2020). It has been reported that social work students studying course work remotely were more anxious about their readiness for placement than on-campus students (Afrouz & Crisp, 2020; Cummings, Chaffin & Cockerham, 2015). It is fair to say that students generally experience anxiety and excitement pre-placement particularly before their first placements, yet little difference in skill outcomes have been found and sometimes online students actually performed better (Afrouz & Crisp, 2020; Beddoe et al., 2018; Cummings, Chaffin & Cockerham, 2015). Taking all these issues into consideration, COVID-19 brought opportunities and challenges in relation to providing field education experiences that enabled students to meet and demonstrate core competencies when they were unable to engage in in-person practice.

Prior to the pandemic and as a result of it, many agencies and universities had experienced shrinking resources that limited their capacity to host placements and made the provision of rich learning environments for students increasingly difficult. In academia, field education programs are already marginalised and seen as cost-intensive activities, a situation further exacerbated by the economic fallout of the COVID-19 pandemic (Craik, 2019). In many countries, the point had been reached where universities as providers of higher education needed to press governments to properly finance social work education as producers of a key and essential workforce, and to ensure meaningful dialogue with professional bodies to review accreditation guidelines and standards to consider different ways in which field education could be offered in the 21st century without compromising quality, skill development or student livelihoods. As Ayala et al. (2018, p. 59) suggested, the development of new sustainable field education models and partnerships require responsiveness to current contextual realities at the micro, mezzo, and macro levels.

By the time a student is eligible for field placement, both the student and the university will have made a significant investment in their education. However, field placements are a pivotal juncture for social work students as they often face personal and institutional challenges prior to, during, and after field placement. Studies have found that social work students juggle mandatory field placements with work, family responsibilities, and other study requirements (McInnis, James & Hartley, 2000; Maidment, 2003; Morley & Dunstan, 2013). Johnstone et al. (2016) and Baglow and Gair (2018) found that unpaid social work placements, in particular, create considerable financial stress for students. Many students in these studies expressed how the limited flexibility in requirements imposed by professional bodies and universities on field placements was a key contributor to financial hardship, often resulting in a need to sacrifice their employment, which in turn, leads to either considerable financial stress or working extensive hours, all while undergoing a full-time field placement. For many students, the stress of managing personal responsibilities with mandated placement hours is challenging (Petra, Tripepi & Guardiola, 2020). COVID-19 related stressors were superimposed on these pre-existing trepidations and challenges in very uncertain and extended situations.

The impact of COVID-19 on field education

In many countries, universities stayed open until measures to control COVID-19 meant campuses had to close (Harper, 2020). On reopening, some universities introduced COVID-19 testing, encouraged physical distancing and other measures, and some found themselves in a cycle of opening and closing, particularly where clusters erupted in the student populations and lecturers fell ill (Andersen et al., 2020; Cheng et al., 2020; Malosh & Masters, 2020). In other countries students experienced disruption to their education while others, for example, California State University System's 23 campuses, ultimately moved to remote teaching for the foreseeable future.

In countries where lockdowns or shelter-in-place conditions were imposed, closures of universities and the majority of agencies occurred with little warning (Blackwell, 2020). Given field education has been mainly achieved during practice-based learning opportunities, immediate concerns were about how to respond to the extended COVID-19 situation where placements were not available or were seriously disrupted. Social work schools, field placement academics and students were confronted by uncertainty about when agencies would reopen and had to plan accordingly. Some students who were placed in hospitals, prisons, and child welfare agencies were expected to continue in-person while adhering to strict COVID-19 safety protocols. During this period, students were anxious about their health in high-risk environments and the health of their families. Students in agencies that closed were also concerned about their progress through their program and the well-being of their clients in lockdown conditions. Agencies had to adapt and introduce different ways of connecting and practising with clients, all of which reduced their capacity to support students. Likewise, students who were able to continue their placements had to grasp tele-social work and connecting virtually in supervision and with the university.

The closure of placements exacerbated existing tensions for students around their studies and created new concerns about their ability to progress through their programs and graduate. COVID-19 impacted student employment, often insecure, rendering some students homeless as they had no income to pay rent or buy food. International students, for example, in Australia, were the most affected and disadvantaged students. Many were already struggling with new environments and cultures and were among the most financially and materially disadvantaged because in Australia the government did not provide support packages for international students (Fronek & Briggs, 2020; Gallagher, Doherty & Obonyo 2020). While many domestic students could return to their parental homes, it was a very different situation for international students who were unable to return to their countries of origin due to international flight cancellations and closed borders (Bilecen, 2020; Fronek et al., 2021a; Harper, 2020). As a result, many international students were left on empty campuses and in locked-down cities without a home base, jobs or financial means of support. Many had no way of paying for reliable internet services, and therefore could not connect with online courses which effectively disrupted their studies further. Anxious for themselves and concerned for fellow students, students also worried about their families living in countries where the pandemic was raging. In addition to being forced to navigate disruption to course work and field placements, the closures of childcare and schools meant that students with school-age children were also tasked with teaching them at home (Bacher-Hicks, Goodman & Mulhern, 2020). Financial and other hardships negatively affected the mental health of many students.

During the pandemic, social work schools were faced with tremendous challenges in supporting students and organising ongoing and effective field education opportunities that allowed students to graduate with social work degrees that met professional requirements. It is well recognised that the need to review and revise how field education is offered is long overdue. The pandemic gave higher education providers and professional bodies a push towards moving more quickly than previously envisaged to different models that allowed students to engage in practice and meet the requirements of their degree.

Innovative social work responses

Lessons learned from previous pandemics and other natural and human disasters provided clues to how social work would respond to this worldwide health emergency. As a discipline, social work has demonstrated its capacity to adapt quickly in significantly changed environmental and social conditions (Maher & Maidment, 2013). The ability of social workers to work effectively within ill-defined changing contexts, such as that presented by the global spread of the COVID-19, while at the same time sitting comfortably with uncertainty, are key attributes needed for contemporary practice environment (Hickson & Lehmann, 2014; Mason, 2011).

How professional social work bodies responded in Australia, the US and New Zealand

In response to the uncertainties caused by the COVID-19 pandemic, most professional social work bodies were flexible in how education standards could be met and made recommendations as to how accredited programs could exercise this flexibility to enable completion of social work placements. Some accrediting bodies, for example, the Australian Association of Social Workers (AASW) and the Council of Social Work Education (CSWE) in the United States, also allowed for flexibility in the minimum number of placement hours required to complete a social work degree. These concessions, although temporary, relieved pressure on students under duress and enabled many to fulfil placement requirements in difficult circumstances.

Another major adjustment was conditions required for work-based placements. Pre-COVID-19 conditions in Australia and the United States meant a student's placement and field education supervisor had to be different to that in their usual role and students were required to demonstrate that they were carrying out a social work student role different to their usual duties. This change allowed students to complete work-based placements with the same supervisor or to conduct both placements in their workplace. In New Zealand, students had previously been able to complete a placement in their usual role provided new learning could be demonstrated pre-pandemic. As a concession during the pandemic, students were able to complete both placements in their workplace.

Worldwide, the social work profession had not prepared for pandemic conditions, but the profession responded nimbly and swiftly to the changed environment. Social work programs across the United States, Australia and New Zealand shared resources and ideas on how to provide creative learning tasks while at the same time ensuring the integrity and rigour of programs. For example, National organisations such as the CSWE and the North American Network of Field Educators and Directors (NANFED) created repositories specific to field education during COVID-19 which was accessible to members.

Innovation in field education

The uncertain context created by the necessary efforts to control the pandemic – lockdowns and physical distancing – alongside diminished resources and risks to health affected practice while at the same time provided opportunities for transformative thinking and creativity to meet these challenges, especially in the field education space. Chappell Deckert and Koenig (2019) describe engaging with uncertainty as the in-between space between a perplexed state and transformation. In that space they insist that uncertainty must be recognised and honoured. Drawing on the core elements of the process described by Chappell Deckert and Koenig (2019, p. 164-165), Table 15.1 shows how these elements of perplexity linked to experiences in social work field education during the COVID-19 pandemic and provides a framework to understand the transformational process for students and social work schools.

TABLE 15.1 Perplexity and uncertainty and social work field education in the COVID-19 pandemic

5 essential elements of perplexity (Chappell Deckert & Koenig, 2019, pp. 164–165)	*Social work field education in the COVID-19 pandemic*
Exposure and immersion into an unfamiliar context	COVID-19 and public health measures – uncertainty linked to health and safety, lockdowns, campus closures, virtual learning – a different world
A critical perspective that examines privilege and power in collaborative relationships	Reflections on working in new ways with self and others; and on macro influences and how the macro impacts the micro
An experience of dissonance or discomfort	Anxiety and stress about life, health, family, work, study, and the future, plus new and unfamiliar modes of learning
Patience and persistence in not knowing	Acknowledging and honouring uncertainty – developing emotional self-regulation and purpose
Transformation of prior understandings by which growth and change occur	Innovation – new ways of thinking, adaptation, professional growth and new approaches

These were the exact conditions that field education academics, agency practitioners and students found themselves in as they grappled with new challenges and opportunities. In field education, responses were needed to support students and address their concerns, to ensure placements could progress albeit in modified and flexible forms, and to prepare educational solutions that would ensure student learning and skill development in different modes of practice and changed conditions.

Within the radically changed educational landscape of the pandemic, agencies and students still offering services, either from the office or from home, turned to tele-social work to assist clients (Reamer, 2020). Although not a new means of service delivery, the profession generally has been reluctant to fully engage with technological tools. Social workers and clients may lack the necessary skills and some clients may have limited access to technology. Social workers have also been concerned about ethical issues such as privacy and confidentiality (Banks et al,, 2020; Reamer, 2020). For example, having a family member within earshot is of particular concern in family violence or child abuse situations.

The announcement of shelter-in-place and the subsequent suspension of placements and changes to service delivery in California meant all in-person placements were suspended. Alongside the flexibility shown by the CSWE, field education academics at California State University Monterey Bay worked with agencies to provide alternative learning opportunities and assessment items that would enable students to meet competencies. Special attention was given to critically reflective learning that focused on the impact of the pandemic on social work and its practice, structural inequality and the skills and insights needed to manage uncertainty at personal and professional levels (Fronek et al. 2021b).

After the implementation of lockdown in New Zealand, placement experiences varied. Maintaining student safety was a key concern, as well as the safety in organisations, and of practitioners and other staff and clients. While some students were able to continue placement by working from home, other placements were immediately suspended. These different arrangements led to inequity across student cohorts which education providers and regulatory bodies sought to mitigate by instigating flexible arrangements (Zachary et al., 2020). Examples from Massey University and the University of Canterbury included developing virtual placements or projects, reducing the number of placement hours required each week or for the entire placement, and allowing students to be situated in more than one learning environment across the placement duration. Despite these measures, a level of inequity was unavoidable, further exacerbating uncertainty for some students.

To address the diversity of placement closures and non-closure placements at Griffith university, four placement combinations were developed ranging from full attendance at an agency, to mixed virtual learning and agency work to full project placements on topics directly related to the agency. Each were designed around the competency standards required (Fronek et al., 2021b). The rapid development of an online alternative placement course allowed students to practice and demonstrate the achievement of core competencies by participating in social work practice using simulated activities and other technological tools in a virtual learning environment. Experiential and simulated learning modules developed provided a safe and effective learning environment for those students unable to attend placement or worked from home. Course content consisted of a series of modules that contained specific topics based on real-life practice encounters. Experiential situations for teaching and learning purposes were created for students to work through in tutor facilitated discussion groups. Two days of weekly placement time were allocated to online interactions over ten weeks. This allowed time for students to undertake the activities in preparation for their virtual tutorial and to complete the simulated and experiential work, research, reading, and reflection. Following each virtual tutorial, the students' submitted their written material to their practice supervisors for discussion in supervision. On the other two days, the students either undertook projects related to their placement agencies or remote client work.

Emergent observations

The COVID-19 pandemic shone a spotlight on key issues such as developing student capacities for managing uncertainty, emotional self-regulation, ethical considerations and bringing fresh emphases on structural disadvantage. Adaptability and creativity in field education escalated issues already under professional scrutiny including what actually constitutes in-person practice in an age of virtual connectivity, the place of alternative placement models in contemporary higher education, and how virtual learning and tele-social work can be viable inclusions in higher education and practice, especially in relation to contemporary challenges in locating suitable placements, and this and future health emergencies.

Simulated learning in virtual environments has certain advantages over opportunistic learning as events can be scheduled, observed, and repeated to consolidate learning. A simulated learning environment also facilitates deliberate practice, enhances transfer of theoretical knowledge to the practice context, and does assist in making the transition from study into the workforce by achieving the required competencies. Social work education has always emphasised in-person learning. However, COVID-19 has changed many aspects of how the world functions and has fast-tracked innovation and the adaptation of technology on many levels. Given the stressors experienced by students in placement semesters and the fiscal position of corporate universities and many agencies, perhaps it is time to revisit the concept of *in-person* in environments increasingly dependent on technologies and to properly evaluate the effectiveness of alternative models.

Examples from Australia, the United States and New Zealand show how educating and supporting students to manage and respond appropriately to uncertainty and adapt quickly to new conditions in crisis situations are components of professional literacy and, indeed, transformational. Students in these examples were highly anxious when agencies first closed. With support, the self-regulation of emotion became a necessary skill as students experienced frustration, anger, worry, and fear, particularly for those students in the US where the pandemic spread exponentially with dire consequences. Student anxiety about their studies eased somewhat with support and when concrete alternatives to completing placements were in place.

Although many students continued to experience personal hardship during the pandemic and beyond, opportunities for students to identify and further develop practice skills in different ways became protective factors which strengthened their capacity to manage in the health emergency. It was helpful for students to carefully consider their own risk and protective factors in response to the evolving situation while being meaningfully engaged whether in continuing placements or educational alternatives. Because COVID-19 lockdowns caused considerable uncertainty and precipitated negative emotions in some people such as stress, boredom, frustration and anger, self-care and the concept of self-compassion as essential components of the social work curriculum became even more important (Pfefferbaum, 2020; Neff, 2003). This permission giving meant many students working from home were able to manage issues such as the blurred boundaries between work and homelife. Taking time to focus on activities that would enhance well-being facilitated boundary setting as they were not always *at-work* and provided the conditions to process the impact on self.

As Chappell, Deckert and Koenig (2019) suggested maintaining a critical perspective that examines privilege and power especially when experiencing dissonance or discomfort can be transformational. For students who are often primarily interested in interpersonal work, turning this lens onto the pandemic environment illuminated causal factors of social problems at the macro level, for example, access to technologies, health and wealth disparities and of racial injustices. Student reflections on these matters in alternative learning situations provided the space for them to delve more deeply into macro level practice and its relationship with micro practice in the amplified context in which students were living and studying (Walter-McCabe, 2020). In California, for example, macro practice became very real as students actively engaged in resource mapping, non-partisan voter registration drives pre-election, and disseminated information about financial and medical resources.

In terms of practice experience, engagement with different forms of service delivery provided opportunities for students in placements to strengthen the skills and attributes needed to respond with flexibility, quickly adapting to diverse digital methods for working with clients as well as undertaking different methods of learning (Zachary et al., 2020). While many students and academics extended their digital literacy skills, others remained challenged by accessibility issues. This was particularly so if the placement organisation did not provide appropriate technology, computers or internet connections (Groton & Spadola, 2020). Communication skills became critical as students needed to interpret and respond to organisational communications and advocate for their own needs and placement requirements.

The rapidly increasing use of tele-social work brings greater awareness of ethical considerations, the skills needed for technological-assisted counselling and other interventions, remote professional supervision, and their inclusion in social work curriculums. Even though many professional associations now provide guidance on technologically enhanced practice and communication and in codes of ethics, these practices are still making their way into curriculums and many social workers have uncomfortable relationships with technology (Banks et al., 2020; Fronek & Chester, 2016; Reamer 2020). A focus on technology invites further in-depth discussion around the particular ethical and boundary issues that come with online practices particularly when engaging with certain vulnerable groups.

Conclusion

The COVID-19 pandemic created new scenarios in higher education and opened avenues for research and evaluation that focuses on sudden transformative shifts, educational needs and future practices. Social work academics and students responded with flexibility and creativity drawing on experiences from prior disasters and health emergencies and acted quickly. Pandemic conditions brought existing debates into greater focus demanding a rethink on contemporary field education practices. A key issue remains in terms of harnessing the lessons learned from this pandemic and how social work professional bodies and higher education institutions should prepare for the next health emergency and the contribution social workers can make to high level preparedness planning with government and educational institutions, and collaborations with agencies in the field.

BOX 15.1

REFLECTIVE QUESTIONS

1. What is your experience of learning skills online?
2. What are some of the differences between tele-social work and working face-to-face?
3. Are there any ethical issues working remotely with clients who have;
    a. been subjected to family violence
    b. their computer in the family room
    c. few technological skills and limited access to technology
4. Are there personal challenges affecting you that you may need to negotiate when conducting tele-social work?

References

Afrouz, R., & Crisp, B. R. (2020). Online education in social work, effectiveness, benefits, and challenges: A scoping review. *Australian Social Work*, 1–13. https://doi.org/10.1080/0312407X.2020.1808030

Andersen, M. S., Bento, A. I., Basu, A., Marsicano, C., & Simon, K. (2020). College openings, mobility, and the incidence of COVID-19 cases. *medRxiv*. https://doi.org/10.1101/2020.09.22.20196048

Ayala, J., Drolet, J., Fulton, A., Hewson, J., Letkemann, L., ...Schweizer, E. (2018). Restructuring social work field education in 21st century Canada. *Canadian Social Work Review*, 35(2), 45–66.

Bacher-Hicks, A., Goodman, J., & Mulhern, C. (2020). *Inequality in household adaptation to schooling shocks: COVID-induced online learning engagement in real time (No. w27555)*. National Bureau of Economic Research. https://www.nber.org/papers/w27555

Baglow, L., & Gair, S. (2018). Australian social work students balancing study, work, and field placement: Seeing it like it is. *Australian Social Work*, 71(1), 46–57.

Banks, S., Tian C., de Jonge, E., Shears, J., Shum, M., ...Weinberg, M. (2020). Practising ethically during COVID-19: Social work challenges and responses. *International Social Work*, 63(5), 569–583.

Beddoe, L., Hay, K., Maidment, J., Ballantyne N., & Walker S. (2018). Readiness to practice social work in Aotearoa New Zealand: Perceptions of students and educators. *Social Work Education*, 37(8), 955–967.

Bilecen, B. (2020). Commentary: COVID-19 pandemic and higher education: International mobility and students' social protection. *International Migration*, 58(4), 263–266.

Blackwell, A. (2020, April 1). Placements closing, online lectures and uncertain futures: COVID-19's impact on social work students. *Community Care*. https://www.communitycare.co.uk/2020/04/01/failed-placements-online-lectures-uncertain-futures-covid-19s-impact-social-work-students/

Bogo, M., Lee, B., McKee, E., Ramjattan, R., & Baird, S. L. (2017). Bridging class and field: Field instructors' and liaisons' reactions to information about students' baseline performance derived from simulated interviews. *Journal of Social Work Education*, 5(4), 580–594.

Chappell Deckert, J., & Koenig, T. L. (2019). Social work perplexity: Dissonance, uncertainty, and growth in Kazakhstan. *Qualitative Social Work*, 18(2), 163–178.

Cheng, S.-Y., Wang, C. J., Shen, A. C.-T., & Chang, S.-C. (2020). How to safely reopen colleges and universities during COVID-19: Experiences from Taiwan. *Annals of Internal Medicine*. https://doi.org/10.7326/M20-2927

Craik, C. (2019). Social work education: Challenges and opportunities. *Australian Social Work*, 72(2), 129–132.

Cummings, S. M., Chaffin, K. M., & Cockerham, C. (2015). Comparative analysis of an online and a traditional MSW program: Educational outcomes. *Journal of Social Work Education*, 51(1), 109–120.

de Oliveira Araújo, F. J., de Lima, L. S. A., Cidade, P. I. M., Nobre, C. B., & Neto, M. L. R. (2020). Impact of SARS-CoV-2 and its reverberation in global higher education and mental health. *Psychiatry Research*, 288. https://doi.org/10.1016/j.psychres.2020.112977

Dewey, J. (1933). *How we think: A restatement of the relation of reflective thinking to the educative process*. Boston: DC Health.

Dewey, J. (1938). *Experience and education*. New York: Collier.

Domakin, A. (2019). Grading individual observations of practice in child welfare contexts: A new assessment approach in social work education. *Clinical Social Work Journal*, 47(1), 103–112.

Egan, R. (2005). Field education as a catalyst for community strengthening strategies: The time is right. *Advances in Social Work and Welfare Education*, 7(1), 35–41.

Fortune, A. E., Lee, M., & Cavazos, A. (2007). Does practice make perfect? *The Clinical Supervisor*, 26(1–2), 239–263.

Fronek, P., & Briggs, L. (2020). Demoralization in the wake of the COVID-19 pandemic: Where to the future for young Australians? *Qualitative Social Work*. https://doi.org/10.1177/1473325020973332

Fronek, P., Briggs, L., Liang, J., Gallagher, H., Doherty, A., Charles, B., & McDonald, S. (2021a). Australian social work academics respond to international students in crisis during COVID-19. *Frontiers in Education*, 6(51). https://doi.org/10.3389/feduc.2021.637583

Fronek, P., Briggs, L., Rondon-Jackson, R., Hay, K., Maidment, J., & Medina-Martinez, K. (2021b). Responding to COVID-19 in social work field education in Australia, New Zealand and the United States. *International Social Work*. https://doi.org/10.1177/00208728211048934

Fronek, P., & Chester, P. (2016). Moral outrage: Social workers in the third space. *Ethics and Social Welfare*, 10(2), 163–176.

Gallagher, H. L., Doherty, A. Z., & Obonyo, M. (2020). International student experiences in Queensland during COVID-19. *International Social Work*. https://doi.org/10.1177/0020872820949621

Groton, D. B., & Spadola, C. E. (2020). Variability, visuals, and interaction: Online learning recommendations from social work students. *Social Work Education*. https://doi.org/10.1080/02615479.2020.1806997

Harper, S. R. (2020). COVID-19 and the racial equity implications of reopening college and university campuses. *American Journal of Education*, 127(1). https://doi.org/10.1086/711095

Hay, K. (2018). 'There is competition': Facing the reality of field education in Aotearoa New Zealand. *Aotearoa New Zealand Social Work*, 30(2), 16–27.

Hickson, H., & Lehmann, J. (2014). Exploring social workers' experiences of working with bushfire-affected families. *Australian Social Work*, 67(2), 256–273.

Johnstone, E., Brough, M., Crane, P., Marston G., & Correa-Velez, I. (2016). Field placement and the impact of financial stress on social work and human service students. *Australian Social Work*, 69(4), 481–494.

Lee, J., Hernandez, P. M., & Marshall, I. (2019). Review of online education in social work programs. *Journal of Evidence-Based Social Work*, 16(6), 669–686.

Maidment, J. (2003), Developing trends in social work field education. *Women in Welfare Education*, (6).http://www.freepatentsonline.com/article/Women-in-WelfareEducation/199990329.html

Maher, P., & Maidment, J. (2013). Social work disaster emergency response within a hospital setting. *Aotearoa New Zealand Social Work*, 25(2), 69–77.

Malosh, R., & Masters, N. (2020, September 2). Campus outbreaks of COVID-19 were almost guaranteed. *The Conversation*. https://theconversation.com/campus-outbreaks-of-covid-19-were-almost-guaranteed-145235

Mason, R. (2011). Confronting uncertainty: Lessons from rural social work. *Australian Social Work*, 64(3), 377–394.

McAllister, C. (2013). A process evaluation of an online BSW program: Getting the student perspective. *Journal of Teaching in Social Work*, 33(4–5), 514–530.

McInnis, C., James, R., & Hartley, R. (2000). *Trends in the first year experience in Australian universities*. Melbourne, VIC: Centre for the Study of Higher Education, University of Melbourne.

Morley, C., & Dunstan, J. (2013). Critical reflection: A response to neoliberal challenges to field. *Social Work Education*, 32(2), 141–156.

National Student Clearinghouse Research Centre. (2020, November 12). *Monthly update on higher education enrolment*. https://nscresearchcenter.org/stay-informed/

Neff, K. (2003). Self-compassion: An alternative conceptualization of a healthy attitude toward oneself. *Self and Identity*, 2(2), 85–101.

Petra, M. M., Tripepi, S., & Guardiola, L. (2020). How many hours is enough? The effects of changes in field practicum hours on student preparedness of social work? *Field Educator*. https://fieldeducator.simmons.edu/wp-content/uploads/2020/05/20-235-1.pdf

Pfefferbaum, B. (2020). Mental health and the Covid-19 pandemic. *The New England Journal of Medicine*, 383, 510–512. https://doi: 10.1056/NEJMp2008017

QS Quacquarelli Symonds. (2020). *The impact of the coronavirus on global higher education*. https://www.qs.com/how-is-covid-19-shaping-the-higher-education-sector/

Reamer, F. C. (2020, April). Tele-social work in a COVID-19 world: An ethics primer. *Social Work Today*. https://www.socialworktoday.com/news/eoe_0420.shtml

Smith, M. K. (2001). John Dewey on education, community-building and change. *Infed Org*. Last updated April 4 2013. http://www.infed.org/thinkers/et-dewey.htm

Smoyer, A. B., O'Brien, K., & Rodriguez-Keyes, E. (2020). Lessons learned from COVID-19: Being known in online social work classrooms. *International Social Work*. https://doi.org/10.1177/0020872820940021

Tija, T., Marshman, I., Beard, J., & Baré, E. (2020). *Australian university workforce responses to COVID-19 pandemic: Reacting to a short-term crisis or planning for longer term challenges?* Melbourne, Australia: L. H. Martin Institute. https://melbourne-cshe.unimelb.edu.au/lh-martin-institute/fellow-voices/australian-university-workforce-responses-to-covid-19-pandemic

Wahler, E. A., Provence, M. A., Helling, J., & Williams, M. A. (2019). The changing role of libraries: How social workers can help. *Families in Society*, 101(1), 34–43.

Walter-McCabe, H. A. (2020). Coronavirus pandemic calls for an immediate social work response. *Social Work in Public Health*, 35(3), 69–72.

Wong, T. W., Gao, Y., & Tam, W. W. S. (2007). Anxiety among university students during the SARS epidemic in Hong Kong. *Stress and Health*, 23(1), 31–35.

Xu, J., Zheng, Y., Wang, M., Zhao, J., Zhan, Q., … Cheng, Y. (2011). Predictors of symptoms of post-traumatic stress in Chinese university students during the 2009 H1N1 influenza pandemic. *Medical Science Monitor*, 17(7), 60–64.

Zachary A., Morris, E. D., Peabody, C., & Carr, K. (2020). Isolation in the midst of a pandemic: Social work students rapidly respond to community and field work needs. *Social Work Education*, 39(6), 1127–1136.

PART III

Preparing for the future

16

SOCIAL INNOVATION AS THE NEED OF THE HOUR IN HEALTH EMERGENCIES

Gokul Mandayam, Samuel Ochieng,
Kelley Bunkers, Siân Long, Yoko Kobayashi
and Karen Smith Rotabi-Casares

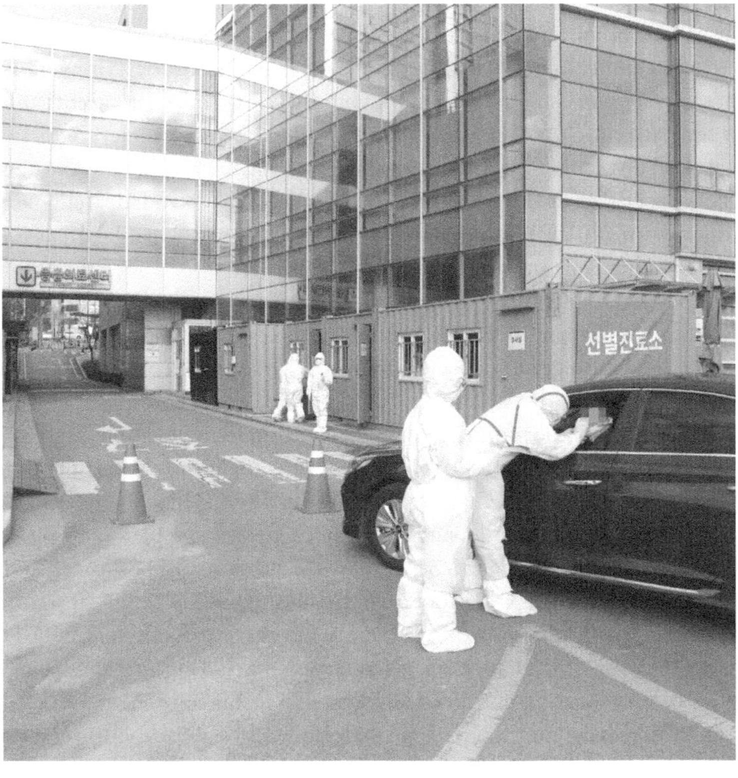

FIGURE 16.0 The first drive-through for mass testing in the world established on 23 February 2020, South Korea

Source: Photograph provided by Kyungpook National University Chilgok Hospital

DOI: 10.4324/9781003111214-19

The COVID-19 pandemic has resulted in a crisis of enormous proportions that has a multidimensional and long-lasting impact on global society. The consequences include increasing poverty levels in countries that already had a low GDP and were suffering multiple problems including high levels of hunger and illiteracy. The pandemic caused disruptions in food production processes, global, domestic and local food supply chains that resulted in huge numbers of people unable to access food (Farzad et al., 2020). This exacerbated health problems, security risks and tensions in many countries (World Bank, 2020). The pandemic also complicated access to educational resources for students globally as regular in-person school dynamics were replaced with online learning. In underdeveloped countries where access to Internet connectivity is a luxury, large swathes of students were excluded from access to education (Farzad et al., 2020). Apart from access to food and education, this pandemic has impacted on many other dimensions of human lives, including health, employment and safety. Creative, new ways of thinking were needed.

While there is still a lot to learn about the spread of the COVID-19 virus and its effective containment among other aspects and impacts of the disease, the incongruity between the successes and failures of different countries in arresting the spread of the virus and reducing deaths go beyond the epidemiological, medical or technical details (Acharya, 2020). Changes in lifestyle were imminent across the globe, and life was undoubtedly going to be different than it was before the pandemic. As COVID-19 continued to devastate society, existing traditional modalities of responding to human needs were unlikely to create a sustainable impact that ensured the well-being of society. Nandan, Bent-Goodley and Mandayam (2019) highlighted that a response to such *wicked problems*, in this case a worrisome and frustrating pandemic, called for a socially innovative approach. Given the inability of traditional approaches to fully address emerging and constantly changing needs and issues caused by the pandemic, the creation of solutions that integrated a social innovation framework in order to achieve sustainable impact is crucial.

Although there is no universal definition of social innovation, Berzin, Pitt-Catsouphes and Gaitan-Rossi (2015) delineate it as the creation and application of new solutions that are more efficient, highly effective and enjoy long-term sustainability as compared to existing solutions that address social problems. These authors identified four distinct themes of social innovation that are innovation and creativity, social entrepreneurship, collaborative partnerships, and the use of technology as exemplified in the following two case examples of India and Kenya. Social innovations from around the globe range from resource rich and high-end technological solutions to resource constrained and low-end technology solutions. Examples include the first drive through testing centre in South Korea, robots in Japan that allow graduating students to experience the graduation ceremony, and community organising in developed and developing countries to meet immediate need.

Such socially innovative approaches have the potential to tackle much of the fallout of this public health crisis efficiently and effectively as they spontaneously create multisectoral partnerships which rapidly bring together government, civil society, and the private sector to not only address pandemic related healthcare concerns, but also address other related societal needs for housing, education, employment, community, civic engagement and safety (Gegenhuber, 2020). The culmination of such an approach produces viable and useful technical and social solutions through the empowerment of stakeholders to take action, learn, and create alongside others.

Historically, global society has struggled to eliminate infectious diseases with country specific modalities of dealing with such diseases as well as strategies promoted by the World Health Organization (WHO). However, the discovery and global diffusion of robust, innovative, scientific solutions that benefit humanity such as the polio vaccine have had significant impact on global well-being. By 2000, 36 Western Pacific countries, including Australia, declared themselves to be polio-free. Europe followed soon after and today, polio is only found in a handful of countries. Dr Jonas Salk developed the first polio vaccine, changing the global landscape of polio disease. Salk's technique remains relevant today, for example, the Chinese COVID vaccine is based on Salk's technique which chemically inactivates the virus (Doherty, 2020). Salk's impact on science, health and society is wide ranging and cannot be underestimated.

It is notable and important that Dr Salk refused to sell or seek profit from his vaccine and instead made it available for free for the benefit of humanity. Medical and scientific innovation has advanced at a rapid pace during the COVID-19 pandemic in efforts to develop vaccines to prevent the disease and effective treatments to treat it. The speed and success of these efforts have relied on private and public cross-sector and expert multidisciplinary collaborations to bring about resultant innovations. Such collaborations have helped address previous struggles in terms of timely responses.

However, not all have followed Salk's example. Deals have been struck and richer countries are paying less than poorer countries. Some vaccine manufacturers are making enormous profits and controlling distribution, while others are charging cost of manufacture only. By mid-2021, the rich were able to purchase vaccinations in countries deprived of adequate supplies or travel to the US to be vaccinated. Over 100 countries supported the unprecedented move of suspending vaccine patents to allow local manufacture in response to the dire situation that developed in India. From the outset, China was manufacturing its own vaccine. Russia's Sputnik-V was released prior to the completion of clinical trials and at that time lacked testing rigour and therefore the safety record of the top contenders approved by January 2021 in richer countries were Oxford AstraZeneca, Moderna and Pfizer BioNTech among some others. Many countries took an emergency approach to vaccination given escalating numbers. In the face of vaccine nationalism, the WHO's COVAX Plan for equitable distribution between countries aimed to ensure the availability of a suite of vaccinations to poorer countries by combining buying power (WHO, 2021). Even these positive advancements highlighted inequities and disadvantages especially in vaccine distribution or, in other words, people's access to innovation. High-tech solutions (vaccine development) and low-tech solutions (local distribution in rural communities) and vice versa must work together.

Utilising a social innovation approach has proven useful in addressing multifaceted societal challenges as stakeholders representing varied sectors including governmental, business, non-governmental organisations (NGOs) and communities jointly examine the challenges through diverse viewpoints before arriving at a comprehensive solution. Cross-sectoral partnerships between government, private and nonprofit organisations can collectively enable the creation of solutions that exemplify the concepts of collective impact and shared value in order to solve complex problems caused by a public health crisis. This emphasises the connectivity that social innovation can bring at multiple levels in planning and response and the important role social workers can play in addressing issues of disadvantage and access. Two very different local and national innovations in India and Kenya that emerged during the pandemic are explored next.

The case of India

India provides a striking example of socially innovative strategies for dealing with the COVID-19 crisis. Although, the nationwide lockdown helped the country to initially arrest the spread of cases, most places in India continued the lockdown scenario in spurts thereafter. The government of India divided the geographic locations across the country into red, orange, and green zones based on the number of cases, with green being the minimum level of cases. The government began to ease restrictions in green zones, while requiring physical distancing to help economic recovery. This was based on the premise that over the course of time, more zones were likely to become COVID-19 free and likely to see a reduction in cases, which would enable people to return to leading a normal routine in daily life. However, the sudden lockdown was not without its failings as the government did not include mechanisms to address how people would cope and comply without access to employment and food during lockdown conditions. Nonetheless, social innovation sought to address these gaps and examples of social innovation should be noted.

Several socially and culturally relevant innovative strategies to address need and build healthcare infrastructure to achieve the goals of reducing mortality and spread of disease were adopted in the country. Strategies to address the problems caused by the pandemic ranged from low-tech interventions grounded in the Indian cultural ethos to high-end technology interventions. Although low-tech solutions may appear simple on the surface, they still require building new collaborations between peoples and sectors to achieve and put innovations into place in a timely way especially in highly bureaucratic societies.

To meet dire need, religious institutions from the Hindu, Sikh, Buddhist, Dawoodi Bohra Muslim and Christian communities volunteered locally to help with providing food, medicines, and temporary shelter to vulnerable communities in urban slum areas that were high contagion areas. (Livemint, 2020). The National Rural Livelihoods Mission (NRLM), a government partnership program, enabled women's self-help groups (SHGs) to produce facemasks and personal protection equipment for hospitals and medical outreach entities, running community kitchens, delivering essential food supplies, educating people about health and hygiene, as well as providing doorstep financial services to people in far-flung communities.

Children's education was abruptly interrupted. With school closures, non-profit organisations partnered with local communities in remote, rural areas with erratic electricity supply, poor telecom infrastructure and no Internet connectivity to provide basic education for children through the use of loudspeakers, radio and SMS text messaging services on non-smart cell phones.

A revival of the historic Indian way of greeting using the folded hand gesture of *Namaste* for welcoming people and the ritualistic ablutions of washing hands and taking a bath when coming from outside, in particular, after visiting the crematorium/burial ground, regained importance in daily life.

Other low-tech innovations included police officers and other officials in rural and smaller towns wearing the costume of Yamaraja, the Hindu god of death, to promote awareness about the dangers of the disease and to enforce the use of protective gear like masks and gloves. Indian Railways converted 20,000 passenger coaches into isolation wards that included key intensive care facilities such as ventilators, as well as bathrooms and other basic facilities to treat COVID-19 patients, to address hospital bed shortages when there was an overflow of patients needing such emergency medical attention. The Indian Government planned for converting hotels, stadiums and open public arenas into quarantine and hospital facilities in metropolitan areas like Mumbai and New Delhi, if needed to create more quarantine facilities and treatment centres.

Several technology intensive innovations were developed to tackle this public health crisis in a population close to 1.3 billion where poverty is rife and people's access to health resources is limited. *Prana-Vayu* (translating to breath of air), a low-cost ventilator, was developed by the Indian Institute of Technology (IIT) Roorkee, a premier technology institute in India. A portable ultraviolet sanitiser device used to sanitise currency notes and gadgets and chemical formulations for disinfecting public spaces were developed by Aqoza Technologies (Kumar, 2020).

The National Informatics Centre of the Indian government's Ministry of Electronics and Information Technology developed a mobile technology application called *Aarogya Setu* (translates to mean "bridge to liberation from the disease") that could be easily downloaded to telephones or any other personal electronic device to identify COVID-19 clusters so that medical services could be targeted to vulnerable communities and monitor the spread of the disease. In the slums of Dharavi in metropolitan Mumbai, the local police force deployed high tech drones that had built-in megaphones connected to the cell phones of police officers stationed near the slums who could dial in and make announcements to communicate with slum dwellers urging them to stay indoors, wear masks and wash their hands frequently.

Indian society experienced considerable psychological and external impacts such as loss of employment during the initial phase of COVID-19 (Varshney et al., 2020). This ushered a sense of urgency among policymakers to consider the psychological and behavioural responses of people while making pandemic-related policies. Furthermore, considering the most affected sections of Indian society – children, women and elderly populations – special counselling and other innovative ways of delivering mental health interventions such as tele-mental health were planned as outreach to these population groups to address the post-pandemic psychological impact and improve emotional well-being and mental health.

Several innovative approaches to address pandemic-related societal issues in the future were being deliberated by the Indian government by the end of 2020. These included simulation-based medical education with the periodic conduct of effective and continuous surveillance studies particularly in arenas where people dealt with animals or worked with viruses in research environments, and the integration of blockchain technology utilisation into healthcare. Aside from these, the government of India also planned to implement a systematic social and digital marketing effort to ensure the proper flow of healthcare information from central to state governments through to rural areas via the village governance structures, timely educational camps or pandemic awareness camps at the village level, and national-level and state-level pandemic exercises or drills. Policies related to internal as well as international migration in the post-COVID era such as online services and working from home as validated by social scientists were being deliberated by the Indian government to help with effective management of the disease and for preparedness for any future pandemic.

Today, there is an urgent need for collective global responsibility as only one individual's intentional or unintentional carelessness can increase the threat to many lives. Yet, beginning in 2020, when the world faced the COVID-19 pandemic, there was an overt focus between the scientific community with other sectors to rapidly develop solutions to address the pandemic, while at the same time, there seemed to be a severe lack in understanding the perceptions, behaviours and needs of individual citizens necessary to bring positive societal change. Advanced research on this aspect may assist with encouraging people to opt for adaptive behaviours in socially innovative ways which meet their needs and are crucial for controlling the severity of public health crisis situations. Towards this end, the Prime Minister's Citizen Assistance and Relief in Emergency Situations Fund (PM CARES Fund), a public charitable trust under the name of the Indian Prime Minister, was set up with the primary objective of being prepared to deal with any kind of future emergency and to provide relief to the affected. This fund also aimed to upgrade healthcare, pharmaceutical facilities and other necessary infrastructure along with funding relevant research and other types of support. As seen in this India example, the novelty of the Sars-CoV-2 virus and the pandemic it caused created unique challenges that underscored the need for socially innovative solutions and strategies to combat this public health crisis.

Next, we turn to Kenya to look closely at a very different innovation, the training of social workers and the social service workforce during the pandemic, with an emphasis on child protection as risks to children worsened in pandemic conditions.

The case of Kenya

As discussed in Chapter 2, Kenya confirmed its first COVID-19 case on 13 March 2020 (Aluga, 2020). The Government of Kenya took proactive action and ordered the closure of Kenya's international airports, introduced a nightly curfew, closed schools and recommended that those who could work from home do so. As the numbers of confirmed COVID-19 cases continued to grow, children were inevitably impacted. The disruption of the education system increased children's exposure to a host of abuses and to psychological impacts. Disruptions to families, friendships, daily routines, schooling and community engagement had negative consequences on children's well-being, development and protection (Odula, 2020; Simba et al., 2020).

Measures to prevent and control the spread of COVID-19 exposed children to protection risks (The Alliance for Child Protection in Humanitarian Action, 2020). Home-based quarantine and isolation measures, while critical to slow the spread of the virus, negatively impacted children and their families in different ways, including limitations around family visits to children in alternative care, court delays, and the rapid and hurried reunification of children in residential institutions with their families (Better Care Network et al., 2020; Goldman et al., 2020; The Alliance for Child Protection in Humanitarian Action, 2020; Wilke, Howard & Goldman, 2020). Children and families who were already living in overcrowded settings, otherwise socially or economically excluded, faced heightened protection and care risks. With schools closed and children at home, tensions within households rose, sometimes resulting in increased levels of harsh discipline and even violence, abuse or neglect against or witnessed by children. COVID-19-related impacts increased risks of child labour, teen pregnancy, and exploitation, documented in the press and increasingly evidenced in global research (Odula, 2020; Peterman & O'Donnell, 2020; World Vision International, 2020). The increased risks to children due to COVID-19 restrictions, posed new challenges for child protection workers in Kenya. While acknowledging the risks that the pandemic brought to children, families and communities, it was important to balance these with concerted efforts to recognise, build upon and leverage the inherent strengths and resilience of children, families and communities.

The response

Recognizing the need for those working with vulnerable children to stay informed about increased risks and reduced safeguards that can and do occur during an emergency, a WhatsApp group for a multiagency COVID-19 response team was formed by Government Children's Officers to share information and ideas to support and protect children and families. As practitioners were unable to report to an office for work, anecdotal stories from the field included workers meeting in *open air offices* to address child protection issues. In response, the Department of Children's Services (DCS) acted so that professionals mandated with child protection responsibilities within the DCS, Charitable Children's Institutions and Statutory Children's Institutions, Probation Hostels, Social Development Officers and Child Protection volunteers could access knowledge and develop the skills necessary to keep children and families safe and respond to child protection issues exacerbated by the requirements in place to manage the pandemic.

Kenya had been investing in strengthening the social service workforce for child protection before the onset of COVID-19. In 2019, the DCS and the Kenya School of Government with the technical support from UNICEF and Maestral International developed a standardised child protection training course for child protection professionals. In December 2019, the first training was implemented at the Kenya School of Government with the intention of further scaling out the professional training through Master Trainers. The training for the second cohort of trainers took place during the pandemic in December 2020 which required new approaches to training and support.

DCS and UNICEF, together with Maestral International, were proactive in designing and delivering a series of 12 webinars that provided child protection practitioners with critical knowledge, information and skills related to child protection practice through the lens of COVID-19. Webinars were delivered in one-hour sessions on Zoom and had two main objectives. Webinars provided up-to-date information on COVID-19 prevention, response and psychosocial support, information about child protection prevention, and response activities relevant to the situation faced by children and families in Kenya in the context of COVID-19. A second objective of the webinars was to facilitate the exchange of experiences and provide a virtual community of practice where child protection professionals could discuss, share, and identify gaps, challenges, practical solutions and action plans in responding to COVID-19 and to debrief about related child protection concerns. These discussions aimed to provide important engagement and online supportive connections with colleagues, which is an important part of self-care.

Each webinar included an average of 447 participants. Five group sessions of the same content were delivered twice weekly, with an average of 89 participants in each session. Two presenters were present for each session. One managed content and the other managed the platform, including the chat function, questions and technology. Given problems with connectivity and lack of familiarity with the virtual platform, challenges with technology did occur and some *Zoom fatigue* was noted towards the end of the 12 sessions. It became clear to facilitators after the first webinar, that participants were eager to connect with colleagues and catch up on work or other topics. To meet this need, an additional 15 minutes was added at the end of each session for a virtual tea break. The facilitators left the webinar open but did not participate nor listen. Anonymous evaluations were provided after each webinar as well as a final evaluation. County Coordinators were of the view that this was the best virtual training they had participated in and that their minds opened to new technical expertise that they needed in response to the pandemic and to where their expertise was most required.

To further extend the core information to communities in which the webinar participants worked, Maestral International drafted a series of 16 short information messages, to be delivered through the Viamo platform direct to the phones of Child Protection volunteers, Chiefs, and other community leaders such as Community Health Workers, religious leaders and Nyumba Kumi (informal community policing) leaders. Through the Viamo platform, an audio script could be sent to ordinary phones. This platform was selected by UNICEF and the DCS in consideration of the level of education of the target audience and limited access to equipment such as smart phones and computers. Internet connectivity would often be an issue.

Each three-minute script was drafted in simple English (to be delivered in English or Kiswahili), introducing the topic and why it was important, describing two to three key messages about the issue, and then ending with a simple quiz that involved answering a Yes/No question on the phone keypad and receiving the response providing the correct answer. The 16 topics focused on the role of community-based actors in sharing information about COVID-19, raising awareness and giving guidance about referrals for child protection and family violence risks, especially for children with disabilities and other vulnerable children, practical guidance on parenting and online safety, stressing the importance of family-based care and prevention of separation and placement into residential care, and including components on mental health and practical tips for managing stress.

Key learnings for policy, programming or workforce response development

One of the key lessons learned from the virtual training, as a social innovation, was the importance of collaboration, planning and coordination for its success. Participation and inclusion in the planning stage and selection of the webinar topics was important to ensure the relevance of topics and a sense of ownership among participants.

Communication from one central place was a key. The DCS established a support team from its headquarters and county level staff provided leadership and support to ensure the smooth running of training and break-out sessions. A database of all participants was developed to ensure a systematic distribution of invitation with zoom links and presentations from the national level. The webinars were successful in mainstreaming the *build back better* concept to ensure the relevance of learning beyond the pandemic. After the first six webinar sessions, all participants were asked to complete action points based on the learning, including a timeline, methods and outputs. These action points were submitted to respective supervisors – County Children's Coordinators – to ensure consolidation at sub-national level. A coordinated approach to action planning at county level was key in making action points more accountable.

Two key challenges were encountered during the webinar series. First, there was a risk that some participants might not fully participate due to multi-tasking during virtual training. This was mitigated by the frequent use of chat box and break-out sessions, as ways to promote continued engagement in the training. Participants were grouped by geographical locations to allow a certain level of monitoring by supervisors. Other challenges related to the fact that officers and most participants were working from home and therefore limited equipment, data bundles and connectivity had to be addressed before the start of the training. UNICEF provided support for airtime of participating officers.

Virtual training is feasible and will continue to be an important learning platform, especially for a professional cadre who has access to the internet and technologies such as computers and smartphones. Since the 12 webinars, which were the first virtual training on child protection for DCS officers, participants have become much more comfortable with virtual learning platforms. Subsequent online trainings have been implemented and have run much more smoothly based on the experiences and learning from the webinar series.

What could be useful in future is to develop a blended or hybrid model which combines the benefits and strength of both virtual and in-person platforms, based on their comparative advantages. Virtual training enables savings in financial and time resources and can reach a much greater number of participants at one time. If the recording of virtual training is made available, it would further increase the reach of the training. At the same time, the advantages of in-person training cannot be dismissed. In-person training offers experiential learning where participants learn by completing activities such as role plays, a mode of delivery more familiar to participants and therefore more comfortable. Human connections and networking which contributed to developing a community of practice are usually created and continued more easily through in-person training. It may, therefore, be useful to explore a blended model where feasible post-pandemic.

Learning from the successful delivery of a series of 12 webinars in Kenya, the Ministry of Gender, Labour and Social Development in Uganda has partnered with UNICEF Uganda to implement a virtual training programme for the child protection workforce, including social service workforce, justice actors, and health providers and counsellors. Adaptions have been made to develop and implement a Training of Trainers designed for key government officials with content and participation decided by a taskforce led by the Ministry of Gender, Labour and Social Development. The Ministry worked closely with the COVID-19 Response Sub-Committee on Gender Based Violence and Violence Against Children to ensure the virtual training programme was coordinated and informed by an overall COVID-19 response.

Conclusion

The social work profession mandates moral and ethical obligations to safeguard the most vulnerable and disenfranchised in society, and therefore deploying timely interventions in the fight against the COVID-19 pandemic and be better prepared for future health emergencies are important to fulfilling these obligations. Social workers are increasingly required to innovate in the midst of complex societal challenges such as health emergencies while adhering to professional values, ethics and commitment towards social justice. Research in social work has underscored the importance of interdisciplinary and cross-sector collaborations, a key feature of social innovation, that enable the creation and implementation of innovative models of practice capable of addressing complex social problems and to ensure more sustainable positive social change (Flynn, 2017).

Social innovations, especially in resource poor environments, are therefore essential in responses to public health emergencies like the COVID-19 pandemic. Some innovations are simple adaptations, while others are more sophisticated and technical with emerging technologies as key. A variety of innovations in two very different contexts with local and national innovations in India and a close look at a national project on the ground in Kenya have been presented. These examples are offered to stimulate thinking on social innovation as responses to human problems in challenging conditions, the key features of which are interdisciplinarity, cross-sectoral and merging the technological and social as essential elements of responses to pandemics and other health emergencies.

Acknowledgement

The authors would like to recognise the leadership and support of the Department of Children's Services (DCS) and UNICEF Kenya. Their continuous support of and belief in the importance of preparing the workforce to address the unique child protection risks resulting from COVID-19 have been crucial to the success of this effort. Our particular gratitude goes to the DCS – Noah Sanganyi, Judy Ndungu, Jecinta Murgor, Jane Muyanga, Marygoretti Mogaka, Maurice Tsuma and Carren Ogoti, and UNICEF – Monika Nylund-Sandvik, Bernard Njue Kiura, Catherine Kimotho, and Haithar Ahmed.

BOX 16.1

REFLECTIVE QUESTIONS

- Why is it important for social workers to understand the importance of social innovation, and to engage in disruptive thinking for the purpose of creating sustainable interventions to address the impact of health emergencies?
- How do we encourage social service organisations across the world to embrace a culture of creative problem-solving and to engage in interdisciplinary practice to better prepare for future health emergencies?
- What were some of the innovations that were undertaken in your community to address quality of life and prevention of the consequences of health emergencies and what features were necessary to develop and action these innovations?
- What is the significance of diversity and culture in developing innovative solutions to help communities grapple with health emergencies?

References

Aluga, M.A. (2020). Coronavirus disease 2019 (COVID-19) in Kenya: Preparedness, response and transmissibility. *Journal of Microbiology, Immunology, and Infection*, 53(5), 671–673.

Acharya, K. (2020, August 20). How to see what the world is teaching us about COVID-19. *Stanford Social Innovation Review*. https://ssir.org/articles/entry/how_to_see_what_the_world_is_teaching_us_about_covid_19#

Berzin, S. C., Pitt-Catsouphes, M., & Gaitan-Rossi, P. (2015). Defining our own future: Human service leaders on social innovation. *Human Service Organizations: Leadership & Governance*, 39(5), 412–425.

Better Care Network, UNICEF, Save the Children, & Alliance for Child Protection in Humanitarian Action. (2020). *Guidance for alternative care provision during COVID-19*. https://www.cpaor.net/sites/default/files/2020-10/Guidance%20for%20alternative%20care%20COVID-19.pdf

Doherty, P. (2020, December 21). Local versus systemic, vaccine versus virus. *Setting it Straight, (38)*. Doherty Institute, The University of Melbourne. https://www.doherty.edu.au/news-events/setting-it-straight/local-versus-systemic-vaccine-versus-virus

Farzad, F. S., Salamzadeh, Y., Amran, A. B., & Hafezalkotob, A. (2020). Social innovation: Towards a better life after COVID-19 crisis: What to concentrate on. *Journal of Entrepreneurship, Business and Economics*, 8(1), 89–120.

Flynn, M. L. (2017). Science, innovation, and social work: Clash or convergence? *Research on Social Work Practice*, 27(2), 123–128.

Gegenhuber, T. (2020, April 29). Countering coronavirus with open social innovation. *Stanford Social Innovation Review*. https://ssir.org/articles/entry/countering_coronavirus_with_open_social_innovation

Goldman, P., van Ijzendoorn, M., Sonuga-Barke, E., & on behalf of the Lancet Institutional Care Reform Commission Group. (2020). The implications of COVID-19 for the care of children living in residential institutions. *The Lancet*. https://doi.org/10.1016/S2352-4642(20)30130-9

Kumar, D. (2020, June 6). Beyond India's coronavirus unlock 1.0: An age of innovation. *Financial Express*. https://www.financialexpress.com/opinion/beyond-indias-coronavirus-unlock-1-0-an-age-of-innovation/1982951/

Livemint. (2020, April 16). Humanity over hate: Religious organizations help out with COVID-19 relief. https://www.livemint.com/mint-lounge/business-of-life/humanity-over-hate-religious-organizations-help-out-with-covid-19-relief-11587041257785.html

Nandan, M., Bent-Goodley, T., & Mandayam, G. (Eds.). (2019). *Social entrepreneurship, intrapreneurship, and social value creation: Relevance for contemporary social work practice*. Washington DC: NASW Press.

Odula, T. (October 20, 2020). From 'role models' to sex workers: Kenya's child labor rises. *AP News*. https://apnews.com/article/virus-outbreak-africa-united-nations-kenya-nairobi-4c0fa9421409d2a8e79045ba896f4db7

Peterman, A., & O'Donnell, M. (2020, September). *COVID-19 and violence against women and children: A second research round up*. Centre for Global Development. https://www.cgdev.org/sites/default/files/covid-19-and-violence-against-women-and-children-second-research-round.pdf

Simba, J., Sinha, I., Mburugu, P., Agweyu, A., Emadau, C., Akech, S., Kithuci, R., Oyiengo, L., & English, M. (2020). Is the effect of COVID-19 on children underestimated in low- and middle-income countries? *ACTA Paediactrica*, 109(10), 1930–1931.

The Alliance for Child Protection in Humanitarian Action. (2020, May). *Technical note: Protection of children during the coronavirus pandemic, Version 2*. https://alliancecpha.org/en/system/tdf/library/attachments/the_alliance_covid_19_tn_version_2_05.27.20_final_2.pdf?file=1&type=node&id=37184

Varshney, M., Parel, J. T., Raizada, N., & Sarin, S. K. (2020). Initial psychological impact of COVID-19 and its correlates in Indian community: An online (FEEL-COVID) survey. *PLoS ONE*, 15(5), e0233874. https://doi.org/10.1371/journal.pone.0233874

Wilke, N. G., Howard, A. H., & Goldman, P. (2020). Rapid return of children in residential care to family as a result of COVID-19: Scope, challenges and recommendations. *Child Abuse & Neglect*, 110 (Part 2). https://doi.org/10.1016/j.chiabu.2020.104712

World Bank. (2020, March 24). *Food security and COVID-19*. https://www.worldbank.org/en/topic/agriculture/brief/food-security-and-covid-19

World Health Organization. (2021). COVAX: Working for global equity access to COVID-19 vaccines. https://www.who.int/initiatives/act-accelerator/covax

WorldVision International. (2020). *COVID-19 aftershocks: Access denied teenage pregnancy threatens to block a million girls across Sub-Saharan Africa from returning to school*. https://www.wvi.org/sites/default/files/2020-08/Covid19%20Aftershocks_Access%20Denied_small.pdf

17

PREPARING FOR THE NEXT HEALTH EMERGENCY

Patricia Fronek and Karen Smith Rotabi-Casares

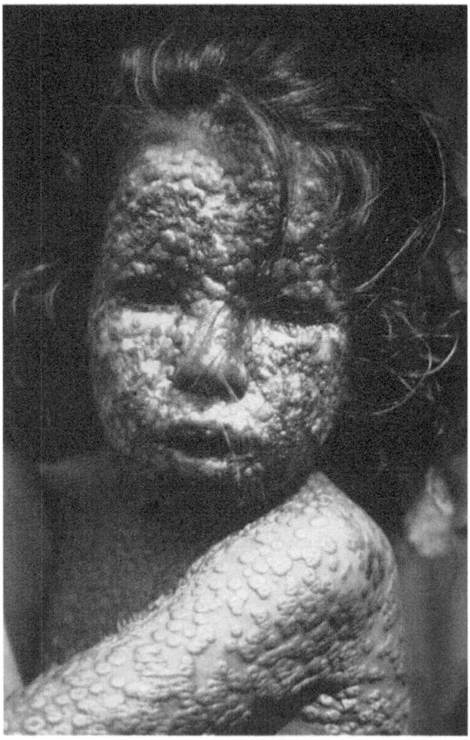

FIGURE 17.0 A child with smallpox in Bangladesh in 1975. Smallpox is the only human disease now eradicated

Source: CDC Public Health Image Library (ID #3266)

DOI: 10.4324/9781003111214-20

Scientists knew a global pandemic was coming but many governments failed to take the warnings seriously enough and the already vulnerable suffered most. As discussed in the bonus chapter with Dr Alan Franklin, the state of the planet is directly linked to the emergence of new diseases. Providing misinformation on climate change is an issue that has been falsely presented in right-wing media as providing a balanced debate when the science is actually very clear. COVID-19 will not be the last novel virus, nor will the next pandemic be 100 years away. In the past 100 years alone, we have seen SARS, MERS, H1N1 and HIV/AIDS alongside dangerous epidemics and outbreaks such as Ebola and Bubonic Plague, and of course seasonal influenza which has seen the lowest rates of infection ever recorded during the COVID-19 pandemic due to mask-wearing and other measures. For some years, the World Health Organization's (WHO's) *Pandemic Influenza Preparedness Plan* has offered guidance to members to prepare national plans and to harmonise national and international plans. In 2020, the *2019 Novel C (2019-nCoV): Strategic Preparedness and Response Plan* was published providing public health measures to support the international community in relation to COVID-19 with regular updates thereafter (WHO, 2020). Plans focus on those measures essential to containing a disease.

Among other documents, *Guidance for All-of-Society Pandemic Readiness* (WHO, 2009) provided guidance at all levels of operation – readiness, response and recovery at local, national, regional and global levels – especially across critical interdependencies such as providers of essential services being equipped with what they need to do their jobs. This guidance went beyond critical healthcare necessitating the importance of issues such as access to food, water, transportation and other issues affecting the well-being of people with particular attention to refugees, migrants, people with disabilities, prisoners and other vulnerable groups, as well as crucial psychosocial support for workers. These attentions were neglected in many countries during the COVID-19 response, and these are the very issues which provide critical junctures with social work practice across multiple fields. Social work is in a unique position to intervene at micro, mezzo and macro levels to address the social determinants of health that are amplified in health emergencies.

In November 2020, The Global Preparedness Monitoring Board (GPMB) published a report that stressed the urgency of global prevention, preparedness and response for the next pandemic as well as learning from the failures highlighted during COVID-19, especially with regards to national, political leadership. The report highlights the link to climate devastation, ongoing inequalities and how those inequalities were exploited during COVID-19, as "there is no health security without social security" for everyone (GPMB, 2020, p. 3).

Preparedness planning

Social workers everywhere responded to human need during COVID-19. Yet, few countries included social work in national or local planning or even consulted with social work professional bodies about the needs of communities, overlooking crucial expertise in readiness, response and recovery. Social workers were responsive to human need in all world regions throughout the pandemic, see Chapter 2. For example, social workers were actively involved in national planning as well as on the ground in Lebanon and throughout Africa in primary, secondary and tertiary roles (Agwu & Okoye, 2021). The WHO guidance specifically highlighted the need for collaboration with civil society and community-based organisations.

Social work is uniquely placed due to intimate practice experience in the daily lives of people and in the organisations that provide services, to forecast practical and psychosocial issues in communities – strengths, risks and vulnerabilities, the complex and often unintended consequences of certain actions, and in identifying where resources will be most needed and to whom they should be distributed. For example, in its simplest form, people must eat. Therefore, a failure to provide food and distribution paths during lockdown to people who must work to eat will invariably mean lockdowns will be breached, and disease will spread in communities. The needs of older people living alone or in institutions, people living in overcrowded and resource-depleted conditions, people with mental illness or disabilities were sorely neglected in many countries during COVID-19. The needs of the vulnerable must be planned for such as in family violence and child protection service delivery to name a few from the many examples explored in this book. Social work in community organising and disaster practice holds knowledge of how communities rally to support each other, their resilience and self-reliance in tragic times, and the supports communities request to strengthen and heal themselves.

Social planning and how to respond is a missing element in many country responses because social work is generally absent from the interdisciplinary planning table. It is our view that social work should have a place at that table, at global, national and local levels. As the co-chairs of GPMB, H. E. Gro Harlem Brundtland and Elhadj As Sy, said "learning without action is pointless" (GPMB, 2020, p. 4). As well as preparing the profession and ourselves, this view poses a significant challenge for the profession in lobbying for inclusion, especially at global and national levels, Pandemic preparedness and response also requires global agreement and commitment to action in social work. The Inclusion of leadership goals and global agreement related to health emergencies in the developing framework for the Global Agenda for Social Work and Social Development 2020–2030 to be further discussed in October 2021, would be an important step (IAASW, ICSW & IFSW, 2020).

Preparing ourselves

Social workers and the profession must also prepare themselves for the larger picture as well as individually. There are gaps in knowledge and preparing for the future highlights a greater need for scientific literacy and including public health social work in professional development and in social work program curriculums. On an individual level, social workers need to understand self-protections, how to protect their client groups and how to stem the spread of a multitude of diseases that negatively affect the health of children, adults and communities. Historically, this knowledge is often designated to social workers working in health or community sectors. However, this pandemic has taught us that all sectors and fields of practice are interconnected with health and affected in health emergencies.

There is another and perhaps more controversial issue that is often left unaddressed in social work. The profession legitimately embraces multiple perspectives and lived experiences in the body of knowledge. However, we often fail to address anti-vax sentiment and, currently, mask-wearing resistance in the ranks of the profession, rare though it may be. Other perspectives such as racism and sexism are rejected as they oppose the profession's value base. Neglecting what needs to be done during COVID-19 does do harm to others which in our view outweighs any tensions with other values. Scientific knowledge comes with certain facts about disease and prevention. Vaccination is part of this story. Conspiracy theories, misinformation and anti-vax sentiments are no longer acceptable in today's world, and we must address these where they exist in our own ranks while acknowledging medical exceptions. Vaccine hesitancy is different. People may be hesitant for a number of reasons which can be addressed by trustworthy and accurate information.

Social work must grapple with ethical dilemmas such as self-determination versus do no harm. Our ethical and value base and even definitions of social work are clear about our obligations to community well-being rather the rampant individualism displayed in many parts of the world today. An ethical decision-making process can grapple with tensions between self-determination, individual rights and human dignity, respect for life and commitments to all people, locally and globally. Although many people may experience little adverse effects from COVID-19, it can certainly kill others or leave them with chronic illness, and future variants could prove to be more contagious and more virulent. For social work, this should indicate a clear position. See Figure 17.1 for a record of some vaccinations Patricia Fronek has received over time.

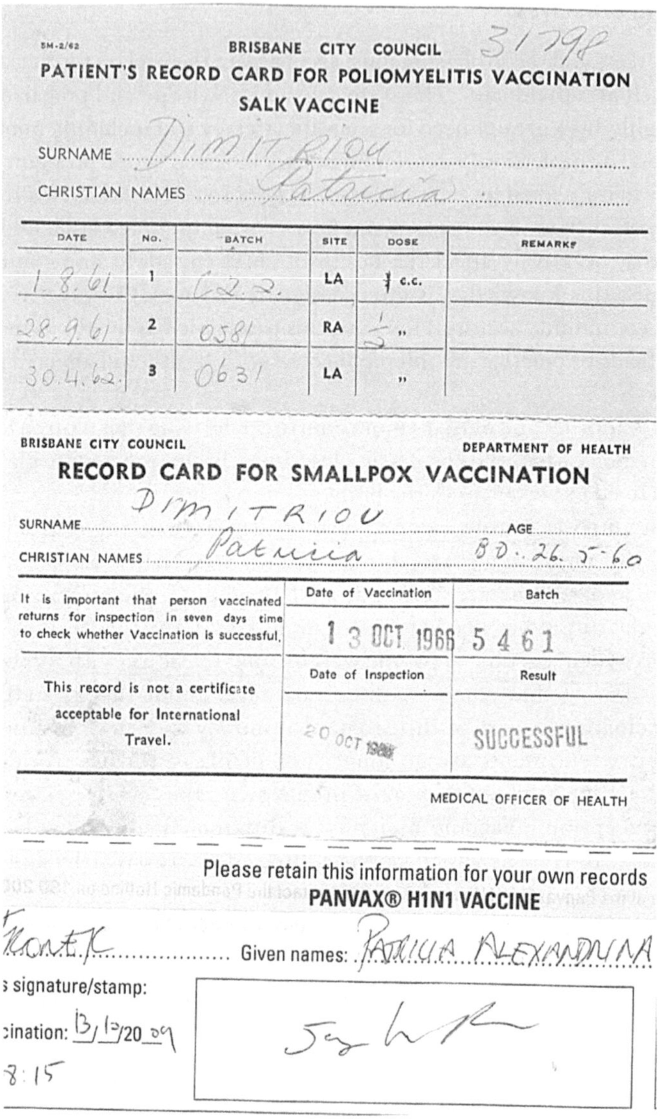

SM-2/62 BRISBANE CITY COUNCIL 31798

PATIENT'S RECORD CARD FOR POLIOMYELITIS VACCINATION

SALK VACCINE

SURNAME Dimitriou

CHRISTIAN NAMES Patricia

DATE	No.	BATCH	SITE	DOSE	REMARKS
1.8.61	1	C2.2.	LA	½ c.c.	
28.9.61	2	0581	RA	½ "	
30.4.62.	3	0631	LA	"	

BRISBANE CITY COUNCIL DEPARTMENT OF HEALTH

RECORD CARD FOR SMALLPOX VACCINATION

SURNAME DIMITRIOU AGE

CHRISTIAN NAMES Patricia BD. 26.5.60

It is important that person vaccinated returns for inspection in seven days time to check whether Vaccination is successful.	Date of Vaccination	Batch
	13 OCT 1966	5461
This record is not a certificate acceptable for International Travel.	Date of Inspection	Result
	20 OCT 1966	SUCCESSFUL

MEDICAL OFFICER OF HEALTH

Please retain this information for your own records

PANVAX® H1N1 VACCINE

Fronek .... Given names: Patricia Alexandra

s signature/stamp:

cination: 13/10/2009

8:15

FIGURE 17.1 Some of Patricia Fronek's vaccinations – against polio, smallpox and H1N1. The editors have had their COVID-19 vaccinations

There are several levels of preparedness planning including: participation in global, national and local interdisciplinary forums; planning and action by professional bodies including driving social work agenda forward; addressing issues of practitioner safety and status during emergencies; preparation of the social work workforce; identifying best practices in fields of practice during health emergencies, particularly lessons learned; and inclusion in social work education. Key questions important in planning are:

- Do we understand the sociopolitical environment and how a health emergency might be managed?
- Have we critically examined past experiences and learnt key lessons?
- Who are the vulnerable in the community and what are their needs in an emergency?
- Have the community and specific vulnerable groups been included in planning?
- Are there any cultural and diversity issues that should be considered?
- How can we continue to deliver services and what training do we need to undertake, offer, and how often?
- Will there be new vulnerabilities created in this emergency?
- What can go wrong and how likely is that risk?
- What are the consequences of possible adverse outcomes and what do we need to do to address them?
- How can we ensure adequate human, material, technological and knowledge resources and with whom do we need to partner to do so?
- Are plans prepared and tailored to specific fields of practice?
- What support might we need in the aftermath for client groups and social workers?
- How might we position ourselves at all planning tables?
- What research has been conducted and how do we disseminate and leverage social work research?

The risks are that memory fades once the crisis is over and when risk seems abstract to individuals or communities, preparedness falls to the wayside (GPMB, 2020). If not directly experienced or seems long ago or far away, the sense of urgency lessens and behaviours are shaped accordingly. Indigenous knowledge offers a lot here, understood through traditional story-telling that keeps cumulative knowledge alive over many, many generations, for example, the prevention and management of bushfires in Australia. Also, as with all disaster training there must be practise exercises and ongoing training. New Zealand and Japan, prone to earthquakes conduct population-wide disaster preparedness training including in schools. Workplaces have fire drills even when there are no fires. Yet, we forget about infectious disease when it abates. It will be especially challenging for social work to maintain attention on health emergencies in those countries that emerged relatively well from the pandemic or experience fewer outbreaks of disease.

Social work as an essential service

As discussed in Chapter 2, the Lebanese Social Workers Syndicate was involved in national planning and response instigating a wide range of prevention and interventions strategies in a resource poor environment. Social workers in many places adapted to new roles such as US social workers undertaking contact tracing roles (Singh, 2020). The flexibility of social work and the profession's capacity to adapt to new roles and changed conditions was discussed in the chapter on hospital social work, social work adaptations in Spain, France, Italy, Romania, Latin America, and many in other regions, as well as the many examples of moving to online service provision.

Social work has a strong and long history in supporting communities in disaster recovery and are often among the first responders in disasters (Harms et al., 2018; Harms et al., 2020; Manning et al., 2007; Plummer et al., 2008: Rowlands, 2013). Pandemic planning and responding share features with other disasters such as the acquired impact of trauma and loss of life, the extended psychosocial and economic aftermath, and the disproportionate impact on the disenfranchised and vulnerable. However, health emergencies, particularly global pandemics, have some key differences. Taking COVID-19 as the example, these relate primarily to five aspects:

- The crisis is extended with little confirmation about when, how and if, it would end combined with the recurring cycle of subsequent waves of infection.
- The social isolation that comes with necessary public health measures such as lockdown and quarantine impede community connectedness and survival capacities that arise in communities in other disasters, especially when communities move in and out of lockdowns and other measures.
- The nature of global emergencies means countries, regions and communities are more reliant on their own resources as neighbouring and allied countries, also affected, are in a lesser position to offer aid, and health and other systems can become overwhelmed for extended periods of time.
- The co-occurrence of natural and other disasters with the pandemic multiplies ill effects and lessens capacities for shorter recoveries.
- The contemporary sociopolitical environment characterised by global inequalities, hypercapitalism, the prioritisation of global economies over lives in many instances, the resurgence of far-right and maverick politics, media monopolies, and the proliferation of conspiracy theories and other populist discourse – aspects that worsened during the COVID-19 pandemic and also occurred historically. Although these issues are present in other kinds of disasters, the status quo is more affected in extended global or wide-spread health emergencies such as COVID-19 due to ongoing economic disruptions and discontent.

These factors suggest that existing disaster planning in social work needs revision to include and address these differences as well as developing strategies to address concurrent disasters such as the hurricanes and fires that occurred during the COVID-19 pandemic. These key differences challenge every layer of the ecological model presented in Chapter 1, disrupting the usual relationships within systems. These disruptions create a marked divergence from how people expect life to be. On top of risks to health and life, people are dramatically affected in different ways depending on privilege or disadvantage as identified in previous chapters which, in turn, affect both positive and negative behaviours.

Hobfoll and colleagues (2007) posed five essential elements of responding to immediate and mid-term trauma events. These are to promote safety, calming, a sense of self and collective efficacy, connectedness and hope. When considering these aspects and how social work responded to COVID-19, these aspects were present and core to many interventions. In terms of safety, there was an information vacuum in the initial stages of the COVID-19 pandemic in many countries and in many cases contradictory and confusing information. The WHO can also be critiqued regarding safety. Instead of erring on the side of caution, precautionary measure such as recommending mask-wearing only eventuated as evidence emerged. A difficult decision at the time and easy to critique in hindsight. However, in future perhaps caution should be exercised immediately as research evidence takes time and might be better served to inform the easing of restrictions.

Social workers and professional bodies took to social media, listservs, websites, blogs and other platforms taking the lead in disseminating information about experiences, safety and social work practices in COVID environments. One example from Spain was the toll-free hotline established to provide social workers with information and emotional support discussed in Chapter 2. Another example was the "Social Workers Helping Each Other" initiative offering personal and professional support to social workers in Italy, a country also impacted badly by COVID-19 (Cabiati, 2021). In July 2020, the Australian Association of Social Workers (AASW) published on the role of social workers in the COVID-19 pandemic (AASW, 2020). Many associations, for example, the AASW, the British Association of Social Workers (BASW) and the National Association of Social Workers (NASW) in the US, provided updates and resources during the pandemic. In other examples, information about end-of-life care, on-line interventions, cancer treatment and family violence were shared.

Calming and self-efficacy, particularly in relation to resilience and coping featured in interpersonal work, while building community support and communities rallying for mutual support featured in many country reports. Engendering hope, even in the midst of loss and bereavement, is one of the many important aspects of helping people manage the enduring nature of pandemics, their psychological responses such as anger or fear, and to counter adverse behavioural responses such as refusal to comply with health measures such as mask-wearing, which should be differentiated from breaking curfews or lockdowns to earn money to provide for families in the absence of adequate safety nets. Truthful and accurate information is important to managing anxiety, and emotional and psychological distress related to the unknown.

During MERS, it was reported that rumours and false information heightened community fears and anxieties (Sim, 2016). The same happened in India during the Bubonic plague in the late 1800s as described by Matthew Ward in Chapter 3. Social isolation and discrimination worsen the impact, and so how social workers address these issues during today's pandemics requires creativity and innovation in developing informal or formal communities of support. When it comes to hope, people generally adapt to adversity and when their goals are thwarted, most people tend to readjust and set new achievable goals within their resources to maintain hope for future outcomes (Snyder, 1994). Shared agency in communities and the mutual support it provides, strongly supports adjustment (and survival) in difficult circumstances even when organised differently such as connecting online. Specific interventions such as Psychological First Aid are useful for concurrent disasters and acute distress; however, at this stage, little is known about its application during a prolonged health emergency (Everly, Barnett & Links, 2012; Saltzman, Hansel & Bordnick, 2020). As well as supporting strengths, coping and resilience, other approaches such as demoralisation in the COVID-19 context should be further explored (Briggs & Fronek, 2019, 2020).

All these factors are important in building trust, an essential goal in transformative leadership during health emergencies.

Social work leadership

The profession will go through a process of evaluating responses to COVID-19 which will be reconsidered, contextualised and revised with the flexibility inherent in the profession. Evaluating what worked well, what didn't and identifying gaps will lead the profession into the future.

Social work leadership is particularly important in this endeavour "given the economic and political influences on how services in health and welfare are actually delivered . . . especially in increasingly market-driven and politicised environments", issues that COVID-19 has laid bare (Fronek, Fowler & Clark, 2011, p. 36). Jonathan Dicken's "Dimensions of State Responses" in Chapter 1 provides a framework to analyse sociopolitical environments and their relationship to health emergency response and its impact that can underscore leveraging activities.

Leadership is an attribute required for all social workers, not just those in particular organisational positions. It's simply about a mental shift that the ability to inspire and empower is part of the social work skill set and not delegated to positional power alone. Leadership drives agenda forward within the profession, interprofessionally and in leveraging governments.

Adapted from a piece by Wilson's (2020) article in the Conversation, Figure 17.2 outlines key leadership practices for planning and response which are framed by the values and principles of the profession to build trust in the expertise and contribution of social work. Four columns are depicted – led by evidence, leverage influence, mobilise collective influence, and support coping – each of which guides social work leadership in health emergencies. The first column highlights the need for scientific literacy and evidence-informed practice relevant to scientific knowledge in addition to best practices in social work. Developing public health social work in health emergencies as a new field of practice requires leadership by professional bodies, universities, practitioners and educators to recognise its importance and its inclusion in all fields of practice and to develop best practices based on critical reviews of unique experiences during COVID-19 and other pandemics. Although the resources to manage its consequences differed, COVID-19 affected everyone regardless of nationality, social status or wealth. Leveraging influence and interprofessional working is a challenging and important aspect of leadership and one where the profession is well versed.

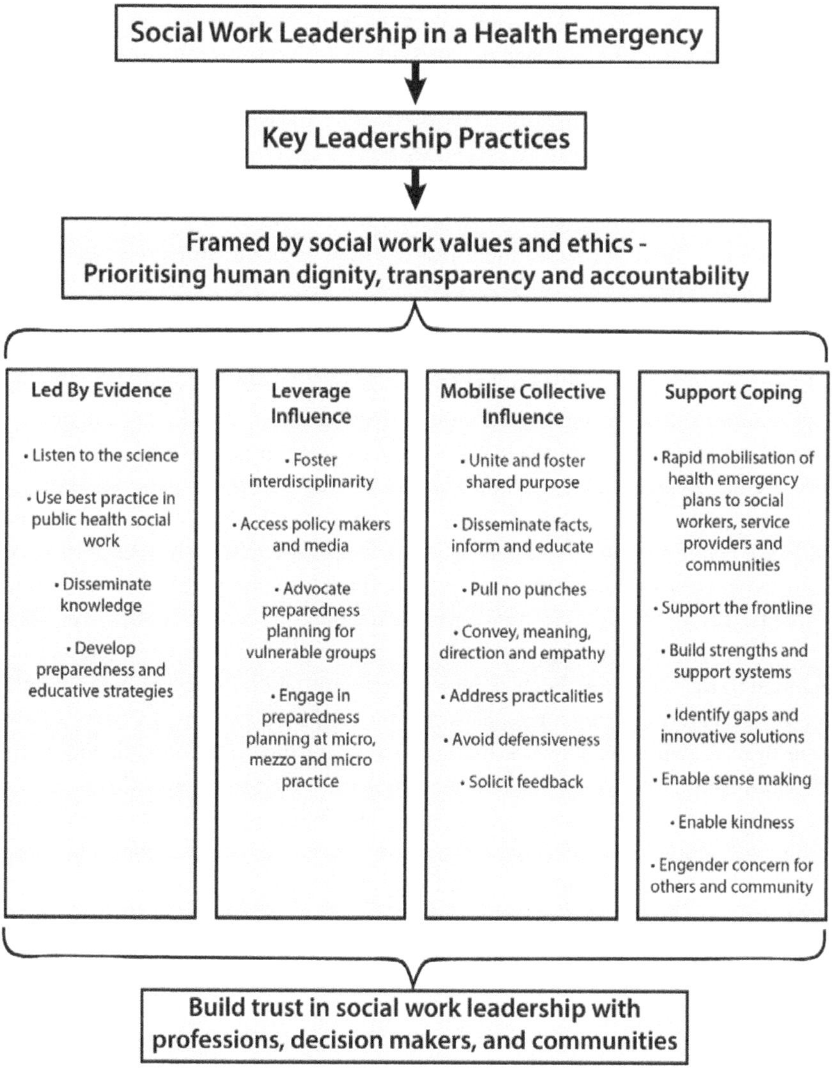

Social Work Leadership in a Health Emergency
Key Leadership Practices
Framed by social work values and ethics - Prioritising human dignity, transparency and accountability
Led By Evidence
• Listen to the science
• Use best practice in public health social work
• Disseminate knowledge
• Develop preparedness and educative strategies
Leverage Influence
• Foster interdisciplinarity
• Access policy makers and media
• Advocate preparedness planning for vulnerable groups
• Engage in preparedness planning at micro, mezzo and micro practice
Mobilise Collective Influence
• Unite and foster shared purpose
• Disseminate facts, inform and educate
• Pull no punches
• Convey, meaning, direction and empathy
• Address practicalities
• Avoid defensiveness
• Solicit feedback
Support Coping
• Rapid mobilisation of health emergency plans to social workers, service providers and communities
• Support the frontline
• Build strengths and support systems
• Identify gaps and innovative solutions
• Enable sense making
• Enable kindness
• Engender concern for others and community
Build trust in social work leadership with professions, decision makers, and communities

Adapted from Wilson, S. (2020, October 23). The reward for good pandemic leadership: Lessons from Jacinda Ardern's New Zealand re-election. The Conversation. https://theconversation.com/the-reward-for-good-pandemic-leadership-lessons-from-jacinda-arderns-new-zealand-reelection-148515

FIGURE 17.2 Social work in a health emergency

The obvious challenge on which to exert influence is the recognition of social work as an essential service where practitioners and students work on the frontline with people directly affected by disease and are exposed to considerable personal risk at the same time. Although social workers have always been well aware of being frontline workers and with many examples of such in the preceding chapters, many governments have failed to recognise this reality, often holding outdated perceptions of social work as charity workers (Healy, 2008;

Walter-McCabe, 2020). Alongside the expansion of neoliberalism, how social work is perceived seems to have declined in recent years in some in some places. For example, one of the editors worked in hospitals during SARS in 2003 and H1N1 in 2009. At that time, social workers were considered frontline and valued members of response teams. All social workers were properly fitted and supplied with masks. In 2020, anecdotal stories emerged that some hospital social workers, even those in emergency departments, were advised mask-wearing was not needed while medical practitioners around them wore the protective equipment needed. In other settings, social workers were given the same consideration as other practitioners and so the picture was mixed. It is not unfair to say in community settings and in many countries, social workers were not provided with what they needed to do their jobs. However, social workers, whether in hospitals, communities or other settings must be recognised, valued and provided the resources to protect themselves, their families and the people with whom they work. Challenges are more profound in those countries with sparse resources.

It is crucial for social work to secure its place at interdisciplinary global, national and local planning tables (as well as in micro, mezzo and macro levels of practice) to share expertise about vulnerabilities, needs and responses for people who have more limited access to resources to weather pandemics and recover from them. We have unique expertise to contribute and improve preparedness and response internal and external to the profession. Such activities also require skills in media engagement as social workers are far from representative in the media especially in discussions about their fields of expertise. These skills are generally missing in social work education.

Mobilising community influence centres on how to engage others, build a shared vision and managing resistance. These leads us to the communication skills and strategies needed to address misinformation or the *infodemic* which commonly occurs in health crises and have done so throughout history whether they were attributed to the gods, a curse or a group of people (WHO, 2018, p. 26). There are many theories relating to misinformation and false beliefs linked to disorders, low level thinking, religiosity or political leanings. One recent study of 660 people in the US, found a more complex and mixed picture (Agly & Xiao, 2020). A key finding was that trust in science and scientists lowered the likelihood of a person accepting misinformation which has implications for planning in terms of addressing misinformation in others whether that be with policymakers, colleagues, in higher education or in practice with client groups. This also means that social workers need to stay abreast of the science and looming risks, for example, accessing trusted websites such as the Global Outbreak Alert and Response Network (GOARN) https://extranet.who.int/goarn/

The final column addresses, issues in practice and the delivery of services, including health promotion and community education, building community and supporting coping rather than a focus on individual deficit. While not ignoring the needs of the particularly vulnerable and access to services, human beings with the right support and interventions are on most occasions able to draw on their own personal resources and do cope even in pandemic conditions. However, when psychosocial and material supports are not there, people do suffer unnecessarily. Mental health can deteriorate when influences are external and outside loci of control and interventions are not properly geared towards need. Natural leaders do emerge in communities as we saw in Chapter 14 in the new social service and Chapter 15 where natural leadership emerged in the community of international students.

Planning for the next pandemic should feature as one of the most significant challenges of this century as consequences for individuals intersects with other social work concerns such as poverty, the climate emergency, inequality, racism and discrimination, and social justice and human rights. Social work must be prepared for the next health emergency, whenever and wherever it next appears.

BOX 17.1

GROUP DISCUSSION

In small groups

- Unpack and discuss what issues social workers and professional bodies need to consider in preparedness planning.
- What do we need to do, individually and collectively, to prepare for the next health emergency?
- Consider how influence can be leveraged and what strategies could be utilised?
- How might you address misinformation?

References

AASW. (2020, July 24). *The role of social workers during the COVID-19 pandemic.* https://www.aasw.asn.au/news-media/2020-2/the-role-of-social-workers-during-the-covid-19-pandemic

Agly, J., & Xiao, Y. (2020). Existence of differential belief profiles of COVID-19 narratives: The role of trust in science. *Research Square.* https://doi.org/10.21203/rs.3.rs-35919/v1

Agwu, P., & Okoye, U. (2021). Social work and COVID-19: A gap in Nigeria's intervention. *International Social Work.* https://doi.org/10.1177/0020872820980799

Briggs, L., & Fronek, P. (2019). Incorporating demoralization into social work practice. *Social Work*, 64(2), 157–164.

Briggs, L., & Fronek, P. (2020). Demoralization in the wake of the COVID-19 pandemic: Whereto the future for young Australians? *Qualitative Social Work.* https://doi.org/10.1177/1473325020973332

Cabiati, E. (2021). Social workers helping each other during the COVID-19 pandemic: Online mutual support groups. *International Social Work.* https://doi.org/10.1177/0020872820975447

Everly, G. S., Barnett, D. J., & Links, J. M. (2012). The Johns Hopkins model of psychological first aid (RAPIDPFA): Curriculum development and content validation. *International Journal of Emergency Mental Health*, 14(2), 95–103.

Fronek, P., Fowler, J., & Clark, J. (2011). Reflecting on reflection, leadership and social work: Social work students ass developing leaders. *Advances in Social Work and Welfare Education*, 13(1), 35–49.

GPMB. (2020). *A world in disorder. Annual Report 2020. Licence: CC BY-NC-SA 3.0 IGO.* Geneva: Global Preparedness Monitoring Board, World Health Organization. https://apps.who.int/gpmb/annual_report.html

Harms, L., Abotomey, R., Rose, D., Woodward Kron, R., Bolt, B., Waycott, J., & Alexander, M. (2018). Postdisaster posttraumatic growth: Positive transformations following the Black Saturday bushfires. *Australian Social Work*, *71*(4), 417–429.

Harms, L., Boddy, J., Hickey, L., Hay, K., Alexander, M., Briggs, L., . . . Hazeleger, T. (2020). Post-disaster social work research: A scoping review of the evidence for practice. *International Social Work*. https://doi.org/10.1177/0020872820904135

Healy, L. M. (2008). Exploring the history of social work as a human rights profession. *International Social Work*, 51(6), 735–748.

Hobfoll, S. E., Watson, P., Bell, C. C., Bryant, R. A., Brymer, M. J., Friedman, M. J., . . . Ursano, R. J. (2007). Five essential elements of immediate and mid-term mass trauma intervention: empirical evidence. *Psychiatry*, 70(4), 283–369

IAASW, ICSW, & IFSW. (2020). Press release – Global agenda for social work and social development [Press release]. https://www.iassw-aiets.org/wp-content/uploads/2021/01/GlobalAgenda-Press-Release-.pdf

Manning, C., Millar, S., Newton, T., & Webb, S. (2007). After the wave – The Centrelink social work response offshore. *Journal of Social Work in Disability & Rehabilitation*, 5(3–4), 81–95

Plummer, C. A., Ai, A. L., Lemieux, C. M., Richardson, R., Dey, S., Taylor, P., . . . Kim, H.-J. (2008). Volunteerism among social work students during hurricanes Katrina and Rita. *Journal of Social Service Research*, 34(3), 55–71.

Rowlands, A. (2013). Disaster recovery management in Australia and the contribution of social work. *Journal of Social Work in Disability & Rehabilitation*, 12(1–2), 19–38.

Saltzman, L. Y., Hansel, T. C., & Bordnick, P. S. (2020). Loneliness, isolation, and social support factors in post-COVID-19 mental health. *Psychological Trauma: Theory, Research, Practice, and Policy*, 12(S1), S55–S57.

Sim, M. (2016). Psychological trauma of Middle East Respiratory Syndrome victims and bereaved families. *Epidemiol Health*, 38. https://doi.org/10.4178/epih.e2016054

Singh, M. (2020, May 1). San Francisco recruits army of social workers, librarians and investigators to track Covid-19. *The Guardian*. https://www.theguardian.com/us-news/2020/may/01/san-francisco-contact-tracing-coronavirus-california

Snyder, C. R. (1994). *You can get there from here: The psychology of hope*. New York: The Free Press.

Walter-McCabe, H. A. (2020). Coronavirus pandemic calls for an immediate social work response. *Social Work in Public Health*, *35*(3), 69–72

Wilson, S. (2020, October 23). The reward for good pandemic leadership: Lessons from Jacinda Ardern's New Zealand reelection. *The Conversation*. https://theconversation.com/the-reward-for-good-pandemic-leadership-lessons-from-jacinda-arderns-new-zealand-reelection-148515

WHO. (2009). *Whole-of-society pandemic readiness: Who guidelines for pandemic preparedness and response in the non-health sector*. Geneva. https://www.who.int/influenza/preparedness/pandemic/2009-0808_wos_pandemic_readiness_final.pdf?ua=1

WHO. (2018). *Managing epidemics: Key facts about major deadly diseases*. Geneva: World Health Organization. https://apps.who.int/iris/handle/10665/272442

WHO. (2020). *2019 Novel coronavirus (2019-nCoV): Strategic preparedness and response plan*. https://www.who.int/publications/i/item/strategic-preparedness-and-response-plan-for-the-new-coronavirus

18

YESTERDAY, TODAY AND TOMORROW

Patricia Fronek and Karen Smith Rotabi-Casares

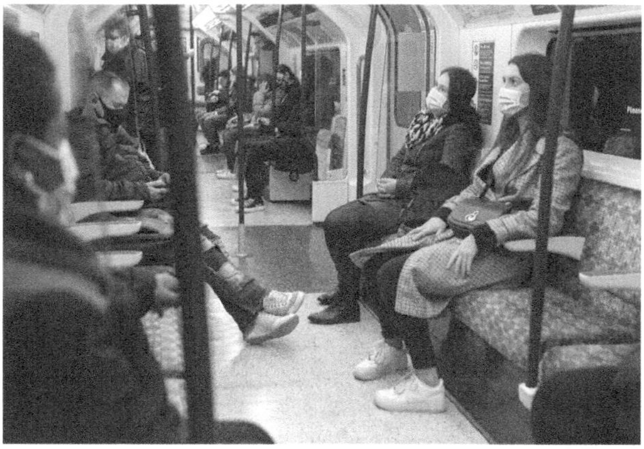

FIGURE 18.0 Living the new normal

Source: Photograph by TheOtherKev

DOI: 10.4324/9781003111214-21

As we conclude this book in mid-2021, the COVID-19 pandemic is far from over and the more infectious Delta variant (B.1.617.2) is dominating, found in 111 countries. The worst-affected countries by the end of June 2021 are the US, India, and Brazil. Globally, over 180,000,000 confirmed cases and almost four million deaths are recorded but likely to be significantly under-estimated (Johns Hopkins Resource Center). Indonesia along with other countries is experiencing escalating numbers worsening the disaster already experienced. One person in ten is left with Long COVID, the chronic conditions that remain (European Observatory on Health Systems and Policies, 2021). Europe, Asia, Oceania, Africa and the Americas remain at risk of more waves of illness. In Europe alone, nine out of ten new infections are predicted to be from the Delta variant by the end of August 2021 (ECDPC, 2021). Although variants are known by a number, they were for a long time called by the country where the virus was first detected. Referring to variants in this way, for example, Trump's *China virus*, incited violence and discrimination against groups of people, therefore variants are now commonly known by the Greek alphabet, for example, Alpha (UK), Beta (South Africa), Gamma (Brazil) and so on (Feil, 2021). Let us hope we don't get to Omega.

People everywhere are expected to adapt to living with this ever-changing virus in what has been called *the new normal*, a term coined long before there was any clarity about what this new normal would actually look like. Working from home is expected to continue in many industries, and new tools such as COVID passports to verify vaccination status are likely to be required into the future. Elimination is no longer possible, and goals to suppress have been dismissed by many governments in a largely unvaccinated world. Tragically, the release of a report by the Independent Panel for Pandemic Preparedness and Response in May 2021 confirmed that the pandemic could have been prevented if world leaders had listened to the science and acted early in the interests of health (The Independent Panel, 2021). The World Health Organization (WHO) predicted that the impact of the pandemic would be worse in 2021, not better, a forecast proving to be correct.

Our analysis identified the successful formula for early containment of SARS-CoV-2 included each of the following mandated actions – immediate, hard lockdowns with the provision of practical support to sustain the population (food and housing), extensive tracing and testing, safe quarantine, physical distancing and hygiene measures – predicated on heeding the science and followed later by the rapid rollout of vaccinations once available. Missing one of these measures at the pandemic's onset led to the unnecessary further spread of the virus, second and third waves, new variants and repeated lockdowns which sorely tested populations creating the environment to abandon elimination and suppression. Virologist, Ian Mackay, applied the Swiss Cheese model, a well-known model of risk management, to COVID-19 explaining how a virus can escape through multiple holes or flaws in the system (Mackay, 2020).

Herd immunity and sufficient vaccination rates in particular have not been reached globally. India is reporting record daily deaths of over 4,000 people, many of whom did not need to die but were faced with few available hospital beds, oxygen and other treatments. Argentina introduced urgent lockdown measures for the first time in response to recording 35,000 cases a day. Indonesia is experiencing yet another wave, worse than the last. The richest US suburbs had quick access to vaccination, while the story was very different for African Americans, Latino and Hispanic populations and other people of colour. People around the world are struggling to breathe and the disease can no longer be kept at bay across Asia and Africa where cases are doubling every three weeks. With the exception of South Africa, Africa's spread was always mooted to be a slow burn and has indeed proved to be so but has ultimately been unable to escape the pandemic. Everywhere the poor remain at highest risk. Unvaccinated populations, vaccine nationalism (countries hoarding vaccines for their population only) and a commitment of some vaccine manufacturers to excessive profit over distribution has ensured new variants, and denial politics continue to override health, dignity and community concerns in many countries.

Children becoming vectors of community transmission have become of more concern with the rise of new variants. In Israel, for example, 85% of the adult population has been vaccinated, and the majority of new cases are under 16 years of age (Mallapaty, 2021). Younger people are now receiving the vaccine. As we noted in Chapter 1, children have always been able to spread the virus but were more likely to be asymptomatic. Concerns remain that children will carry the burden of disease into the future (Mallapaty, 2021).

What is certain is that societal impacts and future changes will necessitate new responses, adaptations and innovations from the social work profession which build on the practice responses and knowledge developed during the pandemic. This brings us to social work in health emergencies and practices that span across theoretical approaches, fields of social work practice and interdisciplinary collaborations.

Public health social work

Public health social work is a relatively new field of practice. As proposed in this book, this field of practice continues to be shaped by the social determinants of health and responses to infectious and other diseases, fitting snugly into the wider transdisciplinary field of public health. Gauffin and Dunlavy (2021, p. 131) define the transdisciplinary nature of public health as the "integration of approaches and the creation of new conceptual frameworks, hypotheses and research strategies", opportunities presented by the COVID-19 pandemic. Conceptually, social work has a dual focus on practice informed by theory and research and the development of theory and knowledge derived from practice, and, as a practice, responds to its environment. Rapid social work responses to human need during COVID-19 thus far have laid the groundwork for new theoretical explanations, research agendas and practice initiatives. Public health social work connects traditional fields of social work practice by rejecting artificial silos. Health cannot be separated from other fields if one considers the social determinants of health and health emergencies. Public health social work also connects practice with other disciplinary knowledges found in health promotion, epidemiology, medicine, and biological and environmental sciences which are explored further in the two bonus chapters.

Social work knowledge has expanded since December 2019 providing opportunities to reflect on what has passed and the path forward for the profession and the people we serve, and to consider the next pandemic. The COVID-19 pandemic has taught us much, or at least reminded us, about how humans behave, and the dangers of segregating human dignity and community responsibility from policy, politics and health strategies. From the beginnings of the social work profession, the impact of inequalities on health including the social, political and ecological factors that play out at a macro level are core to social work's knowledge base. People previously in vulnerable social circumstances suffered more during this and historical pandemics, for example, people living in institutions of all types, people on the move, and those living in poverty. Vulnerable families and those previously at risk of violence and abuse became more vulnerable. Children were at greater risk of all forms of abuse and exploitation and having their rights breached from lack of safety to loss of identity when, for example, parents die or when children are born in a refugee camp without a birth certificate as Justin Lee and Carmen Monico highlighted in Chapter 11.

There was no doubt there would be winners and losers from the start. In our journey through fields of practice, it was evident that older people were considered more disposable based on age, frailty and perceived quality of life. People with disabilities were oft ignored and others such as the poor and victims of all forms of abuse were placed in intractable positions. From the start, social workers everywhere acted to mitigate the crisis, responding to immediate need while navigating drastically changed conditions to support individuals and communities, even at personal risk to themselves and their families. As we read in Section 2, all fields of practice were affected, and although all people were equally affected by disease, inequality and inequities affected access to vaccines, treatment and capacities to isolate safely.

As documented in this book, social workers continue to respond to the needs of communities supporting hope, innovation and strengths with the resources available to them. The chapter on the new social service, where social workers are indelibly embedded in their communities stressed the importance of mobilising communities, and when supported, communities create their own innovative solutions. In all our chapters, social workers recognised the importance of understanding a person in their ecological context and building on strengths and coping capacities. As in other emergency situations, communities do rally together and support each other in antithesis to increased civil conflicts, scapegoating, the politicisation of health, and widening inequalities in health and wealth experienced during COVID-19, also issues documented in pandemic history (Drury, 2018). Most of the world breathed a sigh of relief when Trump lost the

US election, aghast but not entirely surprised when his followers were incited to a lethal infiltration of Congress, and watched as Trump faced his second impeachment, a historical event. Civil unrest made news in the US, throughout Europe, Africa and Asia. The Far Right and white supremacy rallies were held but these groups were reported to also lose political ground. As we read in Matthew Ward's chapter on the history of pandemics, much of our COVID-19 experience has happened before – misinformation, unhelpful behaviours, greed, conflict and civil unrest alongside adaptation, innovation and community strengthening. The need for additional roles especially in the macro social work sphere and in pandemic preparedness and planning have become apparent, especially related to addressing the devastating socioeconomic consequences and social injustices that were, in our view, predictable, and accentuated during the COVID-19 pandemic.

In those areas that had access to technology, working virtually proved to be a significant learning curve for many social workers whether that be in education or service delivery across all fields. Although educating future social workers and delivering social work services remotely poses challenges, a greater focus on technology's utility in serving hard-to-reach populations is required beyond the current health emergency, including how remote practice fits with the future of work. As Pink, Ferguson and Kelly (2021) also highlight such a shift may be as inevitable as it is necessary. An adaptive and reflexive hybrid model of in-person and digital social work has been proposed in child protection practice (Ferguson, Kelly & Pink, 2021), but as we have read in Chapter 6 on child protection in Botswana, the digital divide, access to technology and the skills to confidently use technology cannot be assumed. However, as Chapter 16 on innovation identified, there are many emerging and promising practices that rely on technology for problem solving including digital learning strategies that are relevant to social workers around the world and necessary to engage in public health social work. Technology also presents opportunities to assess novel approaches in higher education as explored in Chapter 15.

Politics and leadership

Political discourse and media reporting have glossed over the substantial holes in social protections left by decades of neoliberalism, hypercapitalism, individualism and consumerism in liberal or neoliberal capitalist economies that are influential on the world stage. Over time inequalities have increased between the disadvantaged and the wealthy in these countries as social protections have decreased or remain underdeveloped. Decades of erosive and divisive ideologies ensured the world fell victim to the perfect storm of *pandemic, politics* and the *planet*. Countries that prioritised economies in the first six months of the pandemic tended to accept greater risks to their population's health and later, opening borders too soon.

Low- and middle-income countries that relied mainly on tourism were in difficult positions as food security became a greater issue for the population. It is clear that countries whether rich or poor needed to take measures to ensure all citizens and non-citizens could eat and be housed when lockdowns are imposed. Decisions and human behaviour at extreme ends of a continuum were shaped by either survival in contexts of poverty and desperation or strong senses of individualism and entitlement, both resulting in further spread of disease. As discussed in Chapter 1, historical analysis and analysis conducted during COVID-19 indicates that prioritising of health is ultimately better for economies which then make better and swifter recoveries. The wait-and-see approaches adopted by some governments served to escalate the emergency to a global pandemic. Few leaders with a softer approach to health measures such as lockdowns or vaccine distribution shifted from their original position even in the face of exponential spread of disease.

The actions of political leaders and the ideologies that informed those actions have probably been the most important influences on how this pandemic impacted humanity. Abbasi (2021) wrote a powerful commentary on *social murder* committed by political leaders who wilfully ignored health advice, the social determinants of health and premeditated the acceptability of lives cut short for the sake of political expediency and economic gain which resulted in millions of global deaths. The concept of social murder, first coined by Engels, refers to the structural advantage the privileged have over the poor. It was older people and people with disabilities who were neglected around the world. As Tarek Zidan highlighted in Chapter 9, families of people with learning disabilities in the UK received "do not resuscitate letters", a concerning state of affairs with a decidedly eugenics flavour. Abbasi (2021) called for accountability and redress for social murder committed during COVID-19 and the role institutions such as the media had in truth telling and critiques.

Alarmingly by mid-2021, political and business discourse especially in industries such as airline travel, tourism and sport, had turned without conscience, to urging the public to make decisions about the number of deaths relatively unvaccinated countries such as Australia would find acceptable for the sake of economic stimulus. Boris Johnson took the lead by experimenting with people's lives by planning to cease all restrictions in July in the face of only two thirds of adults being fully vaccinated and rising numbers of cases infected with the Delta virus. This move has been tagged as the *Big Gamble*, particularly disturbing for the world given the inequities and failures of vaccination distribution, the risk of developing more variants in the UK, unvaccinated children and the global number of deaths, especially in those groups discriminated against or considered expendable. Time will tell if this and other gambles have been *successful* and the cost in lives not great. Ignoring health experts, Japan pushed on with the 2021 Olympics and was forced to declare a state of emergency prior to the opening of the games. Many governments have also failed to address gender issues which had previously compromised responses to Ebola and Zika outbreaks in Africa and South America (Wenham & Davies, 2021). It is important to consider outcomes comparing epidemiological modelling about safe opening of activities and borders at the appropriate time which is subject to changed conditions and pressure to open in a predominantly unvaccinated world.

Governments in countries like France, Hungary, and the Czech Republic suffered from the arrogance of thinking that somehow the impact of the pandemic could be avoided. The leaders in countries such as the US under Trump, Brazil, Belarus and Mexico held complete disregard for their citizens. The damage these leaders caused went beyond endangering the population from allowing large gatherings to actively causing harm by campaigning against mask-wearing, spreading misinformation and false cures. The science was there but many governments chose to ignore the reality until it became obvious that things were out of control. Countries, especially in Europe, allowed porous borders. Other countries that had closed International borders eventually experimented with *safe* country travel bubbles. Countries such as New Zealand that did well dealt with imported infections and focussed on managing outbreaks quickly and efficiently.

Taiwan, an early success story with a total of just over 1,000 infections, felt the consequences of opening too soon. Easing border restrictions when populations are largely unvaccinated meant that even countries once successful in managing COVID-19, experienced an explosion of disease and potentially the development of new variants. Countries that are successfully vaccinating their population have seen a dramatic decrease in illness, hospitalisations and death. Australia with a very low vaccine rate, far below that of comparable countries, left thousands of Australians stranded overseas while allowing many more thousands of unvaccinated non-citizens into the country every month with attendance at a business meeting being the only requirement. Inevitably, the Delta variant entered the country and spread given inadequate federal attention to quarantine facilities and acquiring an adequate number and range of vaccines early. The race to vaccinate sufficient numbers of the world population was on.

Vaccinating the world

Scientists made astounding progress developing effective vaccines within 12 months, work which built on years of previous scientific endeavours. The WHO reported that 246 vaccine projects had been underway from January 2020 and over 50 clinical trials being conducted (VFA, 2021). Vaccines against new variants can be developed quickly but take longer to be approved. Clinical trials with experimental and control groups should be conducted for safety and efficacy on any new vaccine. For example, a new vaccine is tested on a small group of consenting participants in Stage 1. It is then tested on a larger, more diverse group, for example, people with other conditions or older in Stage 2. Finally, a large number of people are vaccinated in Stage 3. Approval by each country's regulatory body follows. Clinical trials are ceased if there are adverse effects attributed to the vaccine. Barriers were broken down to fast track bureaucratic approval of the first vaccines as much as possible while still ensuring scientific efficacy and safety. Laureate Professor Peter Doherty tells us more about vaccination in the last Q&A chapter of this book.

Richer countries were able to obtain more vaccines leaving many poorer countries with very little access. Vaccine nationalism was strongly criticised by the WHO for reasons of equity and world health because as long as the virus was allowed to spread, new variants would arise which could prove to be more deadly, more contagious and be resistant to vaccines (WHO, 2021). In contrast, vaccine altruism recognises that ensuring vaccine access for poorer neighbours protects the world and benefits everyone. In June 2021, the number of people who had received both vaccinations in Australia was 9%, the same percentage of people in low-income countries who had received one vaccination. Planning for vulnerable groups such as older people, people with disabilities and First Australians continued to lag in Australia. In stark contrast, after a devastating start under Trump, the US established a rapid vaccine rollout program under the Biden administration and committed to donating 25 million doses of vaccine mostly through the United Nations' COVAX program and to assist others in targeted donations, for example, in the South Americas, Yemen, Palestine and South Korea. Both countries manufactured vaccines in the country. Access to vaccination remains a global problem. Unfortunately, poorer nations and others lagging are not expected to be sufficiently vaccinated until 2023.

Countries that have thus far done well vaccinating their populations are the Seychelles, Israel, United Arab Emirates, Bahrain, Chile, Uruguay, Mongolia, Serbia and Iceland. Much of Africa remains unvaccinated or data are unavailable. Israel managed to vaccinate half its population with at least one dose in six weeks by the 1st of February except for members of Orthodox communities who opposed vaccinations. Despite the spread of disease in orthodox communities, there is a high trust in medicine and a political commitment to ensuring future generations. Unlike Australia, Israel took early steps to obtain a supply of the vaccine and were willing to pay for it.

The rich can now pay for vaccination or travel to the US to get vaccinated. While this raises very real issues of inequality, others suggest that the more people that get vaccinated the better regardless of how this occurs. Stimulus measures are being used to counter growing vaccine hesitancy such as multi-million-dollar lotteries in some US states. As well as the COVAX program, the Lancet COVID-19 Commission published a statement in February 2021 calling for global cooperation and multi-lateral suppression strategies including rapid and equitable vaccine distribution and the International Federation of Social Workers (IFSW) published an urgent call for vaccine equity in June 2021 (IFSW, 2021; The lancet COVID-19 Commission, 2021).

Behaviour and well-being

The yoyo effect of multiple lockdowns had a significant impact on behaviour especially for people needing to work or were less concerned about their health, especially in countries that had early success in containing the virus but missed one health measure such as early hard lockdowns and in countries where people had less personal experiences of illness. As side effects of vaccines became known and where government messaging was confusing or deceitful, vaccine hesitancy increased, further jeopardising the health of the global population. Leaders such as Trump and Bolsonaro and commentators using alternative broadcasts and other internet tools fuelled the infodemic and conspiracy theories that feed on pre-existing beliefs such as anti-vaccination and anti-government.

As identified in Chapter 2, significant and almost inevitable risks to mental health were touted from the outset of the pandemic. There was a marked focus on deficit rather than strengths, suggesting from the beginning that people were not going to cope. Funding psychological services became the go-to for some politicians as a concrete display of action during the pandemic. This is not to minimise the impact of the pandemic on many people especially those with pre-existing conditions. The compromised well-being of people already marginalised due to loss of life or capacities to earn a living, limited or no access to external resources and healthcare are influences which are not attributable to internal, individual deficits.

As discussed in the previous chapter, a UK study of 14,210,507 primary care found between April and September 2020, they found significant reductions of incidents of depression (43%), self-harm (37.6%) and anxiety (47.8) during lockdown and were one third less by September 2020 (Carr et al., 2021). Another study of 3,342 adults in Scotland found a range of benefits during the 9- to 12-week lockdown which included better sleep, more time with family engaging in new hobbies, and more physical activity (Williams et al., 2021). Although the countries in these studies are comparatively well resourced, they experienced large numbers of infection and deaths. In Chapter 12, Chang and Chiu wrote about the factors that impacted on people's vulnerabilities in Hong Kong and the responses needed from social workers. People with unresolved issues found they resurfaced during COVID-19 and they again sought out assistance including concerns about increases in drug and alcohol use (UN Office on Drugs and Crime, 2021). The resurfacing of unresolved issues was also identified by social workers in Ontario presented in Chapter 5. In Chapter 8, Gabriela Misca, Jan Walker and Gemma Thornton noted that younger people, students, the unemployed and single parents were at greater risk of loneliness during lockdown as well as the marginalised and disadvantaged.

A study by Pirkis et al. (2021) found that many reports in the media of increased suicides due to COVID-19 were not substantiated as in most countries with some exceptions, suicide rates did not change or decreased. A critical perspective would pose questions about distinguishing the range of possible human responses to life-threatening illness and disorders which would require different interventions, similar to differences between grief and depression or depression and demoralisation. Understanding concepts such as demoralisation, emptiness and the normalisation of grief and loss in overwhelming circumstances has relevance to social work practice in conditions of prolonged hardships such as the COVID-19 pandemic (Fronek & Briggs, 2020; Herron & Sani, 2021). As Dorado

Barbé and colleagues (2021) reported from Spain, a country badly affected by COVID-19, not all stress-related conditions are pathological. In their study of professionals, they sought to identify the variables that enhanced resilience. They found higher emotional well-being was correlated with greater resilience and stressed the importance of social workers developing psychosocial interventions that improve well-being suggesting a positive psychology focus, adaptability and self-efficacy, skills that should enhance resilience. The authors quote Guo and Tsui (2010) and Breda and Adrian (2019) who assert that strengths and ecological approaches at multiple levels increase the capacity of people to cope with adversity.

Interestingly, a US study of the electronic health records of 69 million people found associations between pre-existing mental health conditions treated in the preceding 12 months and contracting COVID-19 (Taquet et al., 2021). It should be noted that people with mental illness may also be more likely to live in economically deprived circumstances or other life conditions that puts them at greater physical risk for coronavirus infection. Previous studies of pneumonia found associated risks for people with previously diagnosed ADHD, bipolar disorders, depression and schizophrenia, an association not found in the South Korean context. As the authors point out, there are also cultural aspects of health beliefs to consider. They found first diagnoses especially anxiety, insomnia and dementia were common in 14–90 days after contracting COVID-19, a trend also noted previously in SARs and MERs (Taquet et al., 2021). Public health is now drawing attention to the *syndemic pandemic,* a term first used during the HIV/AIDS pandemic and is now being applied to COVID-19. The syndemic pandemic describes the interactional effects of biological, social and psychological factors that result in two or more diseases clustering together (Bambra et al, 2020; Mendenhall, 2017).

Certainly, stress on individuals and families was exacerbated in lockdown conditions and the chapter on mental health in Hong Kong highlighted multiple factors such as the coexisting crises of political unrest and democratic protests which complicated the well-being of communities. Much is still to be learned about systemic responses to well-being in pandemic conditions. In many places, people were exposed to natural and man-made disasters during the pandemic. Concurrent disasters and loss of life also affected some of the authors in this book such as the experience in Lebanon documented in Chapter 2. The mental and physical well-being of social workers along with other frontline workers should not be neglected and is an area of focus as the world recovers from this latest pandemic. Reporting on research from ground zero during the second wave of the pandemic in Canada, Chapter 5 stressed the importance of support for hospital social workers and developing pandemic guidelines from this experience at multiple levels of governance to prepare for the next health emergency.

The planet

The ecological framework presented in Chapter 1 allows for an understanding of the relationships that connects the three Ps – pandemic, politics and planet. COVID-19 has reinforced what is already taught in social work that people and their social, economic, physical and natural environment are interconnected in mutual influence. Environmental degradation and the present climate emergency provide the conditions for zoonoses and health emergencies as well as natural disasters. For example, the Amazon jungle, vital to cleansing the planet by absorbing carbon, is no longer able to do its job due to deforestation and climate change (Gatti et al., 2021). In the bonus chapter, Alan B Franklin points to human-caused deforestation, agricultural intensification and changed distribution of species and their interconnectedness with disease. The emergence of viruses like SARS-CoV-2 are not a one-hundred-year event and as the natural environment deteriorates, risks of new disease increases hence the prediction that the next pandemic which may be worse than COVID-19 and is not far away. While gains have been made towards addressing the climate emergency, action has not been widely accepted nor adopted at the pace required and the wildlife population continues to be devastated as discussed in Franklin's bonus chapter. As with all aspect of health emergencies, it is those people, particularly women, affected by socioeconomic disadvantage that are most impacted by climate change within and between countries. Environmental and Green social work practice becomes even more important in public health social work.

Dibley, Wetzer and Hepburn (2021) point to the impact of climate change on developing countries' capacities to repay debt totalling 130 billion dollars owed by 100 low- and middle-income countries which they described as a debt tsunami. They highlighted the lack of transparency by lenders and "as of early March 2021, around half of the COVID-19 stimulus funding that wealthy G20 countries had paid to the energy sector – roughly US$250 billion – had gone towards fossil fuels, rather than to cleaner energy sources" (Dibley, Wetzer & Hepburn, 2021, p 184). The short- and long-term impact of the economic and health impact of climate change on people, particularly the poor, has meant even more emphasis is needed in this core area of concern for social workers, particularly in relation to community work and innovation and macro social work to address injustices. In Chapter 14, Joel Izlar poses a radical approach to community organising to address ecosocial crises such as the COVID-19 pandemic.

Actual numbers of COVID cases have been underestimated worldwide and scientific debates about the origin of the virus and how long it has actually been circulating continue while also being weaponised in political arenas. Although considered a zoonotic process the intermediary animal has not been identified and for some, this unanswered question fuels doubt.

What next?

Issues raised in this book stress the need for reflexive social work practice and emphasise the need for transdisciplinary practice. In this global story of practice and innovation, we have presented social work, and indeed public health social work, as having an important contribution to make in policy development, planning and preparedness, practice, research and education alongside colleagues in interconnected disciplines. Today's pandemic had the advantage of cumulative scientific knowledge and the advancement of technology but other lessons such as addressing the climate emergency, the needs of the poor, prioritising health and apolitical leadership were not carried forward, indicating a disconnect from the values social workers hold. Human dignity, social justice and human rights became more important than ever during this historic era.

Privileging economies over people has once again proven wrong-headed with dire social consequences. Even if we put morals and ethics aside and ignore the unwarranted deaths of people, this approach has not worked. It has fuelled a pandemic, prolonged lockdowns, caused yoyo effects and not helped national or global economies – halfway does not cut it. COVID-19 has almost been a social experiment about what not to do. Missteps have also been taken in vaccine distribution. In one experiment, Indonesia badly affected by COVID-19 chose to vaccinate younger people first to ensure the economy thrived which placed people vulnerable to disease at risk of death and illness. Sweden's experiment of relying on herd immunity also resulted in unnecessary deaths.

The WHO has been criticised earning some of those criticisms such as naming a pandemic and recommending mask-wearing a few weeks later than it should. The reality was that global cooperation did not eventuate thanks to politicians like Trump. Trump withdrew US funding from the WHO which Biden later reinstated and rejoined. Without the cooperation of world leaders and a universal approach to pandemic management, no global organisation can fully meet its aims. Even within countries, there were different approaches informed by political ideologies which also determined to what extent health advice was accepted or rejected. Regional cooperation proved important such as the activities of the Association of Southeast Asian Nations (ASEAN) for countries across Asia (Amaya & De Lombaerde, 2021).

We presented examples of social work practice in different fields. None, as it turns out, can function in pandemic conditions without due attention to health and scientific knowledge. It is humans that are destroying our fragile ecosystem, setting the scene for future pandemics and hurting each other. Critical positioning is more important than ever as is the question how can social work raise the global conscience and work with others to do so. Our journey through these terrible times is historic and offers fruitful ground for the advancement of social work and continuing our work towards levelling the playing field by addressing social justice concerns. Teti, Schatz and Liebenberg (2020) pointed out that COVID-19 is not just a medical issue instead it is a phenomenon that has disrupted the social order. They go on to say that what is missing in many disciplines is *the social* and suggests the importance of qualitative research to ensure the social is not overlooked. Social work has an opportunity to ensure this gap is filled. It is clear that social workers everywhere need to share what worked and what didn't, prepare to deal with COVID-19's aftermath and for the next pandemic, and act at all levels of practice and influence.

BOX 18.1

REFLECTION

- What elements of my practice experience and framework might be helpful to understanding and responding to human need in a health emergency?
- How would understanding the perspective of key stakeholders including policy and decision makers enrich or confound my understanding of events that unfold in a health emergency?
- What knowledge will be critical to understanding the next health emergency? Will I have access to this knowledge? If not, how will I gain access to it?
- What resources and opportunities does my practice context, including the institutional environment, offer in responding to a health emergency?

References

Abbasi, K. (2021). Covid-19: Social murder, they wrote – Elected, unaccountable, and unrepentant. *British Medical Journal*. https://doi.org/10.1136/bmj.n314

Amaya, A. B., & De Lombaerde, P. (2021). Regional cooperation is essential to combatting health emergencies in the global south. *Globalization and Health*, 17(9). https://doi.org/10.1186/s12992-021-00659-7

Bambra, C., Riordan, R., Ford, J., & Matthews, F. (2020). The COVID-19 pandemic and health inequalities. *Journal of Epidemiology and Community Health*, 74(11), 964–968.

Breda, V., & Adrian, D. (2019). Reclaiming resilience for social work: A reply to Garrett. *British Journal of Social Work*, 49(1), 272–276.

Carr, M. J., Steeg, S., Webb, R. T., Kapur, N., Chew-Graham, C. A., Abel, K. M., . . . Ashcroft, D. M. (2021). Effects of the COVID-19 pandemic on primary care-recorded mental illness and self-harm episodes in the UK: A population-based cohort study. *The Lancet Public Health*. https://doi.org/10.1016/S2468-2667(20)30288-7

Dibley, A., Wetzer, T., & Hepburn, C. (2021). National COVID debts: Climate change imperils countries' ability to repay. *Nature*. https://www.nature.com/articles/d41586-021-00871-w

Dorado Barbé, A., Pérez Viejo, J. M., Rodríguez-Brioso, M. D. M., & Gallardo-Peralta, L. P. (2021). Emotional well-being and resilience during the COVID-19 pandemic: Guidelines for social work practice. *International Social Work*. https://doi.org/10.1177/0020872820970622

Drury, J. (2018). The role of social identity processes in mass emergency behaviour: An integrative review. *European Review of Social Psychology*, 29(1), 38–81.

ECDPC. (2021, June 23). *Threat assessment brief: Implications for the EU/EEA on the spread of the SARS-CoV-2 Delta (B.1.617.2) variant of concern*. European Centre for Disease Prevention and Control. https://www.ecdc.europa.eu/en/publications-data/threat-assessment-emergence-and-impact-sars-cov-2-delta-variant

European Observatory on Health Systems and Policies. (2021). *In the wake of the pandemic: Preparing for Long COVID (2021)*. https://www.euro.who.int/en/about-us/partners/observatory-old/publications/policy-briefs-and-summaries/in-the-wake-of-the-pandemic-preparing-for-long-covid-2021

Feil, E. (2021, June 1). Coronavirus variants have new names: We can finally stop stigmatising countries. *The Conversation*. https://theconversation.com/coronavirus-variants-have-new-names-we-can-finally-stop-stigmatising-countries-159652

Ferguson, H., Kelly, L., & Pink, S. (2021). Social work and child protection for a post-pandemic world: The re-making of practice during COVID-19 and its renewal beyond it. *Journal of Social Work Practice*. https://doi.org/10.1080/02650533.2021.1922368

Fronek, P., & Briggs, L. (2020). Demoralization in the wake of the COVID-19 pandemic: Whereto the future for young Australians? *Qualitative Social Work*. https://doi.org/10.1177/1473325020973332

Gatti, L. V., Basso, L. S., Miller, J. B., Gloor, M., Gatti Domingues, L., Cassol, H. L. G., . . . Neves, R. A. L. (2021). Amazonia as a carbon source linked to deforestation and climate change. *Nature*, 595(7867), 388–393.

Gauffin, K., & Dunlavy, A. (2021). Finding common ground: How the development of theory in public health research can bring us together. *Social Theory & Health*, 19(2), 127–136.

Guo, W., & Tsui, M. (2010). From resilience to resistance: A reconstruction of the strengths perspective in social work practice. *International Social Work*, 53(2), 233–245.

Herron, S. J., & Sani, F. (2021). Understanding the typical presentation of emptiness: A study of lived-experience. *Journal of Mental Health*. https://doi.org/10.1080/09638237.2021.1922645

IFSW (2021, June 2). *Urgent call for action on equal access to vaccines*. https://www.ifsw.org/ifsw-call-for-action-on-equal-access-to-vaccines/

Mackay, I. M. (2020, December 26). The Swiss cheese infographic that went viral. *Virology Down Under*. https://virologydownunder.com/the-swiss-cheese-infographic-that-went-viral/

Mallapaty, S. (2021, July 8). Will COVID become a disease of the young? *Nature*. https://www.nature.com/articles/d41586-021-01862-7

Mendenhall, E. (2017). Syndemics: A new path for global health research. *The Lancet*, 389(10072), 889–891.

Padma, T. V. (2021, July 5). COVID vaccines to reach poorest countries in 2023 – Despite recent pledges. *Nature*. https://www.nature.com/articles/d41586-021-01762-w

Pink, S., Ferguson, H., & Kelly, L. (2021). Digital social work: Conceptualising a hybrid anticipatory practice. *Qualitative Social Work*. https://doi.org/10.1177/14733250211003647

Pirkis, J., John, A., Shin, S., DelPozo-Banos, M., Arya, V., Analuisa-Aguilar, P., . . . Spittal, M. J. (2021). Suicide trends in the early months of the COVID-19 pandemic: An interrupted time-series analysis of preliminary data from 21 countries. *The Lancet Psychiatry*. https://doi.org/10.1016/S2215-0366(21)00091-2

Taquet, M., Luciano, S., Geddes, J. R., & Harrison, P. J. (2021). Bidirectional associations between COVID-19 and psychiatric disorder: Retrospective cohort studies of 62354 COVID-19 cases in the USA. *The Lancet Psychiatry*, 8(2), 130–140.

Teti, M., Schatz, E., & Liebenberg, L. (2020). Methods in the time of COVID-19: The vital role of qualitative inquiries. *International Journal of Qualitative Methods*. https://doi.org/10.1177/1609406920920962

The Independent Panel. (2021). *COVID-19: Make it the last pandemic*. https://theindependentpanel.org/mainreport/

The Lancet COVID-19 Commission. (2021, February). *Enhancing global cooperation to end the COVID-19 pandemic: Statement of the Lancet COVID-19 Commission*. https://covid19commission.org/enhancing-global-cooperation

UN Office on Drugs and Crime. (2021). *World Drug Report 2021*. https://www.unodc.org/unodc/en/data-and-analysis/wdr2021.html

VFA. (2021, February 1). Vaccines to protect against Covid-19, the new coronavirus infection. *VFA. Die forschenden Pharma-Unternehmen*. https://www.vfa.de/de/englische-inhalte/vaccines-to-protect-against-covid-19

Wenham, C., & Davies, S. E. (2021). WHO runs the world – (not) girls: Gender neglect during global health emergencies. *International Feminist Journal of Politics*. https://doi.org/10.1080/14616742.2021.1921601

WHO. (2021, February 2021). Inside the mammoth undertaking of global vaccine distribution. https://www.who.int/news-room/feature-stories/detail/inside-the-mammoth-undertaking-of-global-vaccine-distribution

Williams, L., Rollins, L., Young, D., Fleming, L., Grealy, M., Janssen, X., . . . Flowers, P. (2021). What have we learned about positive changes experienced during COVID-19 lockdown? Evidence of the social patterning of change. *PLoS One*. https://doi.org/10.1371/journal.pone.0244873

PART IV

Bonus chapters

19

SARS-CoV-2 IN WILDLIFE

Q&A with Alan B. Franklin

Alan B. Franklin

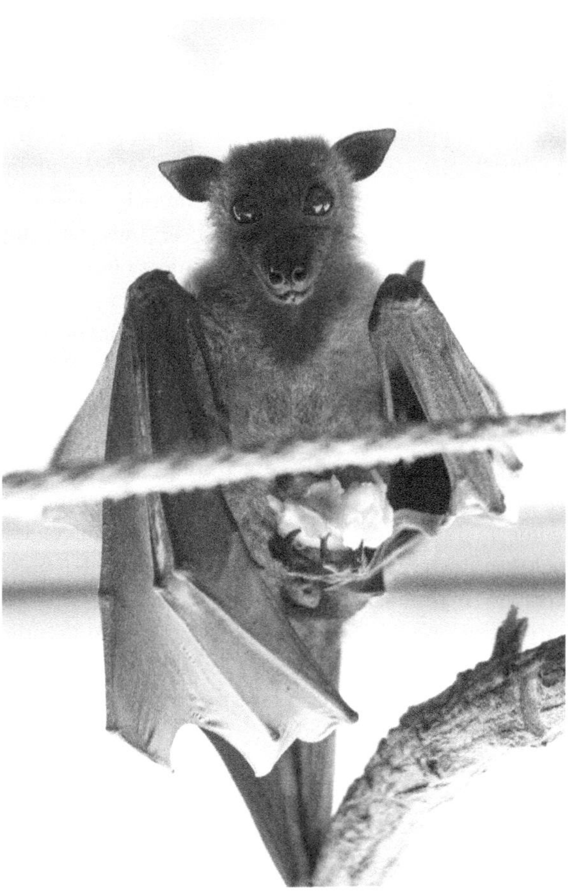

FIGURE 19.0 Viruses can be transferred from wild and domestic animals to humans in a process called zoonosis

Source: Photograph by Johannes Giez on Unsplash

DOI: 10.4324/9781003111214-23

Welcome Dr Franklin and thank you for joining us to help social workers increase their knowledge about the interconnectedness of humans, other mammals and the environment. Let's begin with zoonosis.

Can you explain zoonosis to us and the process that leads to diseases like COVID-19?

Zoonosis is where a disease-causing pathogen is transmitted naturally between vertebrate animals and humans (adapted from Botzler & Brown, 2014; Wobeser 2006). Botzler and Brown (2014) further partition the definition of zoonoses into *zooanthroponoses* (pathogens are transmitted to humans where humans are a dead-end host) and *anthropozoonoses* (pathogens are transmitted from humans to non-humans where the nonhumans are a dead-end host). In both cases, dead-end hosts are where a species serves as a host for the pathogen but does not serve as a source of the pathogen for another host (Botzler & Brown, 2014).

Two types of hosts are of concern in zoonotic pathogen transmission: maintenance and bridge host. *Maintenance*, or reservoir, *hosts* are one or more epidemiologically connected populations where a pathogen is permanently maintained (Haydon et al., 2002). Bridge hosts provide a link between maintenance hosts and target hosts, where the target hosts can be human populations in the case of zoonoses. To be considered a *bridge host*, a species must be competent for the pathogen to replicate within it and it must have infectious contacts with the target host (Caron et al., 2015). Bridge hosts cannot maintain pathogen persistence without additional inputs from maintenance hosts and, therefore, must overlap in time and space with both maintenance hosts and target hosts to effectively link the two. Interspecies transmission from a maintenance host to a non-maintenance host, such as a bridge host, is referred to as *spillover* transmission, and the recipients or secondary hosts as spillover hosts. Such spillover can play important roles in pathogen dynamics (Power & Mitchell 2004) and non-maintenance hosts can ultimately become maintenance hosts if the pathogen evolves within the new host. Nugent (2011) also used the term *spillback* to describe transmission from non-maintenance to maintenance hosts but acknowledged that maintenance transmission in one set of circumstances might be defined as either spillover or spillback, depending on the situation.

There are 1,145 known infectious organisms that are pathogenic to humans, which include viruses, prions, bacteria, fungi, protozoans, and helminths (Taylor et al., 2001). Of these, 61% are zoonotic infectious diseases, making up most of the diseases affecting humans. Of the novel pathogens that have emerged since the 1940s, 75% have been zoonotic and most have emerged from wildlife (Jones et al., 2008). Oftentimes, the pathogens that cause diseases are relatively benign and do not cause disease in their natural hosts. However, when the pathogens jump to another species, these pathogens can become much more virulent in the new host, causing disease that can sometimes have devastating consequences.

What do we know so far about the origins of SARS-CoV-2?

In January 2021, the World Health Organization (WHO) convened a team of scientists to examine the origins of SARS-CoV-2. This team recently released their report (WHO, 2020), which examined four plausible scenarios. These scenarios were:

1. Direct zoonotic transmission where there was transmission of SARS-CoV-2 (or a closely related progenitor) from an animal reservoir host to humans, which was followed by direct person-to-person transmission.
2. Introduction of SARS-CoV-2 from an animal reservoir host to an intermediate animal host, where it then spread among the intermediate host, which was then followed by zoonotic transmission to humans.
3. Similar to scenario 1 or 2 above, BUT introduction of SARS-CoV-2 to humans is through the cold/food chain; cold chain food products serve as the vehicle of introduction and transmission among humans.
4. SARS-CoV-2 is introduced to humans through a laboratory accident where release of the virus is from an accidental infection of laboratory staff by SARS-CoV-2.

Of these scenarios, only scenarios 1 and 2 were considered to be likely, with scenario 2 being assessed as likely to very likely while scenario 1 was considered possible to likely. The other two scenarios were considered to be possible (scenario 3) to extremely unlikely (scenario 4) by the WHO team (WHO-China Study Team, 2021).

Under scenario 1, viruses very closely related to SARS-CoV-2 have been found in insectivorous bats of the genus *Rhinolophus* in China, where COVID-19 was first detected (Lau et al., 2020). However, other wild animal reservoir hosts have been implicated such as the Malayan pangolin (*Manis javanica*) or a member of the weasel family (Mustelidae). The latter potential host is based on the susceptibility of farm-raised mink (*Neovison vison*) to SARS-CoV-2 and their ability to transmit the virus to humans (Oude Munnink et al., 2021).

Scenario 2 also involves a wild animal host but genetic evidence suggested that an intermediate animal host may have been involved because the evolutionary distance between the viruses found in bats and SARS-CoV-2 was estimated to be several decades (Lau et al., 2020). This scenario, where there has been an intermediate amplifying host has been seen in other emerging viruses, such as the original SARS-CoV, MERS-CoV, and Hepinaviruses (Cui, Chen & Fan, 2017). Candidate species for the role of intermediate host include the Malayan pangolin, mustelids and cat (felid) species, which could have been from wild animal farms that supply wet markets in China (WHO-China Study Team, 2021).

Although most agree that SARS-CoV-2 had a wildlife origin, there is some dispute whether it came from direct animal to human transmission or whether a laboratory accident was involved (Bloom et al., 2021). The dispute centres around the Wuhan Institute of Virology, where virologists worked on bat viruses with genetic similarity to SARS-CoV-2. In addition, the Wuhan Centre for Disease Control (CDC) laboratory moved to a new location near the Huanan Market in Wuhan, China, where SARS-CoV-2 was first detected. Bloom et al. (2021) argue that the scenario of an accidental release from a laboratory (scenario 4 above) should have been investigated more heavily by the WHO team and was discounted too readily. Regardless, evidence suggests that SARS-CoV-2 came from wild animals, most likely bats, but how it entered the human population is still largely conjectural and unknown. From the perspective of public health officials, however, understanding how the virus entered the human population is still critical information because it defines how mitigation measures would be shaped to deal with future pandemics.

It seems the process is rather circular, as people have also infected other animals with SARS-CoV-2 – lions in zoos, orangutans in Sumatra, and in mink farms, and we've even infected our pets – but it is said that pets can't give us the virus back? What is the explanation for these transmission paths?

The evidence for spillover of SARS-CoV-2 from humans into novel animal hosts has become increasingly well-documented. For example, whole genome sequencing identified similar strains of SARS-CoV-2 in farmed mink and human workers on those farms, indicating that transmission occurred and the initial introduction from a human worker to the farmed mink was suspected. Human workers on these captive mink farms were subsequently infected from mink carrying SARS-CoV-2 (Oude Munnink et al., 2021).

Spillback of the virus from animals, such as domestic pets, has not been well-documented but could be likely depending on the pet. Such infections will probably be few and very localised because most pets are isolated from others outside their households and would not likely serve as dominant sources of infection other than within their households. For example, the likely scenario is that an infected owner might transmit SARS-CoV-2 to their pet but would also serve as the source of infection to other human members of the household. Thus, pets would serve a very minor role in SARS-CoV-2 infections because the human sources of the infection would infect everyone else within a given household. Therefore, humans would play the dominant role as SARS-CoV-2 sources of infection and household pets serving a minor role. One exception to this would be where pets congregate, such as pet shops, animal shelters and veterinary clinics, where an infected pet can infect other pets from different households and subsequently spread the virus. This may partly explain why one-way transmission from humans to domestic dogs and cats is mostly observed. In coronaviruses similar to SARS-CoV-2, transmission from domestic dogs to humans was recently documented (Vlasova et al., 2021). However, SARS-CoV-2 appears to replicate poorly in domestic dogs, while domestic cats appear to be competent hosts for the virus and are also susceptible to airborne transmission of the virus

(Shi et al., 2020). Thus, Burkholz et al. (2021) and Sharun et al. (2021) argue that viral transfer from humans to farm animals and pets needs to be closely monitored to prevent the establishment of novel viral reservoirs for potential future zoonotic transfer.

Is it true that we can never prevent zoonotic infection and a better focus is on addressing the earliest pathway of transmission?

I am not sure we can never predict zoonotic infection with known pathogens but predictions for most future events are difficult. Nils Bohr, the pioneering physicist, jokingly commented "Prediction is difficult – especially about the future" (Petticrew et al., 2007, p. 106). Especially with unknown pathogens, such as ones that have never been discovered in wild animal hosts, there is a high degree of unpredictability in when, where, and how a zoonotic infection of humans will occur. Pathogen discovery alone will not solve the problem because understanding the host dynamics for those pathogens is critical to assess risk of spillover. Some have developed systems that follow a probabilistic framework to assess the risk of zoonotic spillover for emerging pathogens. For example, Grange et al. (2021) developed a risk assessment framework for 887 wildlife viruses in terms of their potential for spillover into humans. Although imperfect, such a framework can be revised and adjusted as new information becomes available. In addition, such frameworks identify lack of knowledge and can guide where focussed research is needed. However, others argue, and demonstrate to a certain degree, that zoonotic risk assessments are largely inaccurate because of the paucity of data, the uncertainties around current data, and biases in focussing on certain wildlife and domestic animal species (Wille, Geoghegan & Holmes, 2021). For example, ferrets (*Mustela putorius furo*) were found to be competent hosts of SARS-CoV-2 based on experimental inoculations with the virus (Shi et al., 2020). However, there may be genetic barriers for transmission of SARS-CoV-2 from infected humans to ferret (Sawatzki et al., 2021). These contradictory lines of evidence make it difficult to rely solely on studies of host competency but also require transmission studies to develop a complete picture of the process.

Wille, Geoghegan and Holmes (2021) argue that pathogen surveillance of people is required at the human-animal interface, such as people working with raising and slaughtering domestic animals, hunting animals such as bushmeat, to better assess zoonotic transmission. This is similar to focussing on the earliest pathway of transmission from animals to humans. I argue that both approaches have merit and the combination of both would provide increased prevention coverage than each approach considered separately. In addition, surveillance for pathogens of concern in wildlife populations are possible, given political will and financial commitment. An example of large-scale surveillance of wildlife pathogens affecting human and agricultural health is under the National Wildlife Disease Program in the United States (https://www.aphis.usda.gov/aphis/ourfocus/wildlifedamage/programs/nwdp); avian influenza viruses in waterfowl are tracked through a targeted, designed surveillance program that covers the entire US (Bevins et al., 2014).

Thus, it is unlikely that a single approach will prevent future zoonotic pandemics but a combination of approaches in a unified framework will mitigate, but probably not eliminate, the unpredictability of zoonotic outbreaks and pandemics. In all of these and other approaches, the COVID-19 pandemic has spotlighted the need for multi-disciplinary approaches that require collaboration among the human, animal, and environmental sectors (Belay et al., 2017).

A lot of waste goes into sewerage systems including prescribed and illegal drugs. Sewage analysis has been used to detect diseases such as polio or COVID-19. Does this in turn affect marine life and other wildlife?

Even in the most modern countries with sophisticated wastewater treatment plants (WWTP), there are issues with pathogen pollution from sewage. This is more of a problem in developing countries where raw sewage from municipalities is often dumped directly into natural waterways. One example of pathogens from sewage affecting wildlife is infection of southern sea otters (*Enhydra lutris nereis*) with the *Toxoplasma gondii* parasite originating from domestic cat faeces in cat litter that was flushed down toilets, passed through WWTP, and was discharged into the ocean where it subsequently infected sea otter populations (Jessup & Miller, 2011). Avian influenza viruses and some coronaviruses can be detected in effluent from WWTP that is being discharged into the environment (Wigginton, Ye & Ellenberg, 2015). Global surveillance for SARS-CoV-2 in municipalities now includes monitoring of sewage for SARS-CoV-2 RNA, where COVID-19 outbreaks are often detected prior to reports in human individuals (Medema et al., 2020). The basis for this surveillance is that infection with SARS-CoV-2 in humans also causes gastrointestinal symptoms, and the virus is passed through in faeces, which is subsequently detected in wastewater (Kitajima et al., 2020). Based on this, Franklin and Bevins (2020) hypothesised that SARS-CoV-2 released from WWTP had the potential to spillover into wild mammals using aquatic habitats near where WWTP effluent was discharged into the environment. One issue with this hypothesis is whether SARS-CoV-2 remains infective after undergoing the wastewater treatment process. However, a substantial amount of raw sewage is discharged into the environment through accidental spills or when WWTP are overwhelmed during natural disasters, such as hurricanes and floods (Franklin & Bevins, 2020). Such events have the potential to release infective SARS-CoV-2 and other pathogens into the environment where they can theoretically become established in wildlife hosts.

How do changes in climate such as drought and global warming, deforestation, agricultural practices and eco-tourism affect zoonotic transmission from wildlife?

This is a very broad area of interest with some specific examples that all of these factors have contributed to transmission of zoonotic pathogens and increased geographic spread of zoonotic pathogens. For example, climate change has been implicated in the northward geographic expansion of tick-borne zoonotic

Borrelia burgdorferi, the pathogen causing Lyme disease (Brownstein, Holford & Fish 2005), deforestation has been implicated in decreasing wild mammalian species diversity and increasing the prevalence of the zoonotic parasite causing Chagas disease in the remaining small mammal hosts (Vaz, D'Andrea & Jansen 2007), and changes in agricultural practices were considered responsible for the emergence of Nipah virus in human populations (Epstein et al., 2006). A classic example of emergence of a novel zoonotic pathogen in response to anthropogenic changes is with Nipah virus in Malaysia (Epstein et al., 2006). The emergence of Nipah virus from fruit bats (*Pteropus* spp.) coincided with agricultural intensification (Pulliam et al., 2012) that included combining fruit trees with pig farms and where bats feeding on fruits in trees above pig pens dropped partially eaten fruit contaminated with infected saliva into the pig pens (Epstein et al., 2006). Pigs became infected after consuming the virus-contaminated fruit and subsequently infected workers on the farm and in slaughterhouses (Epstein et al., 2006).

In a review of 305 scientific articles, Gottdenker et al. (2014) found that over 56% of the studies documented increased pathogen prevalence and/or transmission in response to human-caused changes. Most of the positive responses were from viral and protozoan pathogens and the principal land use changes associated with those responses were deforestation, agricultural development, and urbanisation. Most of the studies were observational with only seven experimental studies. Thus, inferences about cause and effect were not possible in most cases. However, proposed mechanisms included modified niches for pathogens and/or hosts, changes in host community composition, altered spatial distribution of species, and socio-economic factors that altered human exposure and risk of pathogen transmission. Land use-induced spillover of zoonotic pathogens is considered vitally important to understanding zoonotic disease pandemics (Plowright et al., 2021).

How might we include a planetary health perspective to prevent the emergence and spread of infectious disease and what do we humans need to do differently?

We need to better understand the systems that spawn zoonotic pathogens, such as SARS-CoV-2. Currently, we focus on understanding what species zoonotic pathogens emerge from but pay scant attention to the ecological systems from where these pathogens emerged. This bias is probably because medical and veterinarian scientists initially promoted the concept of *One Health*, which focussed primarily at zoonotic diseases at the human-domestic animal interface. It has since expanded more broadly to include wildlife ecology, with a more encompassing definition for One Health as "... a worldwide strategy for expanding interdisciplinary collaborations and communications in all aspects of health care for people, animals and the environment" and "A collaborative, multisectoral, and transdisciplinary approach (working at the local, regional, national, and global levels) with the goal of achieving optimal health outcomes recognizing the interconnection between people, animals, plants, and their shared environment" (Gibbs, 2014). Thus, One Health attempts to tie together the disparate disciplines that deal with zoonotic diseases into a single collaborative framework. Currently, there is a large effort to incorporate One Health into global programs under the WHO, the Food and Agriculture Organization of the United Nations (see www.fao.org/one-health/en/).

Alan B. Franklin (1 June 2021)

References

Belay, E. D., Kile, J. C., Hall, A. J., Barton-Behravesh, C., Parsons, M. B., Salyer, S. J., & Walke, H. (2017). Zoonotic disease programs for enhancing global health security. *Emerging Infectious Disease*, 23(13), S65–S70.

Bevins, S. N., Pedersen, K., Lutman, M. W., Baroch, J. A., Schmit, B. S., Kohler, D., . . . DeLiberto, T. J. (2014). Large-scale avian influenza surveillance in wild birds throughout the United States. *PLoS One.* https://doi.org/10.1371/journal.pone.0104360

Bloom, J. D., Chan, Y. A., Baric, R. S., Bjorkman, P. J., Cobey, S., Deverman, B. E., . . . D. A. Relman. (2021). Investigate the origins of COVID-19. *Science*, 372(6543), 694–694.

Botzler, R. G., & Brown, R. N. (2014). *Foundations of wildlife diseases.* Oakland, CA: University of California Press.

Brownstein, J. S., Holford, T. R., & Fish, D. (2005). Effect of climate change on Lyme disease risk in North America. *EcoHealth,* 2(1), 38–46.

Burkholz, S., Pokhrel, S., Kraemer, B. R., Mochly-Rosen, D., Carback, R. T., Hodge, T., … Rubsamen, R. (2021). Paired SARS-CoV-2 spike protein mutations observed during ongoing SARS-CoV-2 viral transfer from humans to minks and back to humans. *Infection, Genetics and Evolution*, 93,104897. https://doi.org/10.1101/2020.12.22.424003

Caron, A., Cappelle, J., Cumming, G. S., de Garine-Wichatitsky, M., & Gaidet, N. (2015). Bridge hosts, a missing link for disease ecology in multi-host systems. *Veterinary Research*, 46(1). https://doi.org/10.1186/s13567-015-0217-9

Cui, J.-a., Chen, F., & Fan, S. (2017). Effect of intermediate hosts on emerging zoonoses. *Vector-Borne and Zoonotic Diseases*, 17(8), 599–609.

Epstein, J. H., Field, H. E., Luby, S., Pulliam, J. R. C., & Daszak, P. (2006). Nipah virus: Impact, origins, and causes of emergence. *Current Infectious Disease Reports*, 8(1), 59–65.

Franklin, A. B., & Bevins, S. N. (2020). Spillover of SARS-CoV-2 into novel wild hosts in North America: A conceptual model for perpetuation of the pathogen. *Science of the Total Environment*, 733,139358. https://doi.org/10.1016/j.scitotenv.2020.139358

Gibbs, E. P. J. (2014). The evolution of One Health: A decade of progress and challenges for the future. *Veterinary Record*, 174(4), 85–91.

Gottdenker, N. L., Streicker, D. G., Faust, C. L., & Carroll, C. R. (2014). Anthropogenic land use change and infectious diseases: A review of the evidence. *EcoHealth*, 11(4), 619–632.

Grange, Z. L., Goldstein, T., Johnson, C. K., Anthony, S., Gilardi, K., Daszak, P., . . . Mazet, J. A. K. (2021). Ranking the risk of animal-to-human spillover for newly discovered viruses. *Proceedings of the National Academy of Sciences,* 118(15). https://doi.org/10.1073/pnas.2002324118

Haydon, D. T., Cleaveland, S., Taylor, L. H., & Laurenson, M. K. (2002). Identifying reservoirs of infection: A conceptual and practical challenge. *Emerging Infectious Diseases*, 8(12), 1468–1473.

Jessup, D. A., & Miller, M. A. (2011). The trickle-down effect: How toxoplasmosis from cats can kill sea otters. *The Wildlife Professional*, 5, 62–64.

Jones, K. E., Patel, N. G., Levy, M. A., Storeygard, A., Balk, D., Gittleman, J. L., & Daszak, P. (2008). Global trends in emerging infectious diseases. *Nature*, 451, 990–994. https://doi.org/10.1038/nature06536

Kitajima, M., Ahmed, W., Bibby, K., Carducci, A., Gerba, C. P., Hamilton, K. A., Haramoto, E., & Rose, J. B. (2020). SARS-CoV-2 in wastewater: State of the knowledge and research needs. *Science of the Total Environment,* 739. https://doi.org/10.1016/j.scitotenv.2020.139076

Lau, S. K. P., Luk, H. K. H., Wong, A. C. P., Li, K. S. M., Zhu, L., He, Z., . . . Woo, P. C.Y. (2020). Possible bat origin of severe acute respiratory syndrome coronavirus 2. *Emerging Infectious Diseases*, 26(7), 1542–15.

Medema, G., Heijnen, L., Elsinga, G., Italiaander, R., & Brouwer, A. (2020). Presence of SARS-Coronavirus-2 RNA in sewage and correlation with reported COVID-19 prevalence in the early stage of the epidemic in the Netherlands. *Environmental Science & Technology Letters,* 7(7), 511–516.

Nugent, G. (2011). Maintenance, spillover and spillback transmission of bovine tuberculosis in multi-host wildlife complexes: A New Zealand case study. *Veterinary Microbiology*, 151 (1-2), 34–42.

Oude Munnink, B. B., Sikkema, R. S., Nieuwenhuijse, D. F., Molenaar, R. J., Munger, E., Molenkamp, R., . . . Koopmans, M. P. G. (2021). Transmission of SARS-CoV-2 on mink farms between humans and mink and back to humans. *Science*, 371(6525), 172–177.

Petticrew, M., Cummins, S., Sparks, L., & Findlay, A. (2007). Validating health impact assessment: Prediction is difficult (especially about the future). *Environmental Impact Assessment Review,* 27(1), 101–107.

Plowright, R. K., Reaser, J. K., Locke, H., Woodley, S. J., Patz, J. A., Becker, D. J., Oppler, G., Hudson, P. J., & Tabor, G. M. (2021). Land use-induced spillover: A call to action to safeguard environmental, animal, and human health. *The Lancet Planetary Health*, 5(4), e237–e245. https://doi.org/10.1016/S2542-5196(21)00031-0

Power, A. G., & Mitchell, C. E. (2004). Pathogen spillover in disease epidemics. *The American Naturalist,* 164, S79–S89. https://doi.org/10.1086/424610

Pulliam, J. R. C., Epstein, J. H., Dushoff, J. S., Rahman, S. A., Bunning, M., Jamaluddin, A. A., . . . Daszak, P. (2012). Agricultural intensification, priming for persistence and the emergence of Nipah virus: A lethal bat-borne zoonosis. *Journal of the Royal Society Interface*, 9(6), 89–101.

Sawatzki, K., Hill, N. J., Puryear, W. B., Foss, A. D., Stone, J. J., & Runstadler, J. A. (2021). Host barriers to SARS-CoV-2 demonstrated by ferrets in a high-exposure domestic setting. *Proceedings of the National Academy of Sciences,* 118(18). https://doi.org/10.1073/pnas.2025601118

Sharun, K., Dhama, K., Pawde, A. M., Gortázar, C., Tiwari, R., Bonilla-Aldana, D. K., . . . Attia, Y. A. (2021). SARS-CoV-2 in animals: Potential for unknown reservoir hosts and public health implications. *Veterinary Quarterly*, 41(1), 181–201.

Shi, J., Wen, Z., Zhong, G., Yang, H., Wang, C., Huang, B., . . . Bu, Z. (2020). Susceptibility of ferrets, cats, dogs, and other domesticated animals to SARS – Coronavirus 2. *Science*, 368(6494), 1016–1020.

Taylor, L. H., Latham, S. M., & Woolhouse, M. E. J. (2001). Risk factors for human disease emergence. *Philosophical Transactions of the Royal Society of London, Series B. Biological Sciences*, 356(1411), 983–989.

Vaz, V. C., D'Andrea, P. S., & Jansen, A. M. (2007). Effects of habitat fragmentation on wild mammal infection by Trypanosoma cruzi. *Parasitology,* 134(Pt. 12), 1785–1793.

Vlasova, A. N., Diaz, A., Damtie, D., Xiu, L., Toh, T-H., Lee, J. S-Y., Saif, L. J., & Gray, G. C. (2021,). Novel canine coronavirus isolated from a hospitalized pneumonia patient, East Malaysia. *Clinical Infectious Diseases.* https://doi.org/10.1093/cid/ciab456

Wigginton, K. R., Ye, Y., & Ellenberg, R. M. (2015). Emerging investigators series: The source and fate of pandemic viruses in the urban water cycle. *Environmental Science: Water Research & Technology*, 1(6), 735–746.

Wille, M., Geoghegan, J. L., & Holmes, E. C. (2021). How accurately can we assess zoonotic risk? *PLoS Biology*, 19. https://doi.org/10.1371/journal.pbio.3001135

Wobeser, G. A. (2006). *Essentials of disease in wild animals.* Ames, IA: Blackwell Publishing.

WHO. (2020). *Report of the WHO-China joint mission on coronavirus disease 2019 (COVID-19).* Geneva, Switzerland: WHO.

WHO-China Study Team. (2021). *WHO-convened global study of origins of SARS-CoV-2: China Part.* Geneva, Switzerland: WHO.

20

COVID-19

Q&A with Peter C. Doherty

Peter C. Doherty

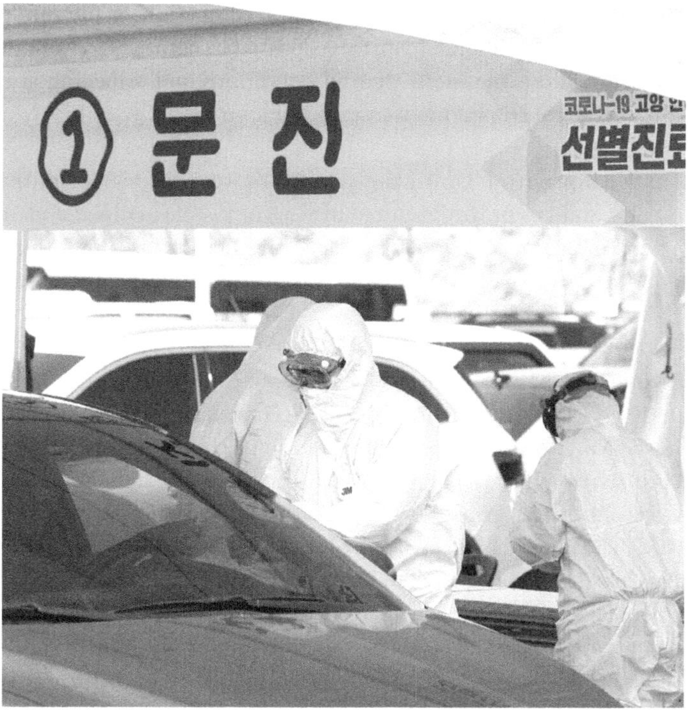

FIGURE 20.0 Drive-through testing in Goyang City, South Korea

Source: Photograph provided by Goyang City Council

DOI: 10.4324/9781003111214-24

Welcome Professor Doherty and thank you for joining us to help social workers increase their knowledge about the COVID-19 pandemic.

Professor Doherty, what is SARS-CoV-2 and should we be concerned about new variants?

The SARS-CoV-2 coronavirus has likely long been maintained in nature in one or other species of bat and has recently crossed over into us, perhaps via an intermediate host. This virus causes the severe, acute respiratory (SARS) disease we call COVID-19. The initial suspicion was that a pangolin had been infected with SARS-CoV-2 by contact with bat droppings or by eating, say, fruit that had been partly consumed by bats. Then, the virus transmitted from pangolins to people in, perhaps, one of the Asian live animal markets that sell wild animals for human consumption and possible use in traditional medicines. That idea was based on the confirmed transmission scenario for the related SARS-CoV-1 virus from 2002–2003 that had gone from bats, to Himalayan civet cats to humans. However, though closely related viruses have been found in bats, SARS-CoV-2 has not been recovered from them, so there is no final proof of this speculation. Also, though SARS-CoV-2 was first detected in Wuhan, and the "Seafood Market" – which also sells wild mammals captured in nature – was an early focus of virus dissemination, the moist, humid conditions and crowding at that site could simply have contributed to the spread of a virus that was already circulating between humans.

What is a coronavirus? Up to the year 2000, two coronaviruses that cause common colds and croup had been circulating in people across the planet since first detected, and named – by Scottish electron microscopist June Almeida – in the 1960s. After 2000, five more have crossed (likely from bats) into humans. The original SARS/CoV-1 in 2002 – that virus *burnt out* and is no longer infecting people – two more common cold CoVs in 2004 (one in the Netherlands, and one in Hong Kong), the MERS virus in 2012 (bats, to camels, to people), and SARS-CoV-2 in 2019. The last four viruses are still circulating in human populations, MERS in the Middle East and parts of Asia, and the other three across the planet.

The coronaviruses have a complex RNA genome – the influenza ('flu) viruses and HIV are also RNA viruses – which, with 30,000 base pairs, is two to three times larger than either the 'flu viruses or HIV. With an inbuilt *proof reading* mechanism, the CoVs throw off many fewer mutants than either 'flu or HIV but, with so many people across the planet infected, mutants are slowly emerging. So far, the main *antibody escape mutant* (vaccines work by promoting a very specific antibody response) of concern – generally referred to as the South African variant – is at least partly controlled by vaccination. Also, it will be an easy matter to reformulate the current vaccines (which will need little further testing) to deal with this. That will, though, require additional *shots*. Considering the current 'flu vaccines, which are a mix of separate vaccines specific for three or four different viruses, it is possible that, if SARS-CoV-2 continues to circulate beyond 2021, we may be *jabbed* with a vaccine that covers a range of mutants.

Given what we now know about SARS-CoV-2, why is washing hands, physical distancing and mask wearing so important for practitioners like social workers who are also engaged on the frontline in institutions and communities with vulnerable people and the sick?

The original SARS-CoV-1 virus was shown to survive very well on surfaces (called *fomites* by public health doctors) like door handles and lift buttons and, under experimental conditions, infectious SARS-CoV-2 can still be found on refrigerated plastic (e.g., food wrapping) for more than 48 hours. Still, there's little evidence that SARS-CoV-2 has infected people in this way, though there have been suspicions (in both China and NZ) of import on frozen foods. Mainly, though, the hand washing requirement reflect that, generally without being conscious of doing so, we constantly touch our faces, and nose picking is not unknown! That could, for instance, lead to an infected person who is blowing out infected mucus (snot) unconsciously transmitting the disease to someone else by shaking hands.

Physical distancing and masking reflects that the main means of transmission (beyond hand to face) is thought to be due to the inhalation of microdroplets of mucus containing infectious virus that have been coughed, spluttered or just breathed out by others. Whether we call this aerosol or droplet spread is of little relevance to most of us and, no doubt of interest to social workers, it's intriguing that respiratory physicians and aerosol engineers use these terms differently. The doctors were describing fine particle *mucus clouds* comprised of droplets less than five microns (one 200,000th of a metre) in diametre as aerosols, while the engineers were referring to those less than 50 microns as aerosols – two science subcultures divided by a common language.

What the infectious disease physicians have been finding to be particularly encouraging is that the implementation of these measures to limit COVID-19 has also led to a big drop in the incidence of 'flu and other respiratory virus infections. So long as pre-schools were shut, that also applied to the endemic sniffles and croups suffered by infants that they generally pass onto their parents who, after the passage of the years, are no longer immune as a consequence of their own childhood exposure. With the end of lockdowns in Melbourne, my impression from talking with younger colleagues is that this is pretty much gone back to normal!

There has been a lot written about immunity and its decline after recovering from COVID-19. Can you explain this decline and the role of the body in developing its own immunity and can it sometimes go into overdrive?

Immunology, along with neuroscience, is perhaps the most complex of all the laboratory-based (versus behavioural) sciences. If you want a more detailed understanding of how immunity works, go to my *Setting it Straight* articles on the Peter Doherty Institute website. Basically, after infection or vaccination (the terms vaccination and immunisation are interchangeable), we would, after about 10–12 days, expect to start finding highly specific, protective (neutralising) antibodies (also called immunoglobulins, Igs) in the blood. The vaccines mimic infection but, unlike the virus, they don't go on to infect other cells or other people and do minimal damage to us. They can, though, reproducing what we would normally expect for the early stage of any developing immune response, make us feel drowsy and a bit *off* for a day or two.

That's due to the production of molecules, called cytokines and chemokines, that are characteristic of the early, non-specific *innate* immune response. These natural chemicals spill over into the blood and can affect the brain directly. And they are important for setting up the lymph nodes (the axillary lymph nodes, e.g., are the *glands* under your armpit) as the *nurturing microenvironments* where the virus-specific, *adaptive immune* response develops. Called a *reactogenic response*, I'll be happy to endure that transient discomfort if it occurs when I am eventually vaccinated, as it will tell me that I am responding.

When people talk about the immune response going into dangerous *overdrive*, what's generally being referred to is the *cytokine storm* effect that was first identified for severe influenza and can emerge late in the course of disease when people fail to make a strong virus-specific adaptive response, the virus is not eliminated and these innate – and rather toxic molecules (they cause vascular leakage for example) – are massively overproduced as part of a compensatory mechanism. The intensive care physicians have been countering this in COVID-19 by treating with the old, and cheap, drug dexamethasone. Some patients have also benefitted from dosing with monoclonal antibodies that block the action of the cytokine IL-6, with the difference that this is very expensive therapy!

With regard to waning immunity we know that, after a single encounter, people can be circulating protective antibodies to yellow fever virus (following immunisation) or a particular influenza virus variant (following infection) for as long as 50 years. The doctors don't rely on that for yellow fever, though, and recommend a ten-yearly booster shot for those who are travelling to regions where they might be exposed to infected mosquitoes. On the other hand, kids infected with a particular parainfluenza virus (another RNA virus) can be reinfected with the same virus in subsequent years, with less severe symptoms every year. Then, when they grow up and become parents, they can be infected again. We suspect that the common cold CoVs may be a bit like this, but we have no idea how vaccines would behave in this regard. The reason: the common colds and croups are caused by more than 100 different viruses, people recover anyway, and it has been too daunting a task to contemplate immunisation. With SARS-CoV-2, time has been short, and we are just beginning what will be a very comprehensive experiment!

Scientists have been exploring why some populations appear to have more resistance to COVID-19, looking at factors like previous exposure to other diseases, previous vaccinations and even Neanderthal genes. Do we have any firm findings that shed light on this question?

The neanderthal gene hypothesis is intriguing and, once we have the disease under control and are at a less pressing stage regarding the science associated with that, we will no doubt be doing detailed genomic studies on large numbers of people who have had diverse clinical outcomes. These cohorts are currently being setup and approved for human experimentation (likely just taking blood samples from time to time) by various university and research institute ethics committees.

Otherwise, it is clear that some of the molecular structures (epitopes) recognised by killer T lymphocytes (their job is to search and destroy the virus-producing cellular factories) are shared between SARS-CoV-2 and some of the common cold CoVs (*Setting it Straight* for November 2020). These *primed killers* aren't immediately available following infection but, if we do have immune memory in that population, they will turn on fast and eliminate the virus more quickly. This may be part of the explanation for the extremely varied disease course with COVID-19.

Apart from such biological considerations, it's also important to take into account the mean age of human populations (African societies tend to have more young people), cultural factors that influence, e.g., compliance with social distancing and masking, and the status of local public health systems. Some well-organised, but poorer societies, have long emphasised preventive medicine via good public health practices, and may have done well with COVID-19 as a consequence. Then there's also the issue of how people define *case numbers*. In Australia, we count everyone who has tested positive by PCR, and we have been testing just about everyone with a sniffle in times when the virus is circulating. In other countries, they may only be counting people who present to a doctor with significant symptoms. This is one reason why death rates relative to diagnosed *cases* can be greatly divergent.

Currently there are three main available vaccines – Oxford-AstraZeneca, Moderna and BioNTech-Pfizer. What are the differences, do differences matter and how do we know which one to have?

They all target the SARs-CoV-2 spike protein and deliver the gene sequences that make the protein that, expressed on the surface of an invading virus particle, is the target of the protective antibody response. In the case of the Pfizer and Moderna vaccines, the product is mRNA – the RNA form that stays in the cytoplasm and is *translated* to make protein. Both are encased in a protective layer of lipid (fat) which, when injected, is taken up (pinocytosed) by our cells. Prior to inoculation, the Pfizer vaccine is very temperature sensitive and requires a –70°C cold chain though, once thawed, it can be held in an ordinary chest or *fridge freezer* for a day or two.

With the AstraZeneca product, the SARS-CoV-2 RNA is copied to DNA (using a reverse transcriptase) which is then incorporated into the incomplete DNA of a replication-defective, chimpanzee adenovirus (ChAd9). The packaging ChAd9 *vector* infects our cells, the virus particle breaks down and the DNA is released to enter the cell nucleus. There it is transcribed by the cell's molecular machinery to make mRNA, which in turn goes to the cytoplasm and makes protein. Neither product can be transmitted to other cells, be copied into our genomes, or in any way revert to an infectious form (see *Setting it Straight* for February/March 2021). In practice, recent results from public Health Scotland and Public Health England have been showing that both types of vaccines are working well, in fact, better than expected from the clinical trials. Enormous numbers of people have now been given these vaccines, including 50 million Americans (and half the population of Israel) who have received the mRNA product.

Will we have an evolution-proof vaccine in the future?

Maybe, but unlikely: we have been trying to make such vaccines against both 'flu and HIV for several decades. Still, it's always possible that there will be a breakthrough.

What is your perspective on the challenges and ethical considerations of vaccine distribution?

Ethics, apart from the ethics of experimentation, is hardly my field, and I expect that most social workers would be more familiar with the nuances than I am. My thinking on this reflects the over-simplification typical of most laboratory scientists, who have full control of an experimental system.

My perception is that what the Australian authorities are doing re vaccination is both correct and ethical in every sense. Everyone will have access to free vaccine, with those at greatest risk, or in frontline healthcare and quarantine roles being vaccinated first. While I don't think government-mandated vaccination for all citizens is either workable or a good idea, I do think that employers running aged care facilities, hospitals and so forth should be able to require that all staff with any level of patient or public contact must either be vaccinated or find employment in some other setting. That should also be true for airlines and cruise ships when it comes to carrying passengers. In addition, any customer at a hotel, bar or store should have the right to know that anyone they contact in those settings has been vaccinated. The *rights* in this matter are, in my opinion, weighted towards the collective interests of society at large and not solely applicable to those who refuse vaccination.

Vaccines may not prevent all transmission, but it is likely true that those who are vaccinated will both be less likely to transmit and at a much lower risk of contracting infection that spreads beyond the upper airways. This is war. To date (March 2021), more American have died of COVID-19 than in all wars during the 20th century. To my mind, vaccination is a collective responsibility.

It seems most countries first waited for evidence (which takes time) before instigating cautionary measures. One wonders how events would have unfolded if caution had come first, and the easing of restrictions followed the evidence as it emerged. In a hypothetical world and given the speed and volume of human movement around the globe, what would have happened if the world had universally and immediately

instituted a hard lockdown for a few weeks (and ensured people had food and maintained their housing), conducted extensive and effective testing, contact tracing and quarantine, and mandated physical distancing, mask-wearing and other protective measures?

We have already learned a great deal from this pandemic, especially as we have seen different *experiments* unfold in different countries. There are now, as a consequence, a spectrum of varied data sets from a diversity of approaches that should provide an extraordinary resource for (among others) further analysis by public health doctors, medical scientists, economists, policy wonks and those in the behavioural sciences. We know what works in this type of setting, but are we capable of acting on that information? Personally, unless we modify our profiles of international air travel and immediate public health responsiveness across the planet, my perception is that we will face further and worse pandemics in the not too distant future.

As a specific recommendation, my widely-stated position is that all nations need to agree that, whenever we see a repeat of an outbreak like the one that happened in Wuhan, we have prior global agreements that we will immediately stop all passenger air travel out of that local region and, perhaps, from that Nation State until the situation is resolved. Though expensive, that would be infinitely less economically and socially damaging than what has happened with COVID-19.

My second recommendation stems from the fact that any vaccine must be very specific for the pathogen in question and, though we can start making *product* very quickly, the need for careful safety and efficacy trials means that there will be at least a 12-month delay before we start to roll-out these preventives. As a consequence, I am arguing that we need a massive, global initiative to produce and trial specific antiviral drugs against all classes of viruses that are potential pandemic threats. We already have these for all the influenza viruses (they have to be used very early in the infection) and for the HIV type viruses – these drugs are stopping massive numbers of people from progressing to AIDS. We need comparable products for the coronaviruses, the henipaviruses (Nipah and Hendra), the filoviruses (Marburg and Ebola) and the arenaviruses (Lassa and Junin), at least. Most of these names may be unfamiliar to you, but they are all bad pathogens that are *lurking* out there. And, to avoid the emergence of drug-resistant mutants, we need two of these drugs (therapeutics) that target different molecular pathways for each virus class. How would we use them? As soon as the cause of an outbreak is identified, anyone who tests positive would be treated immediately. That would likely save their lives and prevent the ongoing spread of the pathogen.

The third point is that we need to do a much better job of educating people. Many, including a number of reporters in the Australian media initially, at least, seemed to be ignorant of the difference between a drug (an introduced therapeutic, or treatment that acts immediately) and a vaccine, which stimulates our own immune response to prevent, or limit, an infection and is delayed (3–4 weeks) in effect. Having grown up in a distant era – I was a small child during WW2- It is my deep conviction that we must return to a societal perception that emphasises collective responsibility and shared fates. Even philosophers like Hume did not endorse the idea that individual freedom overrides all else! As a species, we triumphed through evolution by acting together to solve big problems. A hole in the bottom of a boat in the ocean is not solely the responsibility for the people at that end of the boat! And we also need people to stretch their minds a little and grasp the linked ideas of probability and relative risk.

What is your advice on what social workers need to know to prepare for the next health emergency?

We know how to protect ourselves and have discussed some of that above. One area where we all need your help is when it comes to countering the ready acceptance of disinformation in some communities, along with the distrust of advice from those who know what they are talking about. Clearly, the medical and public health communities have a lot to learn about effective messaging.

What do you think a post-COVID world will look like?

Your guess is as good as mine. There is enormous potential for learning from what happened here, but are we capable of taking advantage of that? With challenge comes opportunity! As professionals, the more that we explore those opportunities, then take what we learn and incorporate it in both practice and in general awareness, the greater the potential for human wellbeing. And we should all bear in mind that humanity, in fact life on this planet, faces an even greater challenge, anthropogenic climate change. In some senses, COVID-19 has been a trial run for what is to come. Can we learn?

Peter C. Doherty (5 March 2021)

INDEX

Italicized and **bold** pages refer to figures and tables respectively.

For Product Safety Concerns and Information please contact our EU representative GPSR@taylorandfrancis.com Taylor & Francis Verlag GmbH, Kaufingerstraße 24, 80331 München, Germany